A Functional Medicine Monograph

MUSCULOSKELETAL PAIN:
Expanded Clinical Strategies

Alex Vasquez, DC, ND

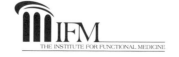

THE INSTITUTE FOR FUNCTIONAL MEDICINE

A Nonprofit Educational Organization
www.functionalmedicine.org
©2008 The Institute for Functional Medicine

Musculoskeletal Pain: Expanded Clinical Strategies

Alex Vasquez, DC, ND

Disclaimer

This publication is intended only for use as an educational tool to broaden the knowledge and perspective of health practitioners. Nothing herein is intended to substitute for an individualized, thoughtful decision process by patients and providers. Clinically related material is not presented as a prescription for treatment, but rather as an indicator of the kind of information clinicians may want to consider in making treatment decisions for their patients. Neither the publisher, the authors, the editors, nor the reviewer assume any liability for any injury and/or damage to persons or property arising from the information to be found in this publication.

Project Team

Allison Templet, Project Manager and Editor

Sheila Quinn, Planning and Content Development

Michael W. Loes, MD, Technical Reviewer

Mary Smith, Cover Design

D. Kari Luraas, Interior Design and Layout

Lynn Siefken, Illustrations

Peer and Editorial Review

Julian Vickers, DC, FIACN

Mark Grosman, DC

Tim Irving, DC

Ronald D'Agostino, DO

Leslie Axelrod, ND, LAc

Tamara Sachs, MD

Chris Meletis, ND

Bob Sager, MD, DABFM

Heather A. Kahn, MD

Deirdre Orceyre, ND, LAc

Zachary Watkins, DC, DACBI

ISBN-10: 0-9773713-6-0

ISBN-13: 978-0-9773713-6-5

Contents

Contents

Continuing Medical Education General Information

Accreditation Statement

The Institute for Functional Medicine (IFM) is accredited by the Accreditation Council for Continuing Medical Education (ACCME) to provide continuing medical education (CME) for physicians.

Commercial Support

This CME activity is supported by educational grants from Doctor's Data Inc., Genova Diagnostics, InnoVision Health Media Inc., Metagenics, Inc., Metametrix Clinical Laboratory, Nordic Naturals, Inc., SpectraCell Laboratories, Inc., Thorne Research, Inc., TID*health*, Vital Nutrients, Vitamin Research Products, and Xymogen.

Continuing Education Credit Designations

For MDs and DOs, IFM designates this educational activity for a maximum of 6 *AMA PRA Category 1 credit(s)™*. Physicians should only claim credit commensurate with the extent of their participation in the activity.

Release date: May 22, 2008
Expiration date: May 22, 2011
Medium: Monograph

Method of Participation

To obtain CME credit for your participation in this activity:

1. Please read this monograph.
2. Complete the online evaluation, which will be sent to you via e-mail after purchase of the monograph; if you have any questions about accessing or completing the evaluation, contact IFM Client Services by e-mailing client_services@fxmed.com or calling 800-228-0622.

Statement of Need

Gap analysis and needs assessments conducted by IFM demonstrate an urgency for education and new approaches in treating chronic musculoskeletal pain. Musculoskeletal pain disorders are a major cause of human suffering, healthcare expenses, and lost productivity, yet conventional treatments for these disorders often have high rates of inefficacy and iatrogenesis in addition to their high costs. Education is needed to improve prevention, assist physicians in developing strategies for pain conditions, and provide an integrated, evidence-based model of care that includes not only drugs and surgery, but also manual therapies, nutritional and dietary approaches, botanical medicines, and acupuncture.

Learning Objectives

- Evaluate and, when appropriate, utilize comprehensive assessment procedures in the diagnosis of pain disorders.
- Assess environmental and lifestyle influences that may contribute to chronic musculoskeletal pain, including proinflammatory, nutrient-deficient diets, heavy metal toxicity, lack of exercise, and stress.
- Incorporate dietary interventions, nutritional supplements, botanical medicines, and manipulative therapies (massage and manipulation) to enhance the management of pain.
- Improve patient outcomes by applying functional medicine principles to the treatment of migraine, low back pain, fibromyalgia, and rheumatoid arthritis.

Purpose Statement

The purpose of this monograph is to provide healthcare professionals with functional medicine assessment and management strategies for chronic pain conditions, as well as a review of the evidence that supports these strategies.

Who Should Participate?

Any practitioner who cares for patients with chronic musculoskeletal pain, including primary care and specialist physicians.

Objectivity and Independence

It is the policy of IFM that all CME activities sponsored by IFM shall provide independent, balanced, objective, and scientifically rigorous presentations that are free of commercial bias. In accordance with ACCME Essential Areas and policies, IFM is totally responsible for all decisions on key components of activity development, including the development of activity goals and objectives, promotional material, content, faculty selection and approval, activity evaluation, and maintenance of physicians' credits.

Policy on Disclosure

As a sponsor accredited by ACCME, it is the policy of IFM to require all planners, authors, and editors to disclose (1) the existence of any relevant financial relationships with the supporters of this activity or manufacturer(s) of any commercial product(s) or services(s) that are discussed in their presentation, and (2) references in their presentations to unlabeled or unapproved use of drugs or devices. Disclosures are provided below.

Author Disclosure Statements

Alex Vasquez, DC, ND, OMSII, is the online Forum consultant for the Institute for Functional Medicine. He also indicated that he receives an honorarium from the Institute for Functional Medicine and an honorarium/salary from Biotics Research Corporation.

Content Planner Disclosure Statements

David Jones, MD, is President and Director of Medical Education of the Institute for Functional Medicine.

Dan Lukaczer, ND, is Associate Director of Medical Education of the Institute for Functional Medicine.

Sheila Quinn has indicated she has no financial relationships with any relevant commercial supporter or with the manufacturer of any commercial product or provider of any commercial service relevant to this activity.

Allison Templet is project editor and coordinator at the Institute for Functional Medicine.

Preface

"Criticism may not be agreeable, but it is necessary. It fulfils the same function as pain in the human body. It calls attention to an unhealthy state of things."

Sir Winston Churchill

The best health care seeks always to alter the unhealthy states that cause or contribute to pain and thereby bring relief to suffering patients. When we seek relief of pain without addressing underlying causes, however, we have not completed our efforts on behalf of our patients. Until we do, self-criticism is healthy and useful (although, indeed, not agreeable). Functional medicine provides concepts and tools for staying on the path of healing until all that can be done for the patient has been tried. We look for underlying common pathways of disease to locate points of leverage where a comprehensive treatment plan can help to normalize multiple systems.

Alex Vasquez, DC, ND, OMSII, an experienced clinician, teacher, and author (and The Institute for Functional Medicine's Forum consultant), has created a masterful exploration of how chronic musculoskeletal pain can be understood and ameliorated. Dr. Vasquez empowers practitioners to learn a new model—a way to identify and treat the dysfunctions and dysregulations that cause and perpetuate the pain associated with many chronic diseases, not just those discussed here. He also encourages each of us to look beyond our own knowledge base to understand and utilize the skills of many different disciplines, whether we are conventional physicians who refer patients to chiropractors, naturopathic physicians, and massage therapists, or alternative practitioners who work in tandem with conventionally trained colleagues. Pain crosses all organ-system boundaries, necessitating an integrated model of care that includes not only drugs and surgery, but manual therapies (manipulation and massage), nutritional and dietary approaches, botanical medicine, and acupuncture. Dr. Vasquez is a knowledgeable guide to the evidence for a wide variety of therapeutic approaches.

Every clinician knows, and the research cited here demonstrates, that we have not yet achieved great success in alleviating many kinds of pain. We have countless drugs that provide temporary relief, but at a very high cost (both financially and in the side effects that accompany most pain-relieving drugs). There is every reason, therefore, to pursue other approaches that will help us improve both the effectiveness and the cost-effectiveness of care. In addition to learning a different approach to assessment and treatment, we must also understand the many environmental and lifestyle influences that contribute to chronic musculoskeletal pain—such as the standard American diet (proinflammatory, nutrient deficient), heavy metal toxicity, lack of exercise, and stress—so that we can help our patients alter the triggers and mediators of their conditions. Without that level of change, we and they are forever enmeshed in a cycle of relapse and further treatment.

Dr. Vasquez provides an excellent introduction to the use of the Functional Medicine Matrix Model, a tool that can help clinicians collect, organize, and prioritize a great deal of patient data more effectively. He provides extensive information on assessment strategies and nutritional, botanical, and manipulative therapies for musculoskeletal pain. He provides a useful review of conventional treatments, as well. He then discusses four cornerstone conditions that exemplify the functional medicine applications of this knowledge: fibromyalgia, migraine, rheumatoid arthritis, and low back pain—conditions that many millions of Americans suffer from and that entail very high costs, both for conventional treatments that are often lifelong and for lost work and productivity. Finally, he presents cases that show the real-life use of the integrative therapeutics he recommends.

All of this is done within the context of what he calls "two fundamental premises of functional medicine":

1. Chronic diseases are a manifestation of chronic dysfunction.
2. Dysfunction can result from a wide range of interconnected genotropic, metabolic, nutritional, microbial, inflammatory, toxic, environmental, and psychological influences.

Indeed, these two premises highlight the areas in which a new kind of analytical and critical thinking is required of a functional medicine practitioner. It's no longer sufficient to name the disease and prescribe palliative pharmaceuticals. If we hope to significantly improve patient pain (and many other complaints), we must utilize a multifactorial, integrated model to look for and address the interconnections and underlying dysfunctions that characterize chronic disease. A huge challenge for us all!

Many thanks to Dr. Vasquez for this stimulating monograph. Thanks also to Allison Templet, project manager and editor, and to Michael W. Loes, MD, the monograph's technical reviewer.

David S. Jones, MD
President and Director of Medical Education
The Institute for Functional Medicine

Chapter 1

Overview of Musculoskeletal Pain and Introduction to the Functional Medicine Matrix Model

Introduction

Musculoskeletal disorders are extremely prevalent and represent a major cause of human suffering, healthcare expenses, and lost productivity, yet patients with these disorders face a series of difficult and often insurmountable obstacles to getting the relief they seek. Many standard medical interventions show high rates of inefficacy and iatrogenesis in addition to their high costs,[1,2,3] and pervasive deficiencies in musculoskeletal knowledge exist among healthcare providers[4,5,6,7,8] (with exceptions [9]).Further, many standard medical textbooks deprioritize nutritional and other nonsurgical and nonpharmacological interventions despite proof of efficacy shown in replicable, high-quality clinical trials published in top-tier medical journals. For example, many painful neuromusculoskeletal disorders can be alleviated and often effectively treated with nutritional interventions, but physicians trained only in standard medicine receive little to no training in nutrition and are therefore generally unable or unwilling to use these science-based interventions to help their patients.[10] In addition, despite the more than 800 articles documenting the role of nutritional interventions in the direct or adjunctive treatment of rheumatoid arthritis, the 17th edition of *The Merck Manual* published in 1999 reports that "food and diet quackery is common and should be discouraged."[11]

Combined, these factors present a picture of a field of medicine that is clearly in need of a pervasive paradigm shift in both physician training and patient management in order to improve the effectiveness and cost-effectiveness of care.[12] Functional medicine provides this paradigm shift. By incorporating evidence-based medicine into a conceptual framework that facilitates pattern recognition, functional medicine allows the effective prevention and treatment of disease based on an appreciation of human physiology as a highly interconnected and interdependent biological system (rather than marginally related organ systems). The power of this approach is evident in research documenting tremendous reductions in disease severity, mortality, and healthcare expenses when patients are enrolled in integrative treatment protocols for various conditions; many examples of such research will be cited in this monograph. A description of functional medicine from The Institute for Functional Medicine (IFM) is provided in Table 1.1, while a more comprehensive explanation is provided in the *Textbook of Functional Medicine*.[13]

Since approximately 1 of every 7 (14% of total) visits to primary healthcare providers is for the treatment of musculoskeletal pain or dysfunction,[14][15] every healthcare provider needs to have: (1) knowledge of important concepts related to musculoskeletal medicine, (2) the ability to recognize urgent and emergency conditions, (3) the ability to competently perform orthopedic examination procedures and interpret laboratory assessments, and (4) the knowledge and ability to design and implement effective treatment plans and to coordinate patient management. Clinicians utilizing a functional medicine approach to patient care must be knowledgeable in the details of integrative physiology and nutritional biochemistry and must possess the clinical acumen necessary to ensure safe and expedient patient care. These traits are of particular necessity when a serious condition is presented. Life-threatening and limb-threatening neuromusculoskeletal problems are notorious for presenting under the guise of an apparently benign complaint such as fatigue, headache, or simple joint pain.

Table 1.1—Principles of Functional Medicine

Functional medicine is a science-based field of health care that is grounded in the following principles:

- **Biochemical individuality**, which describes the importance of individual variations in metabolic function that derive from genetic and environmental differences among individuals.
- **Patient-centered** medicine, which emphasizes *patient care* rather than *disease care*, following Sir William Osler's admonition that "it is more important to know what patient has the disease than to know what disease the patient has."
- **Dynamic balance** of internal and external factors.
- **Web-like interconnections** of physiological factors in the human body, which functions as an orchestrated network of interconnected systems, rather than individual systems functioning autonomously and without effect on each other. For example, we now know that immunologic dysfunctions can promote cardiovascular disease, that dietary imbalances can cause hormonal disturbances, and that environmental exposures can precipitate neurological syndromes such as Parkinson's disease.
- **Health as a positive vitality**—not merely the absence of disease.
- **Promotion of organ reserve** as the means to enhance health span.

Functional medicine is grounded in scientific principles and information widely available in medicine today, combining research from various disciplines into highly detailed, yet clinically relevant models of disease pathogenesis and effective clinical management.

Source: http://www.functionalmedicine.org/about/whatis.asp

The purpose of this monograph is to provide healthcare professionals with an overview of the functional medicine assessment and management strategies that are applicable to painful neuromusculoskeletal disorders, as well as an examination of the research that supports these strategies. Chapter 1 will review the state of the evidence and present the functional medicine teaching tools and clinical models that are based on that evidence. Chapter 2 will provide an overview of assessments and treatments used by functional medicine practitioners treating pain conditions; special attention will be given to the abundant research supporting interventions such as diet; fatty acid, vitamin, and mineral supplements; protein and amino acids; botanicals; and physical medicine. A practical clinical approach to 4 common conditions (migraine, low back pain, fibromyalgia, and rheumatoid arthritis) will follow in Chapters 3, 4, 5, and 6. Finally, Chapter 7 will provide clinical case reports that illustrate how this complex array of possible interventions is applied to the challenge of effectively identifying and treating patients in pain.

In recognition of the diversity of this document's readership (inclusive of students, recent graduates, experienced professionals, academicians, and policy makers), this monograph on pain will necessarily review some basic concepts; however, this document alone cannot replace professional training in musculoskeletal medicine, nor does it include protocols for patient management and differential diagnosis for each of the neuromusculoskeletal problems seen in clinical practice. This text should be used in conjunction with the clinician's previous professional training, other textbooks, and best judgment for the delivery of personalized care for each individual patient, including those who present with similar or identical diagnoses. Supportive texts include *Current Medical Diagnosis and Treatment* edited by Tierney et al,[16] *Orthopedic Physical Assessment* by Magee,[17] and *Integrative Orthopedics* and *Integrative Rheumatology* by Vasquez.[18,19] Further, clinicians can note that this monograph is written primarily for routine outpatient management of chronic pain conditions and not acute emergency department situations.

Background

Historically, prevailing views of disorders of pain and inflammation were conceptually similar to those of most other diseases. Our clinical predecessors did the best they could to understand, describe, and treat the health problems that their patients presented, and the paradigm from which these clinical entities were viewed and addressed was shaped by the social, religious, and scientific views and limitations of their time. However, these premodern clinicians lacked a molecular and physiological understanding of disease origination, and they were restrained by metaphysical and simplistic models of cause and effect. The models they devised for the understanding and treatment of disease generally appear unsatisfactory today in light of the advances in our understanding of disparate yet interrelated fields such as psychoneuroimmunology, molecular biology, nutrigenomics, environmental medicine, and toxicology.

Despite these advances, we as a society and as healthcare providers still carry many of these previous conceptualizations and misconceptualizations with us. Though we feel that our views and interventions are much more precise and objective, the generalized and phenomenalistic approaches that typified premodern medicine still permeate some aspects of clinical care today. For example, we still use the term *stroke* to describe acute cerebrovascular insufficiency, although the term originated from the view that affected patients had been "struck" by the gods or fates, perhaps as a form of punishment for some ethical or religious transgression. Even today, some patients and clinicians interpret health and disease as a form of punishment or as an extension of a spiritual or intrapersonal shortcoming. However, advancing science allows us to disassemble complex events that were previously experienced as *phenomena*, that is, as undecipherable and enigmatic events that overwhelmed comprehension.

Whereas the advancement of our scientific knowledge often leads us to discard previous models and interventions, occasionally modern science helps us to better understand previous interventions that may have been prematurely or unduly discarded. For example, Hippocrates' admonition to "let thy food be thy medicine, and thy medicine be thy food" experienced decades of devaluation when dietary, nutritional, and other natural interventions were misbranded as quackery. On the contrary, simple, natural interventions such as therapeutic fasting and augmentation of vitamin D3 status (via nutritional supplementation or exposure to ultraviolet-B radiation) have shown remarkable safety and efficacy in the mitigation of chronic hypertension, musculoskeletal pain, and autoimmunity.[20,21,22,23,24,25,26] Furthermore, the appropriate use of vitamin supplements helps prevent chronic disease by numerous mechanisms including modulation of gene transcription, enhancement of DNA repair and stability, and enhancement of metabolic efficiency.[27,28,29]

State of the Evidence

This monograph will provide a representative survey of current research in the use of dietary, nutritional, and integrative therapeutics commonly utilized in the clinical management of disorders characterized by pain and inflammation. A "blanket statement" to cover all the different assessments and interventions described herein would be necessarily inaccurate, and therefore, each intervention will be considered on the merits of its own rationale, safety, effectiveness, and cost-effectiveness. These considerations must ultimately be viewed within the context of the individual patient's condition and the overall cohesion and comprehensiveness of the treatment plan.

While all clinicians can appreciate the importance of protocols and clinical practice guidelines, we must also perpetually stress the importance of tailoring treatment to the patient's unique combination of biochemical individuality, comorbid conditions, drug use, personal goals, and willingness to participate in a health-promoting lifestyle. Standardized protocols and practice guidelines are founded on the fallacy of disease homogeneity and the irrelevance of physiological, psychosocial, and biochemical individuality. As the advancement of biomedical science provides the means for and underscores the importance of customized treatments for each patient, so too has the standard of care begun to shift in the direction of patient individuality. Failure to utilize nutritional interventions when such interventions are clinically indicated is inconsistent with the delivery of quality health care and may be considered malpractice.[30,31,32]

A clinician who is unaware of the political forces that shape healthcare policy and research is analogous to a captain of an oceangoing ship not knowing how to use a compass, sextant, or coastline map. Medical science and healthcare policy are influenced by a myriad of powerful private interests motivated by their own goals, at times different from the stated goals of medicine, which purports to hold paramount the patient's welfare. Scientific objectivity and the guiding ethical principles of informed consent, beneficence, autonomy, and non-malfeasance are subject to different interpretations depending on the lens through which a dilemma is viewed. This gives rise to a disarrayed tug-of-war between factions and private interests, with paradigmatic victory often being awarded to those with the best marketing campaigns and political influence while less importance is given to safety, efficacy, and the economic burden to consumers.[33,34,35,36,37,38,39,40] To be ignorant of such considerations is to be blind to the nature of research, policy, and our own biased inclinations for and against particular paradigms, assessments, and interventions. Research articles and sources of authority must be approached with an artist's delicacy and with a willingness to consider new information that may contradict deeply rooted beliefs.

Understanding the Multifaceted Nature of Disease Pathogenesis: The Functional Medicine Matrix Model as Paradigm and Clinical Tool

Functional medicine offers extremely useful tools for helping clinicians grasp a multidimensional, decipherable view of disease and its corresponding treatment in order to facilitate higher clinical efficacy, improved patient outcomes, and more favorable safety and cost-effectiveness profiles. These include the Functional Medicine Matrix Model, which is both a teaching tool and a clinical method. When viewed as a diagram, the web of intrinsic and extrinsic influences at play in a given disease process or individual patient can be appreciated, revealing how imbalance or disruption in one area or system can lead to problems in another. Such a tool can help us bridge the gaps between nutritional status, neurotransmitter synthesis, pain sensitivity, immune function, and mitochondrial bioenergetics, as described in this monograph.

Over the course of many years, discussions, and reconsiderations, the faculty at IFM elucidated 8 preeminent systems or loci for clinicians to consider when working with any chronic health disorder. These *core clinical imbalances* are described below, with particular consideration of neuromusculoskeletal pain and inflammation. Interested readers are directed to IFM's monographs on topics including depression and gastrointestinal inflammation/dysbiosis to see how this model is applied to disease states in different organ systems.

1. Hormonal and Neurotransmitter Regulation

Hormonal imbalances are particularly relevant to the discussion of chronic pain caused by inflammation, and such pain is characteristic of autoimmune diseases such as rheumatoid arthritis. Often clinically subtle but nonetheless of extreme importance, these hormonal influences on painful inflammation are worthy of their own detailed discussion. Rectification of endocrinologic imbalances (*orthoendocrinology*) will be discussed in this monograph (see *Clinical Focus: Rheumatoid Arthritis*) and has been detailed with broader clinical applicability elsewhere by this author.[19]

While most clinicians are aware that neurotransmitters can either transmit pain signals or dampen their reception, many are not aware that neurotransmitter status is somewhat malleable and can

> **Clinical Pearl:**
>
> Patients with autoimmune neuromusculoskeletal inflammation generally display a complete or partial pattern of hormonal disturbances typified by elevated estrogen and prolactin and lowered testosterone, DHEA, and cortisol; appropriate therapeutic correction of these imbalances can safely result in disease amelioration.

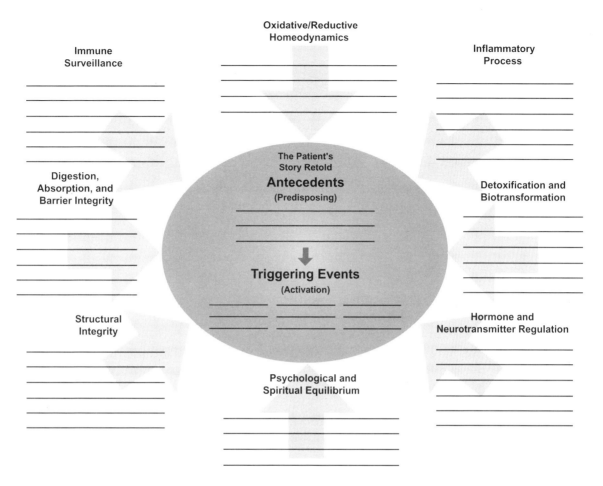

Figure 1.1—The Functional Medicine Matrix Model
©2007, The Institute for Functional Medicine

be modulated with nutritional supplementation and botanical medicines, as well as massage. The examples considered here are the tryptophan-serotonin-melatonin and the phenylalanine-epinephrine-enkephalin pathways.

- Tryptophan and 5-hydroxytryptophan (5-HTP) are prescription and nonprescription nutritional supplements that are the amino acid precursors for the formation of the neurotransmitter serotonin and, subsequently, the pineal hormone melatonin. Biochemically, these conversions are linear as follows: tryptophan → 5-HTP → serotonin → melatonin. Tryptophan depletion and low levels of serotonin are consistently associated with depression, anxiety, exacerbation of eating disorders, and increased sensitivity to acute and chronic pain. Serotonergic pathways are impaired by chronic stress due to increased utilization of serotonin (e.g., serotonin-dependent cortisol release) and increased hepatic degradation of tryptophan by cortisol-stimulated tryptophan pyrrolase.[41] Certainly part of the benefit from 5-HTP supplementation is derived from the increased formation of melatonin, as the biological effects of melatonin extend beyond its sleep-promoting role to include powerful antioxidation, anti-infective immunostimulation,[42] and preservation of mitochondrial function, a benefit which is of particular relevance to the treatment of fibromyalgia.[43]
- The conditionally essential fatty acids found in fish oil modulate serotonergic and adrenergic activity in the human brain.[44] Given the role of serotonin and norepinephrine in the central processing of pain perception,[45] a reasonable hypothesis holds that the pain-relieving activity of fish oil supplementation[46] is partly due to central modulation of pain perception and is not wholly due to modulation of eicosanoid production and inflammatory mediator transcription as previously believed.

- Vitamin D3 supplementation may also augment serotonergic activity,[47] and this mechanism may partly explain the mood-enhancing and pain-relieving benefits of vitamin D3 supplementation.
- Supplementation with DL-phenylalanine (DLPA; racemic mixture of D- and L-forms of the amino acid phenylalanine derived from synthetic production) has long been used in the treatment of pain and depression.[48] The nutritional L-isomer is converted from phenylalanine to tyrosine to L-dopa to dopamine to norepinephrine and epinephrine. Augmentation of this pathway promotes resistance to fatigue, depression, and pain. The synthetic D-isomer augments pain-relieving enkephalin function by inhibiting enkephalin degradation by the enzyme carboxypeptidase A (enkephalinase); the resultant augmentation of enkephalin levels is generally believed to underlie the analgesic and mood-enhancing benefits of DLPA supplementation.
- Therapeutic massage is yet another means to modulate neurotransmitter synthesis for the alleviation of pain. In a study of patients with chronic back pain, massage increased serotonin and dopamine levels (measured in urine).[49]

2. Oxidative-Reductive Homeodynamics

Oxidative stress results from chronic, systemic inflammation as seen in painful disorders such as rheumatoid arthritis. This imbalance contributes to the perpetuation and exacerbation of inflammatory diseases via expedited tissue destruction, alterations in gene transcription, and resultant enhancement of inflammatory mediator production.[52] Immune activation increases production of reactive oxygen species (ROS), or free radicals. Oxidative stress increases activation of proinflammatory transcription factors and increases spontaneous oxidative modification of endogenous proteins such as cartilage matrix, which then undergo expedited degradation or immunologic attack. Thus, a vicious cycle of oxidation and inflammation exacerbates and perpetuates various inflammation-associated diseases, resulting in therapeutic recalcitrance and autonomous disease progression.[53,54]

> **Clinical Pearl:**
> Therapeutically, supplementation with 5-HTP augments serotonin and melatonin synthesis and has specific applicability in the alleviation of depression and pain syndromes such as fibromyalgia and headache, including migraine, tension headaches, and juvenile headaches.[50,51]

A rational clinical approach to breaking this vicious, pathogenic cycle can include simultaneous antioxidation and immunomodulation, the former with diet optimization and nutritional supplementation and the latter with allergen avoidance, hormonal correction, xenobiotic detoxification, and specific phytonutritional modulation of proinflammatory pathways. Severe and acute inflammation can and often should be suppressed pharmacologically, but sole reliance on pharmacological immunosuppression leaves the patient vulnerable to iatrogenic immunosuppression and the well-known increased risk for cardiovascular disease, infection, and clinical malignancy; in addition, this reliance fails to address the underlying biochemical and immunologic imbalances that underlie all chronic inflammatory and autoimmune diseases.

The contribution of mitochondrial dysfunction to chronic recurrent or persistent pain is most plainly demonstrated in migraine and fibromyalgia (see *Clinical Focus: Migraine* and *Clinical Focus: Fibromyalgia*). An important characteristic of migraine is mitochondrial dysfunction, the severity of which correlates positively with the severity of the headache syndrome.[55] In fibromyalgia, numerous abnormalities in cellular bioenergetics are noted, which correlate clinically with the lowered lactate threshold, persistent muscle pain, reduced functional capacity, and subjective fatigue that characterize the disorder.[56] Nutritional preservation and enhancement of mitochondrial function was termed *mitochondrial resuscitation* by Bland in the 1990s, and clinical implementation of such an approach generally includes, in addition to diet and lifestyle modification, supplementation with coenzyme Q10, niacin, riboflavin, thiamin, lipoic acid, magnesium, and other nutrients and botanical medicines that enhance production of adenosine triphosphate (ATP).[57]

3. Detoxification and Biotransformation

As our environment becomes increasingly polluted and as researchers and clinicians mature and expand their appreciation and knowledge of the adverse effects of xenobiotics (toxic metals and chemicals), healthcare providers will need to attend to their patients' detoxification capacity and xenobiotic load as a component of the prevention and treatment of disease. Many clinicians are now aware of the association of xenobiotics in prototypic diseases such as Parkinson's disease,[58,59] adult-onset diabetes mellitus,[60,61,62,63] and attention-deficit hyperactivity disorder.[64,65,66] The role of xenobiotic exposure and impaired detoxification in neuromusculoskeletal pain and inflammatory disorders is more subtle and is generally mediated through the resultant immunotoxicity that manifests as autoimmunity. Occasionally, clinicians will encounter patients with musculoskeletal symptomatology that defies standard diagnosis and treatment but that responds remarkably and permanently to empiric clinical detoxification treatment; such a case will be presented in Chapter 7 of this monograph. The numerous roles of xenobiotic exposure in the genesis and perpetuation of chronic health problems and the role of clinical detoxification in the treatment of such problems has been detailed elsewhere by Crinnion,[67,68,69,70,71] Rea,[72] Bland,[73,74] Vasquez,[19,75] and others.[76,77]

4. Immune Imbalances

Immune imbalances have an obvious role in musculoskeletal inflammation when discussed in the context of autoimmune diseases such as rheumatoid arthritis, ankylosing spondylitis, and systemic lupus erythematosus (SLE). While the standard medical approach to this pathophysiology has focused almost exclusively on the pharmacological suppression of resultant inflammation and tissue destruction, other approaches such as naturopathic medicine and functional medicine have emphasized the importance of determining and addressing the underlying causes of such immune imbalance. Clinicians of all disciplines must appreciate the role of pharmacological immunosuppression in the treatment of inflammatory exacerbations as seen with giant cell arteritis or neuropsychiatric lupus; however, they should also appreciate that sole reliance on immunosuppression for long-term management of inflammatory disorders can result in therapeutic failure insofar as it does not correct the underlying cause of the disease and creates dependency upon perpetual immunosuppression, with its attendant costs (not uncommonly in the range of $50,000 per year) and adverse effects, including infection and increased risk for cancer.

> **Clinical Pearl:**
>
> The role of xenobiotic exposure and impaired detoxification in neuromusculoskeletal pain and inflammatory disorders is generally mediated through the resultant immunotoxicity that manifests as autoimmunity.

Rather than presuming that immune dysfunction and the resultant inflammation and autoimmunity are results of spontaneous generation, astute clinicians seek to identify and correct the causes of these immune imbalances (when possible). In this way, clinicians can lessen or obviate the need for chronic, polypharmaceutical treatment with anti-inflammatory and immunosuppressive agents. It is proposed that secondary immune imbalances (distinguished from primary congenital disorders) generally arise from 1 or more of 5 main problems: (1) habitual consumption of a proinflammatory diet, (2) food allergies and intolerances, (3) microbial dysbiosis, including multifocal poly-dysbiosis, (4) hormonal imbalances, and (5) xenobiotic exposure and accumulation resulting in immunotoxicity via bystander activation and enhanced processing of autoantigens, as well as haptenization and neoantigen formation.[19] These influences may act singularly or, when combined, may be additive and synergistic. Each of these problems will be reviewed in Chapter 2, *Overview of Clinical Approach, Assessments, and Therapeutics*, as well as in the clinical focus subsections, particularly rheumatoid arthritis.

5. Inflammatory Process

Inflammatory imbalances may be distinguished from immune imbalances insofar as inflammatory imbalances connote disorders of inflammatory mediator production in the absence of the immunodysfunction typical of allergy, autoimmunity, or immunosuppression. Here again, long-term consumption of a proinflammatory diet[78] is a primary consideration because it oversupplies inflammatory precursors such as arachidonate and undersupplies anti-inflammatory phytonutrients such as vitamin D, zinc, selenium, and the numerous phytochemicals that reduce activation of inflammatory pathways.[79,80,81,82]

Three of the best examples of correctable inflammatory imbalances are those due to vitamin D deficiency, fatty acid imbalances, and overconsumption of simple sugars and saturated fats.

- Vitamin D deficiency is a serious health problem that spans nearly all geographic regions and socioeconomic strata. Adverse effects include systemic inflammation[83] and chronic musculoskeletal pain,[84] which both resolve quickly upon correction of the nutritional deficiency. (For more information on Vitamin D, see *Vitamin and Mineral Supplements* in Chapter 2.)
- Overconsumption of arachidonic acid and underconsumption of alpha-linolenic acid (ALA), gamma-linolenic acid (GLA), eicosapentaenoic acid (EPA), docosahexaenoic acid (DHA), and oleic acid subtly yet powerfully shift nutrigenomic tendency and precursor availability in favor of enhanced systemic inflammation. Correction of this imbalance has consistently proven to be of significant clinical value in the management of chronic inflammatory disorders.[85,86] (For more information, see *Fatty Acid Supplements* in Chapter 2.)
- Measurable increases in systemic inflammation and oxidative stress follow glucose challenge,[87] consumption of saturated fatty acids as found in cream,[88] and consumption of fast food breakfasts, which trigger the prototypic inflammatory activator nuclear factor-kappa B (NF-κB) for enhanced production of inflammatory mediators.[89]

This triad (vitamin D deficiency, fatty acid imbalance, and overconsumption of sugars and saturated fats) is typical of the Western/American pattern of dietary intake, and the molecular means and clinical consequences of such dietary choices are evident in the burgeoning epidemics of metabolic and inflammatory diseases.

6. Digestion, Absorption, and Barrier Integrity

The grouping of digestive and absorptive considerations suggests that the alimentary tract and its accessory organs of the liver, gall bladder, and pancreas will be the focus of these core clinical imbalances. In addition, microbiological imbalances (gastrointestinal dysbiosis) are important and frequent clinical considerations. Impaired digestion begins neither in the stomach nor in the mouth, but it stems rather from any socioeconomic milieu that deprives people of the means to prepare wholesome, health-promoting meals and the time to consume those meals in a relaxed, parasympathetic-dominant mode. Poor dentition, xerostomia, hypochlorhydria, cholestasis or cholecystectomy, pancreatic insufficiency, mucosal atrophy, altered gut motility, and bacterial overgrowth of the small bowel are important and common contributors to impaired digestion and absorption; clinicians should consider these frequently and implement treatment with a low threshold for intervention. The relevance of these problems to pain and the musculoskeletal system is generally that of malnutrition and its macro- and micronutrient consequences. Sunlight-deprived individuals must rely on dietary sources of vitamin D, which are hardly adequate for the prevention of overt deficiency; any impairment in digestion, emulsification, or absorption of this fat-soluble vitamin can readily lead to hypovitaminosis D and its resultant musculoskeletal consequences of osteomalacia and unremitting pain.[90]

Consumption of foods to which the individual is sensitized (food allergies) can trigger migraine and other chronic headaches,[91,92] as well as generalized musculoskeletal pain and arthritis.[93,94,95.] Avoidance of the offending foods result in amelioration or complete remission of the painful syndrome at low cost and high efficacy without reliance on expensive or potentially harmful or addictive pain-relieving drugs. Occasionally, gluten enteropathy (celiac disease) presents with arthritic pain and chronic synovitis; the pain and inflammation remit on a gluten-free diet.[96]

Alterations in intestinal microbial balance or an individual's unique response to endogenous bacteria can lead to systemic inflammation, arthritis, vasculitis, and musculoskeletal pain. Eradication of the occult infection or mucosal colonization often results in marked reductions in systemic inflammation and its clinical complications. Interested readers are directed to the excellent review by Noah[97] on the relevance of dysbiosis and its treatment relative to psoriasis. (For a discussion of clinical nuances and molecular mechanisms of gastrointestinal dysbiosis based on previous reviews by this author, [98] see *Laboratory Assessment* in Chapter 2.)

7. Structural Integrity

Molecular structural imbalances lie at the heart of the concept of biochemical individuality, a term originated by Roger J. Williams[99] in 1956, and this concept was soon expanded into the theory and practice of orthomolecular medicine, pioneered by Linus Pauling and colleagues.[100,101] Pauling is considered by many authorities to be the original source of the concept of molecular medicine because he coined the phrase *molecular disease* after his team's discovery in 1949 that sickle cell anemia resulted from a single amino acid substitution that caused physical deformation of the hemoglobin molecule in hypoxic conditions.[102] (One of Pauling's students, Jeffrey Bland, continued this legacy with the organization of functional medicine and the founding of IFM.[103])

> **Clinical Pearl:**
>
> Dysbiosis can occur at sites other than the gastrointestinal tract, most importantly the nasopharynx and genitourinary tracts.

Single nucleotide polymorphisms (SNPs; pronounced "snips") are DNA sequence variations that can result in amino acid substitutions rendering the final protein (e.g., structural protein or enzyme) abnormal in structure and therefore function. This aberrancy may cause clinical disease (depending on the severity and importance of the variation), and consequences of the dysfunction may be occult, subtle, or obvious. One of the most powerful and effective means for treating diseases resultant from SNPs is high-dose vitamin supplementation, and this forms the scientific basis for megavitamin therapy, as elegantly and authoritatively reviewed by Bruce Ames et al.[104] SNP-induced alterations in enzyme structure reduce affinity for vitamin-derived coenzyme binding; this reduced affinity can be overpowered by administration of high doses of the required vitamin cofactor, increasing tissue concentrations of the nutrient and promoting binding of the enzyme with its ligand for the performance of enzymatic function.

> **Clinical Pearl:**
>
> The scientific rationale for nutritional therapy is derived in part from the recognition that altered enzymatic function due to altered enzyme structure can often be corrected by administration of supra-dietary doses of nutrients.

Relatedly, the structure and function of cell membranes are determined by their composition, which is influenced by dietary intake of fatty acids and which influences production of prostaglandins and leukotrienes. This is an important aspect of the scientific rationale for the use of specific fatty acid supplements in the prevention and treatment of inflammatory musculoskeletal disease. Cell membrane structure and function can also be altered by systemic oxidative stress; the concomitant alterations in intracellular ions (e.g., calcium) and receptor function, along with activation of transcription factors such as NF-κB, contribute to widespread physiological impairment, which creates a vicious cycle of inflammation, metabolic disturbance, and additional free radical generation.[105,106]

Somatic dysfunction, musculoskeletal disorders, and inefficient biomechanics contribute to pain, increased production of inflammatory mediators, and the expedited degeneration of tissues such as collagen and cartilage matrix. Physicians trained in clinical biomechanics and physical medicine appreciate the subtle nuances of musculoskeletal structure-function relationships and address these problems directly with physical and manual means rather than ignoring the physical problem and treating only its biochemical sequelae. Concepts of biomechanics, palpatory diagnosis, and manual therapies will be reviewed later in this monograph.

8. Psychological and Spiritual Equilibrium

The connections between physical pain and psycho-emotional status and events are worthy of thorough discussion, despite the fact that conventional clinical practices have typically marginalized these considerations or considered them only long enough to substantiate psychopharmaceutical intervention. A survey of the literature makes clear the interconnected nature of pain, inflammation, psycho-emotional stress, depression, social isolation, and nutritional status; though a complete discussion is beyond the scope of this monograph, a brief exemplification of these concepts is provided here.

Stressful and depressive life events promote the development, persistence, and exacerbation of disorders of pain and inflammation through nutritional, hormonal, immunologic, oxidative, and microbiological mechanisms. Stated most simply, the perception of stressful events and the resultant neurohormonal cascade result in expedited metabolic utilization and increased urinary excretion of nutrients (e.g., tryptophan and zinc, magnesium, retinol, respectively), which sum to affect nutritional imbalances and depletion, particularly when the stress response is acute or prolonged.[107,108,109]

Specific to the consideration of pain, the depletion of tryptophan (and thus serotonin and melatonin) leaves the patient vulnerable to increased pain from lack of antinociceptive serotonin and to increased inflammation due to impaired endogenous production of anti-inflammatory cortisol, the adrenal release of which requires serotonin-dependent stimulation.[41] Severe stress, inflammation, and drugs used to suppress immune-mediated tissue damage (e.g., cyclosporine) increase urinary excretion of magnesium,[110] and the eventual magnesium depletion renders the patient more vulnerable to hyperalgesia, depression, and other central nervous system and psychiatric disorders.[111,112] Furthermore, experimental and clinical data have shown that magnesium deficiency leads to a systemic proinflammatory state associated with oxidative stress and increased levels of the nociceptive and proinflammatory neurotransmitter substance P.[113] Stress increases secretion of prolactin, a hormone that plays an important pathogenic role in chronic inflammation and autoimmunity.[114,115]

An abundance of experimental and clinical research supports the model that chronic psycho-emotional stress reduces mucosal immunity, increases intestinal permeability, and allows for increased intestinal colonization by microbes. These microbes then stimulate immune responses that cross-react with musculoskeletal tissues and result in the clinical manifestation of autoimmunity and painful rheumatic syndromes, which appear clinically as variants of acute and chronic reactive arthritis (formerly Reiter' syndrome[116]) in susceptible patients.[19,117,118,119,120,121,122,123] Interestingly, intestinal bacteria have been shown to become more virulent when their host is stressed, whereas previously these same bacteria may have been incapable of causing disease.[124,125] Psycho-emotional stress also reduces mucosal immunity and increases colonization in locations other than the gastrointestinal tract. Microbial colonization of the genitourinary tract (genitourinary dysbiosis[19]) appears highly relevant in the genesis and perpetuation of rheumatoid arthritis.[122,126,127,128] Stressful life events also lower testosterone in men, and the resultant lack of hormonal immunomodulation can increase the frequency and severity of exacerbations of rheumatoid arthritis[129]; resultant inflammation further suppresses testosterone production and bioavailability,[130] leading to a self-perpetuating cycle of hypogonadism and inflammation. Thus, by numerous routes and mechanisms, psycho-emotional stress increases the prevalence, persistence, and severity of musculoskeletal inflammation and pain.

Psychiatric codiagnoses are common among patients with painful neuromusculoskeletal disorders, and when the prevailing medical logic cannot solve the musculoskeletal riddle, the disorder is often ascribed to its accompanying mental disorder. The "appropriate" treatment from this perspective is the prescription of psychoactive drugs, generally of the antidepressant class. Science-based explanations are needed to expand clinicians' consideration of new possibilities that may someday prevail over commonplace suppositions that idiopathic pain is caused by its associated depression and both should be treated with antidepressant drugs. Alternatives to this hypothesis include the following:

- **Pain, inflammation, and depression are final common pathways for nutritional deficiencies and imbalances.** Research in various fields has shown that Western/American lifestyle and diet patterns diverge radically from human physiological expectations and human nutritional requirements[131]—modern diets are a "setup" for musculoskeletal pain and depression. For example, we now know that the epidemic problem of vitamin D deficiency leads to musculoskeletal pain,[132] as well as depression,[133] and that supplementation with physiological doses of vitamin D results in an enhanced sense of well-being[134] and alleviation of musculoskeletal pain and depression while providing other major collateral benefits.[135] In addition, musculoskeletal pain and depression are both alleviated by corrective fatty acid intervention such as fish oil supplementation as a source of EPA and DHA.[136,137] Also relevant to this discussion are the pain-sensitizing effects of epidemic magnesium deficiency.[138] Therefore, correction of nutritional imbalances may be considered more rational in the co-management of pain and depression than sole reliance on antidepressant and anti-inflammatory drugs; the latter have their place in treatment, but neither addresses the primary cause of the problem and both have important adverse effects and significant costs, in contrast to the safety, affordability, and collateral benefits derived from nutritional supplementation.

- **Pain, inflammation, and depression are final common pathways of physical inactivity.** Exercising muscle elaborates cytokines ("myokines") with anti-inflammatory activity; a sedentary lifestyle fails to stimulate this endogenous anti-inflammation and is therefore relatively proinflammatory.[139] Further, exercise has antidepressant benefits mediated by positive influences on neurotransmission, growth factor elaboration, endocrinologic function, self-image, and social contact.[140] Patients with musculoskeletal pain should be encouraged to exercise to the extent possible given the individual's capacity and type of injury. Thus, a prescription for exercise might supersede the prescription of drugs in patients with concomitant depression and pain. Exercise prescriptions must consider frequency, duration, intensity, variety, safety, enjoyment, accountability, and objective measures of compliance and progress, as well as appropriate combinations of components that emphasize aerobic fitness, strengthening, flexibility, muscle balancing, and coordination.
- **Pain and depression are final common pathways of inflammation.** Several proinflammatory cytokines are psychoactive and cause depression, social withdrawal, impaired cognition, and sickness behavior.[141] As an alternative to the use of antidepressant drugs, correction of the underlying inflammatory disorder by natural, pharmacological, or integrative means may subsequently promote restoration of normal affect and cognitive function.
- **Pain, inflammation, and depression are final common pathways for hormonal deficiencies and imbalances.** Deficiencies of thyroid hormones, estrogen (insufficiency or excess), testosterone, cortisol, and DHEA can cause depression and impaired neuro-emotional status. Hormonal aberrations are common in patients with chronic musculoskeletal pain, particularly of the inflammatory and autoimmune types. Clinical trials have shown that administration of thyroid hormones, testosterone, DHEA, and cortisol and suppression of prolactin can each provide anti-inflammatory, analgesic, and antidepressant benefits among appropriately selected patients. Thus, identification and correction of hormonal imbalances might supersede the prescription of antidepressant drugs in patients with concomitant depression, inflammation, and pain.

Our cultural and scientific advancements in the knowledge of how the brain functions have been paradoxically paralleled by social trends showing increasing depression and social isolation; the typical American has only 2 friends and no one in whom to confide.[142] In the United States, violent injuries are epidemic, and the level of firearm morbidity and mortality is far higher than anywhere else in the industrialized world.[143] This does to some extent beg the question of the value of scientific knowledge of the mind within a social structure that is increasingly violent and fragmented. Further, depression resulting from social isolation would be better served by physicians' admonition for increased social contact than by drugs that inhibit neurotransmitter reuptake.

Conclusion

The functional medicine approach to chronic disease management and health promotion rests upon a foundation of competent patient management, then extends to consider the well-documented contributions of the core clinical imbalances that have allowed the genesis and perpetuation of the problem(s) under consideration. The attainment of wellness, the success of preventive medicine, and the optimization of socio-emotional health cannot be attained by pharmacological suppression of the manifestations of dysfunction that result from nutritional and neuroendocrine imbalances, xenobiotic accumulation, sedentary lifestyles, social isolation, and mucosal microbial colonization. Instead, the functional medicine approach addresses these problems directly. These core clinical imbalances must remain foremost in the mind of the physician committed to the successful, ethical, and cost-effective long-term prevention and management of chronic health disturbances, particularly those characterized by inflammation and pain.

References

1. Moseley JB, O'Malley K, Petersen NJ, et al. A controlled trial of arthroscopic surgery for osteoarthritis of the knee. *N Engl J Med*. 2002;347:81-88.
2. Kolata G. Arthritis surgery in ailing knees is cited as sham. *New York Times*. July 11, 2002:A1.
3. Rosner AL. Evidence-based clinical guidelines for the management of acute low-back pain: response to the guidelines prepared for the Australian Medical Health and Research Council. *J Manipulative Physiol Ther*. 2001;24:214-220.
4. Freedman KB, Bernstein J. Educational deficiencies in musculoskeletal medicine. *J Bone Joint Surg Am*. 2002;84-A:604-608.
5. Joy EA, Hala SV. Musculoskeletal curricula in medical education: Filling in the missing pieces. *The Physician and Sportsmedicine*. 2004;32:42-45.
6. Matzkin E, Smith ME, Freccero CD, Richardson AB. Adequacy of education in musculoskeletal medicine. *J Bone Joint Surg Am*. 2005;87-A(2):310-314.
7. Schmale GA. More evidence of educational inadequacies in musculoskeletal medicine. *Clin Orthop Relat Res*. 2005;437:251-259.
8. Stockard AR, Allen TW. Competence levels in musculoskeletal medicine: comparison of osteopathic and allopathic medical graduates. *J Am Osteopath Assoc*. 2006;106:350-355.
9. Humphreys BK, Sulkowski A, McIntyre K, Kasiban M, Patrick AN. An examination of musculoskeletal cognitive competency in chiropractic interns. *J Manipulative Physiol Ther*. 2007;30:44-49.
10. Adams KM, Lindell KC, Kohlmeier M, Zeisel SH. Status of nutrition education in medical schools. *Am J Clin Nutr*. 2006;83:941S-944S.
11. Beers MH, Berkow R, eds. *The Merck Manual of Diagnosis and Therapy*. 17th ed. Whitehouse Station; Merck Research Laboratories; 1999: 419.
12. Hyman M. Paradigm shift: the end of "normal science" in medicine understanding function in nutrition, health, and disease. *Altern Ther Health Med*. 2004;10:10-15, 90-94.
13. Jones DS, ed. *Textbook of Functional Medicine*. Gig Harbor, Wash: The Institute for Functional Medicine; 2005.
14. American College of Rheumatology Ad Hoc Committee on Clinical Guidelines. Guidelines for the initial evaluation of the adult patient with acute musculoskeletal symptoms. *Arthritis Rheum*. 1996;39:1-8.
15. Vasquez A. Musculoskeletal disorders and iron overload disease: comment on the American College of Rheumatology guidelines. *Arthritis Rheum*. 1996;39:1767-1768.
16. Tierney ML. McPhee SJ, Papadakis MA, eds. *Current Medical Diagnosis and Treatment*. New York, NY: Lange Medical Books. Updated annually
17. Magee DJ. *Orthpedic Physical Assessment*. 4th ed. W.B. Saunders;2002.
18. Vasquez A. *Integrative Orthopedics*. 2nd ed. Fort Worth, Tex; Integrative and Biological Medicine Research and Consulting; 2007.
19. Vasquez A. *Integrative Rheumatology*. 2nd ed. Fort Worth, Tex; Integrative and Biological Medicine Research and Consulting; 2007.
20. Goldhamer A, Lisle D, Parpia B, Anderson SV, Campbell TC. Medically supervised water-only fasting in the treatment of hypertension. *J Manipulative Physiol Ther*. 2001;24:335-339.
21. Goldhamer AC. Initial cost of care results in medically supervised water-only fasting for treating high blood pressure and diabetes. *J Altern Complement Med*. 2002;8:696-697.
22. Pfeifer M, Begerow B, Minne HW, Nachtigall D, Hansen C. Effects of a short-term vitamin D(3) and calcium supplementation on blood pressure and parathyroid hormone levels in elderly women. *J Clin Endocrinol Metab*. 2001;86(4):1633-1637.
23. McCarty MF. A preliminary fast may potentiate response to a subsequent low-salt, low-fat vegan diet in the management of hypertension - fasting as a strategy for breaking metabolic vicious cycles. *Med Hypotheses*. 2003;60:624-633.
24. Hyppönen E, Läärä E, Reunanen A, Järvelin MR, Virtanen SM. Intake of vitamin D and risk of type 1 diabetes: a birth-cohort study. *Lancet*. 2001;358:1500-1503.
25. Fuhrman J, Sarter B, Calabro DJ. Brief case reports of medically supervised, water-only fasting associated with remission of autoimmune disease. *Altern Ther Health Med*. 2002;8:112, 110-111.
26. Holick MF. Vitamin D deficiency: what a pain it is. *Mayo Clin Proc*. 2003;78:1457-1459.
27. Fletcher RH, Fairfield KM. Vitamins for chronic disease prevention in adults: clinical applications. *JAMA*. 2002;287:3127-3129.
28. Heaney RP. Long-latency deficiency disease: insights from calcium and vitamin D. *Am J Clin Nutr*. 2003;78:912-919.
29. Ames BN. The metabolic tune-up: metabolic harmony and disease prevention. *J Nutr*. 2003;133(5 Suppl 1):1544S-1548S.
30. Heaney RP. Vitamin D, nutritional deficiency, and the medical paradigm. *J Clin Endocrinol Metab*. 2003;88:5107-5108.
31. Berg A. Sliding toward nutrition malpractice: time to reconsider and redeploy. *Am J Clin Nutr*. 1993;57:3-7.
32. Cobb DK, Warner D. Avoiding malpractice: the role of proper nutrition and wound management. *J Am Med Dir Assoc*. 2004;5:H11-16.
33. Drug-company influence on medical education in USA [Editorial]. *Lancet*. 2000;356:781.
34. Topol EJ. Failing the public health: rofecoxib, Merck, and the FDA. *N Engl J Med*. 2004;351:1707-1709.
35. Wenban AB. Inappropriate use of the title "chiropractor" and term "chiropractic manipulation" in the peer-reviewed biomedical literature. *Chiropr Osteopat*. 2006;14:16.
36. Trever W. *In the Public Interest*. Los Angeles, Calif: Scriptures Unlimited; 1972.
37. McGlynn EA, Asch SM, Adams J, et al. The quality of health care delivered to adults in the United States. *N Engl J Med*. 2003;348:2635-2645.
38. Brennan TA, Leape LL, Laird NM, et al. Incidence of adverse events and negligence in hospitalized patients: results of the Harvard Medical Practice Study I. 1991. *Qual Saf Health Care*. 2004;13:145-151; discussion 151-152.
39. Whitaker R. The case against antipsychotic drugs: a 50-year record of doing more harm than good. *Med Hypotheses*. 2004;62:5-13.

40. Zhang F, Swanson SM, van Breemen RB, et al. Equine estrogen metabolite 4-hydroxyequilenin induces DNA damage in the rat mammary tissues: formation of single-strand breaks, apurinic sites, stable adducts, and oxidized bases. *Chem Res Toxicol*. 2001;14:1654-1659.

41. Sandyk R. Tryptophan availability and the susceptibility to stress in multiple sclerosis: a hypothesis. *Int J Neurosci*. 1996;86:47-53.

42. Gitto E, Karbownik M, Reiter RJ, et al. Effects of melatonin treatment in septic newborns. *Pediatr Res*. 2001;50:756-760.

43. Acuna-Castroviejo D, Escames G, Reiter RJ. Melatonin therapy in fibromyalgia. *J Pineal Res*. 2006;40:98-99.

44. Hibbeln JR, Ferguson TA, Blasbalg TL. Omega-3 fatty acid deficiencies in neurodevelopment, aggression and autonomic dysregulation: opportunities for intervention. *Int Rev Psychiatry*. 2006;18:107-118.

45. Wise TN, Fishbain DA, Holder-Perkins V.Painful physical symptoms in depression: a clinical challenge. *Pain Med*. 2007;8(Suppl 2):S75-S82.

46. Goldberg RJ, Katz J. A meta-analysis of the analgesic effects of omega-3 polyunsaturated fatty acid supplementation for inflammatory joint pain. *Pain*. 2007;129:210-223.

47. Lansdowne AT, Provost SC. Vitamin D3 enhances mood in healthy subjects during winter. *Psychopharmacology (Berl)*. 1998;135:319-323.

48. Russell AL, McCarty MF. DL-phenylalanine markedly potentiates opiate analgesia: an example of nutrient/pharmaceutical up-regulation of the endogenous analgesia system. *Med Hypotheses*. 2000;55:283-288.

49. Hernandez-Reif M, Field T, Krasnegor J, Theakston H. Lower back pain is reduced and range of motion increased after massage therapy. *Int J Neurosci*. 2001;106:131-145.

50. Turner EH, Loftis JM, Blackwell AD. Serotonin a la carte: supplementation with the serotonin precursor 5-hydroxytryptophan. *Pharmacol Ther*. 2006;109:325-338.

51. Birdsall TC. 5-Hydroxytryptophan: a clinically-effective serotonin precursor. *Altern Med Rev*. 1998;3:271-280.

52. Hitchon CA, El-Gabalawy HS. Oxidation in rheumatoid arthritis. *Arthritis Res Ther*. 2004;6:265-278.

53. Tak PP, Zvaifler NJ, Green DR, Firestein GS. Rheumatoid arthritis and p53: how oxidative stress might alter the course of inflammatory diseases. *Immunol Today*. 2000;21:78-82.

54. Kurien BT, Hensley K, Bachmann M, Scofield RH. Oxidatively modified autoantigens in autoimmune diseases. *Free Radic Biol Med*. 2006;41:549-556.

55. Lodi R, Kemp GJ, Montagna P, et al. Quantitative analysis of skeletal muscle bioenergetics and proton efflux in migraine and cluster headache. *J Neurol Sci*. 1997;146:73-80.

56. Park JH, Phothimat P, Oates CT, Hernanz-Schulman M, Olsen NJ. Use of P-31 magnetic resonance spectroscopy to detect metabolic abnormalities in muscles of patients with fibromyalgia. *Arthritis Rheum*. 1998;41:406-413.

57. Pieczenik SR, Neustadt J. Mitochondrial dysfunction and molecular pathways of disease. *Exp Mol Pathol*. 2007;83:84-92.

58. Corrigan FM, Wienburg CL, Shore RF, Daniel SE, Mann D. Organochlorine insecticides in substantia nigra in Parkinson's disease. *J Toxicol Environ Health A*. 2000;59:229-234.

59. Fleming L, Mann JB, Bean J, Briggle T, Sanchez-Ramos JR. Parkinson's disease and brain levels of organochlorine pesticides. *Ann Neurol*. 1994;36:100-103.

60. Fujiyoshi PT, Michalek JE, Matsumura F. Molecular epidemiologic evidence for diabetogenic effects of dioxin exposure in U.S. Air force veterans of the Vietnam war. *Environ Health Perspect*. 2006;114:1677-1683.

61. Lee DH, Lee IK, Song K, et al. A strong dose-response relation between serum concentrations of persistent organic pollutants and diabetes: results from the National Health and Examination Survey 1999-2002. *Diabetes Care*. 2006;29:1638-1644.

62. Lee DH, Lee IK, Jin SH, Steffes M, Jacobs DR Jr. Association between serum concentrations of persistent organic pollutants and insulin resistance among nondiabetic adults: results from the National Health and Nutrition Examination Survey 1999-2002. *Diabetes Care*. 2007;30:622-628.

63. Remillard RB, Bunce NJ. Linking dioxins to diabetes: epidemiology and biologic plausibility. *Environ Health Perspect*. 2002;110:853-858.

64. Rauh VA, Garfinkel R, Perera FP, et al. Impact of prenatal chlorpyrifos exposure on neurodevelopment in the first 3 years of life among inner-city children. *Pediatrics*. 2006;118:e1845-1859.

65. Cheuk DK, Wong V. Attention-deficit hyperactivity disorder and blood mercury level: a case-control study in chinese children. *Neuropediatrics*. 2006;37:234-240.

66. Nigg JT, Knottnerus GM, Martel MM, et al. Low blood lead levels associated with clinically diagnosed attention-deficit/hyperactivity disorder and mediated by weak cognitive control. *Biol Psychiatry*. 2008;63:325-331.

67. Crinnion WJ. Results of a decade of naturopathic treatment for environmental illnesses: A review of clinical records. *Journal of Naturopathic Medicine*. 1997;7:21-27.

68. Crinnion WJ. Environmental medicine, part 1: The human burden of environmental toxins and their common health effects. *Altern Med Rev*. 2000;5:52-63.

69. Crinnion WJ. Environmental medicine, part 2: Health effects of and protection from ubiquitous airborne solvent exposure. *Altern Med Rev*. 2000;5:133-143.

70. Crinnion WJ. Environmental medicine, part 3: Long-term effects of chronic low-dose mercury exposure. *Altern Med Rev*. 2000;5:209-223.

71. Crinnion WJ. Environmental medicine, part 4: Pesticides-biologically persistent and ubiquitous toxins. *Altern Med Rev*. 2000;5:432-447.

72. Rea WJ, Pan Y, Johnson AR. Clearing of toxic volatile hydrocarbons from humans. *Bol Asoc Med P R*. 1991;83:321-324.

73. Bland JS, Barrager E, Reedy RG, Bland K. A medical food-supplemented detoxification program in the management of chronic health problems. *Altern Ther Health Med*. 1995;1:62-71.

74. Minich DM, Bland JS. Acid-alkaline balance: role in chronic disease and detoxification. *Altern Ther Health Med*. 2007;13:62-65.

75. Vasquez A. Diabetes: Are toxins to blame? *Naturopathy Digest*. 2007;2. Available at: http://www.naturopathydigest.com/archives/2007/apr/diabetes.php.

76. Kilburn KH, Warsaw RH, Shields MG. Neurobehavioral dysfunction in firemen exposed to polycholorinated biphenyls (PCBs): possible improvement after detoxification. *Arch Environ Health*. 1989;44:345-350.

77. Cecchini M, LoPresti V. Drug residues store in the body following cessation of use: impacts on neuroendocrine balance and behavior: use of the Hubbard sauna regimen to remove toxins and restore health. *Med Hypotheses*. 2007;68:868-879.

78. Seaman DR. The diet-induced proinflammatory state: a cause of chronic pain and other degenerative diseases? *J Manipulative Physiol Ther*. 2002;25:168-179.

79. Vasquez A. Reducing pain and inflammation naturally, part 1: New insights into fatty acid biochemistry and the influence of diet. *Nutritional Perspectives*. October 2004:5, 7-10, 12, 14.

80. Vasquez A. Reducing pain and inflammation naturally, part 2: New insights into fatty acid supplementation and its effect on eicosanoid production and genetic expression. *Nutritional Perspectives*. January 2005:5-16.

81. Vasquez A. Reducing pain and inflammation naturally, part 3: Improving overall health while safely and effectively treating musculoskeletal pain. *Nutritional Perspectives*. April 2005;28:34-38, 40-42.

82. Vasquez A. Reducing pain and inflammation naturally, part 4: Nutritional and botanical inhibition of NF-kappaB, the major intracellular amplifier of the inflammatory cascade. A practical clinical strategy exemplifying anti-inflammatory nutrigenomics. *Nutritional Perspectives*. July 2005:5-12.

83. Timms PM, Mannan N, Hitman GA, et al. Circulating MMP9, vitamin D and variation in the TIMP-1 response with VDR genotype: mechanisms for inflammatory damage in chronic disorders? *QJM*. 2002;95:787-796.

84. Al Faraj S, Al Mutairi K. Vitamin D deficiency and chronic low back pain in Saudi Arabia. *Spine*. 2003;28:177-179.

85. James MJ, Gibson RA, Cleland LG. Dietary polyunsaturated fatty acids and inflammatory mediator production. *Am J Clin Nutr*. 2000;71(Suppl 1):343S-348S.

86. James MJ, Proudman SM, Cleland LG. Dietary n-3 fats as adjunctive therapy in a prototypic inflammatory disease: issues and obstacles for use in rheumatoid arthritis. *Prostaglandins Leukot Essent Fatty Acids*. 2003;68:399-405.

87. Mohanty P, Hamouda W, Garg R, Aljada A, Ghanim H, Dandona P. Glucose challenge stimulates reactive oxygen species (ROS) generation by leucocytes. *J Clin Endocrinol Metab*. 2000;85:2970-2973.

88. Mohanty P, Ghanim H, Hamouda W, Aljada A, Garg R, Dandona P. Both lipid and protein intakes stimulate increased generation of reactive oxygen species by polymorphonuclear leukocytes and mononuclear cells. *Am J Clin Nutr*. 2002;75:767-772.

89. Aljada A, Mohanty P, Ghanim H, et al. Increase in intranuclear nuclear factor kappaB and decrease in inhibitor kappaB in mononuclear cells after a mixed meal: evidence for a proinflammatory effect. *Am J Clin Nutr*. 2004;79:682-690.

90. Basha B, Rao DS, Han ZH, Parfitt AM. Osteomalacia due to vitamin D depletion: a neglected consequence of intestinal malabsorption. *Am J Med*. 2000;108:296-300.

91. Grant EC. Food allergies and migraine. *Lancet*. 1979;1(8123):966-9

92. Millichap JG, Yee MM. The diet factor in pediatric and adolescent migraine. *Pediatr Neurol*. 2003;28:9-15.

93. van de Laar MA, Aalbers M, Bruins FG, van Dinther-Janssen AC, van der Korst JK, Meijer CJ. Food intolerance in rheumatoid arthritis. II. Clinical and histological aspects. *Ann Rheum Dis*. 1992;51(3):303-306

94. Golding DN. Is there an allergic synovitis? *J R Soc Med*. 1990;83:312-314.

95. Hvatum M, Kanerud L, Hällgren R, Brandtzaeg P. The gut-joint axis: cross reactive food antibodies in rheumatoid arthritis. *Gut*. 2006;55:1240-1247.

96. Bourne JT, Kumar P, Huskisson EC, Mageed R, Unsworth DJ, Wojtulewski JA. Arthritis and coeliac disease. *Ann Rheum Dis*. 1985;44:592-598.

97. Noah PW. The role of microorganisms in psoriasis. *Semin Dermatol*. 1990;9:269-276.

98. Vasquez A. Reducing pain and inflammation naturally, part 6: Nutritional and botanical treatments against "silent infections" and gastrointestinal dysbiosis, commonly overlooked causes of neuromusculoskeletal inflammation and chronic health problems. *Nutritional Perspectives*. January 2006:5-21.

99. Williams RJ. *Biochemical Individuality: The Basis for the Genetotrophic Concept*. Austin and London: University of Texas Press; 1956.

100. Pauling L. On the orthomolecular environment of the mind: Orthomolecular theory. In: Williams RJ, Kalita DK, eds. *A Physician's Handbook on Orthomolecular Medicine*. New Cannan; Keats Publishing; 1977: 76.

101. Pauling L, Robinson AB, Teranishi R, Cary P. Quantitative analysis of urine vapor and breath by gas-liquid partition chromatography. *Proc Natl Acad Sci U S A*. 1971;68:2374-2376.

102. Pauling L, Itano HA, Singer SJ, Wells IC. Sickle cell anemia, a molecular disease. *Science*. 1949;110:543-548.

103. Bland JS. Jeffrey S. Bland, PhD, FACN, CNS: functional medicine pioneer. *Altern Ther Health Med*. 2004;10:74-81.

104. Ames BN, Elson-Schwab I, Silver EA. High-dose vitamin therapy stimulates variant enzymes with decreased coenzyme binding affinity (increased K(m)): relevance to genetic disease and polymorphisms. *Am J Clin Nutr*. 2002;75:616-658.

105. Evans JL, Maddux BA, Goldfine ID. The molecular basis for oxidative stress-induced insulin resistance. *Antioxid Redox Signal*. 2005;7(7-8):1040-1052.

106. Joseph JA, Denisova N, Fisher D, et al. Membrane and receptor modifications of oxidative stress vulnerability in aging. Nutritional considerations. *Ann N Y Acad Sci*. 1998;854:268-276.

107. Stephensen CB, Alvarez JO, Kohatsu J, Hardmeier R, Kennedy JI Jr, Gammon RB Jr. Vitamin A is excreted in the urine during acute infection. *Am J Clin Nutr*. 1994;60:388-392.

108. Ingenbleek Y, Bernstein L. The stressful condition as a nutritionally dependent adaptive dichotomy. *Nutrition*. 1999;15:305-320.

109. Henrotte JG, Plouin PF, Lévy-Leboyer C, et al. Blood and urinary magnesium, zinc, calcium, free fatty acids, and catecholamines in type A and type B subjects. *J Am Coll Nutr*. 1985;4:165-172.

110. DiPalma JR. Magnesium replacement therapy. *Am Fam Physician*. 1990;42:173-176.

111. Murck H. Magnesium and affective disorders. *Nutr Neurosci*. 2002;5:375-389.

112. Hashizume N, Mori M. An analysis of hypermagnesemia and hypomagnesemia. *Jpn J Med*. 1990;29:368-372.

113. Weglicki W, Quamme G, Tucker K, Haigney M, Resnick L. Potassium, magnesium, and electrolyte imbalance and complications in disease management. *Clin Exp Hypertens*. 2005;27:95-112.

114. Imrich R. The role of neuroendocrine system in the pathogenesis of rheumatic diseases (minireview). *Endocr Regul*. 2002;36:95-106.

115. Orbach H, Shoenfeld Y. Hyperprolactinemia and autoimmune diseases. *Autoimmun Rev*. 2007;6:537-542.

116. Panush RS, Wallace DJ, Dorff RE, Engleman EP. Retraction of the suggestion to use the term "Reiter's syndrome" sixty-five years later: the legacy of Reiter, a war criminal, should not be eponymic honor but rather condemnation. *Arthritis Rheum*. 2007;56:693-694.

117. Tlaskalová-Hogenová H, Stepánková R, Hudcovic T, et al. Commensal bacteria (normal microflora), mucosal immunity and chronic inflammatory and autoimmune diseases. *Immunol Lett*. 2004;93(2-3):97-108.

118. Collins SM. Stress and the gastrointestinal tract IV. Modulation of intestinal inflammation by stress: basic mechanisms and clinical relevance. *Am J Physiol Gastrointest Liver Physiol*. 2001;280:G315-G318.

119. Hart A, Kamm MA. Review article: mechanisms of initiation and perpetuation of gut inflammation by stress. *Aliment Pharmacol Ther*. 2002;16:2017-2028.

120. Farhadi A, Fields JZ, Keshavarzian A. Mucosal mast cells are pivotal elements in inflammatory bowel disease that connect the dots: stress, intestinal hyperpermeability and inflammation. *World J Gastroenterol*. 2007;13:3027-3030.

121. Yang PC, Jury J, Söderholm JD, Sherman PM, McKay DM, Perdue MH. Chronic psychological stress in rats induces intestinal sensitization to luminal antigens. *Am J Pathol*. 2006;168:104-114.

122. Rashid T, Ebringer A. Ankylosing spondylitis is linked to *Klebsiella*: the evidence. *Clin Rheumatol*. 2007;26:858-864.

123. Samarkos M, Vaiopoulos G. The role of infections in the pathogenesis of autoimmune diseases. *Curr Drug Targets Inflamm Allergy*. 2005;4:99-103.

124. Alverdy J, Holbrook C, Rocha F, et al. Gut-derived sepsis occurs when the right pathogen with the right virulence genes meets the right host: evidence for in vivo virulence expression in *Pseudomonas aeruginosa*. *Ann Surg*. 2000;232:480-489.

125. Wu L, Holbrook C, Zaborina O, at al. *Pseudomonas aeruginosa* expresses a lethal virulence determinant, the PA-I lectin/adhesin, in the intestinal tract of a stressed host: the role of epithelia cell contact and molecules of the Quorum Sensing Signaling System. *Ann Surg*. 2003;238:754-764.

126. Ebringer A, Rashid T. Rheumatoid arthritis is an autoimmune disease triggered by *Proteus* urinary tract infection. *Clin Dev Immunol*. 2006;13:41-48.

127. Erlacher L, Wintersberger W, Menschik M, et al. Reactive arthritis: urogenital swab culture is the only useful diagnostic method for the detection of the arthritogenic infection in extra-articularly asymptomatic patients with undifferentiated oligoarthritis. *Br J Rheumatol*. 1995;34:838-842.

128. Ebringer A, Rashid T, Wilson C. Rheumatoid arthritis: proposal for the use of anti-microbial therapy in early cases. *Scand J Rheumatol*. 2003;32:2-11.

129. James WH. Further evidence that low androgen values are a cause of rheumatoid arthritis: the response of rheumatoid arthritis to seriously stressful life events. *Ann Rheum Dis*. 1997;56:566.

130. Karagiannis A, Harsoulis F. Gonadal dysfunction in systemic diseases. *Eur J Endocrinol*. 2005;152:501-513.

131. O'Keefe JH Jr, Cordain L. Cardiovascular disease resulting from a diet and lifestyle at odds with our Paleolithic genome: how to become a 21st-century hunter-gatherer. *Mayo Clin Proc*. 2004;79:101-108.

132. Plotnikoff GA, Quigley JM. Prevalence of severe hypovitaminosis D in patients with persistent, nonspecific musculoskeletal pain. *Mayo Clin Proc*. 2003;78:1463-1470.

133. Wilkins CH, Sheline YI, Roe CM, Birge SJ, Morris JC. Vitamin D deficiency is associated with low mood and worse cognitive performance in older adults. *Am J Geriatr Psychiatry*. 2006;14:1032-1040.

134. Vieth R, Kimball S, Hu A, Walfish PG. Randomized comparison of the effects of the vitamin D3 adequate intake versus 100 mcg (4000 IU) per day on biochemical responses and the wellbeing of patients. *Nutr J*. 2004;3:8.

135. Vasquez A, Manso G, Cannell J. The clinical importance of vitamin D (cholecalciferol): a paradigm shift with implications for all healthcare providers. *Altern Ther Health Med*. 2004;10:28-36.

136. Kiecolt-Glaser JK, Belury MA, Porter K, Beversdorf DQ, Lemeshow S, Glaser R. Depressive symptoms, omega-6:omega-3 fatty acids, and inflammation in older adults. *Psychosom Med*. 2007;69:217-224.

137. Simopoulos AP. Omega-3 fatty acids in inflammation and autoimmune diseases. *J Am Coll Nutr*. 2002;21:495-505.

138. Park JH, Niermann KJ, Olsen N. Evidence for metabolic abnormalities in the muscles of patients with fibromyalgia. *Curr Rheumatol Rep*. 2000;2:131-140.

139. Petersen AM, Pedersen BK. The anti-inflammatory effect of exercise. *J Appl Physiol*. 2005;98:1154-1162.

140. Cotman CW, Berchtold NC, Christie LA. Exercise builds brain health: key roles of growth factor cascades and inflammation. *Trends Neurosci*. 2007;30:464-472.

141. Wilson CJ, Finch CE, Cohen HJ. Cytokines and cognition: the case for a head-to-toe inflammatory paradigm. *J Am Geriatr Soc*. 2002;50:2041-2056.

142. McPherson M, Smith-Lovin L, Brashears ME. Social isolation in America: Changes in core discussion networks over two decades. *American Sociological Review*. 2006;71:353-375.

143. Preventing firearm violence: a public health imperative. American College of Physicians. *Ann Intern Med*. 1995;122:311-313.

Chapter 2

Overview of Clinical Approach, Assessments, and Therapeutics

Introduction to Clinical Approach

This chapter will provide a representative overview of patient management considerations, clinical assessments, and therapeutic interventions that are commonly used in the practice of functional medicine, specifically with regard to the treatment of conditions characterized by musculoskeletal pain. This approach is founded on the presupposition that pain occurs due to one or more pathophysiological causes and that pain is most effectively treated by addressing the causative factor(s); this contrasts to the *pharmacocentric* view that pain is a target for suppression independent from its cause(s). The practice and art of patient-centered healthcare delivery necessitates the skillful, individualized selection of appropriate assessments and interventions drawn from the clinician's repertoire of knowledge and experience; these acquisitions are readily available via diligent study and persistent practice. Also required are the willingness and discipline to see each new patient, with all of his or her problems and characteristics, and each clinical encounter as an opportunity to develop a more intricate comprehension of the patterns and web-like interconnections of the factors that promote health and disease. Eventually, complexity becomes simplicity, and what was previously impossible becomes routinely attainable.

Each clinician must weigh his or her own unique abilities against the seriousness of each condition being treated; when the scale tips toward doubt or uncertainty, the clinician should institute an appropriate referral for specialist management or co-management. Referral to a neurologist or neurosurgeon should be implemented when neurological deficits are noted, and patients with systemic autoimmune diseases should generally be co-managed with an internist or rheumatologist in the event that a sudden inflammatory exacerbation leads to a potentially catastrophic complication such as cerebral vasculitis or transverse myelitis. When dealing with potentially limb-threatening or life-threatening conditions, clinicians should recall the rule "when in doubt, send (refer) them out" for the sake of ensuring patient safety and avoiding medicolegal complications.

Commonly Employed Assessments in Functional Medicine

The practice of functional medicine begins with competent and comprehensive patient assessment and the exclusion or management of urgent problems. Thereafter, a customized treatment plan is tailored by the clinician to fit the patient's needs, goals, desires, limitations, and other individual nuances.

History

Effective clinical management of the patient with neuromusculoskeletal pain and dysfunction begins with a detailed understanding of the patient's current physical, biochemical, and psycho-emotional status. The process of collecting the patient's history is a dynamic process that requires clear, open-ended questions from the clinician couched in a manner that demonstrates authentic empathy and facilitates the building of rapport and trust. Patient interviews are not merely a data collection tool; they can be a creative, enjoyable, comforting opportunity to build rapport and to establish meaningful connection with another human being. This connection can be truthfully established only if the clinician is first in touch with his or her own humanity and feelings.

Intake forms and interpersonal dialogue form the patient history, which includes the chief complaint, associated problems, psychosocial history, past medical/health history, and family history. Clinicians learn these skills early in their clinical training, and the details of history taking are reviewed in clinical textbooks such as *Bates' Guide to Physical Examination and History Taking*[1] and will not be reiterated here. Clinicians should ask a broad range of open-ended questions because when it comes to understanding our patients there is no such problem as too much information. Whereas the purpose of the standard medical interview is the determination of the diagnosis, the functional medicine interview includes yet extends beyond the diagnosis to arrive at an understanding of how this particular constellation of dysfunctions has coalesced in this patient at this time in order to manifest ill health and disease.[i]

The importance of *details* and the *review of systems* require emphasis. The success or failure of the functional medicine approach depends on the clinician's understanding of the disease manifestation in a particular patient regardless of the codified diagnosis. While certain generalizations can be made about the genesis and perpetuation of certain disease states—for example, the quintet of dysbiosis, proinflammatory diet, dysendocrinism, xenobiotic immunotoxicity, and psycho-emotional factors in chronic pain in general and autoimmunity in particular—the successful clinician remains vigilant for nuances that hold the key to therapeutic efficacy *for each individual patient*. Every disease in every patient has one or more underlying causes. Except in rare instances of clearly defined *genotropic* disease of "inborn errors," the clinician absolutely must proceed with determination to discover and correct the underlying factors that have contributed to the manifestation of the disease even when genotropic contributions may be a part of the constellation of influences that have led to the disease. Genetic *predispositions* must never be confused with genetic *causes*. Because of the interconnected nature of the functional medicine interventional approach, the purpose of the history is not simply to arrive at a diagnosis but rather to arrive at an understanding of how the patient's genes, history, lifestyle, emotional climate, toxic exposures, and other factors are interwoven to create the status of health dysfunction currently presenting.

To summarize, the goal of history taking is to achieve a comprehensive, multidimensional view of each of the patient's diagnoses and clinically relevant characteristics, particularly those related to biochemical individuality and the psycho-emotional qualities that guide health-seeking (or disease-seeking) behaviors. At the end of the interview, the clinician should have enough data and insight to recount the antecedents, triggers, events, and therapeutic basis to the patient in such a manner that the patient hears his or her own story, starting from before the onset of the illness and extending to the immediate future and anticipated therapeutic outcome.

Physical Examination (standardized, basic)

The physical examination is either generalized or focused, depending on whether the purpose of the visit is an extended, comprehensive evaluation (especially for a new patient) or a focused examination when working with an established patient or when time limitations or urgency mandate expediency. Generally, all patients should at minimum receive a screening examination of the heart, lungs, abdomen, and nervous system. Patients with musculoskeletal

---

[i] The Institute for Functional Medicine (IFM) offers supplemental history and intake forms which facilitate the overall assessment and development of the resultant treatment plan. The forms are generally available from IFM at the Applying Functional Medicine in Clinical Practice (AFMCP) programs. Members of the IFM Forum can access forms at http://www.functionalmedicine.org/membercommunity/ifmtoolkit.asp

complaints should additionally receive a more detailed neuroorthopedic examination pursuant to their chief complaint. Potential emergencies such as atlantoaxial instability, vertebral fracture, cauda equina syndrome, acute compartment syndrome, septic arthritis, and malignant disease must always be considered.

Physical Examination (detailed, functional)

In addition to the refinement of the musculoskeletal diagnosis, this more detailed examination can include the identification of nuances overlooked in routine, standardized examinations. For example, the observations of follicular hyperkeratosis, delayed Achilles return, and a diagonal ear crease strongly suggest vitamin A deficiency,[2] hypothyroidism,[3] and atherosclerotic cardiovascular disease,[4,5] respectively. Many patients with apparently normal findings on a standard physical and orthopedic examination can be found to have subtle aberrations in musculoskeletal structure and function when assessed with more detailed palpatory assessments. Examples of these subtle yet significant abnormalities and nuances include myofascial trigger points (MFTP), pelvic postural asymmetry, sacral base unleveling, limb length discrepancies, myofascial restrictions, and segmental motion restrictions or hypermobility in the peripheral and axial skeleton.

Didactic and practical training for the detection of these problems is not included in allopathic graduate training but is a mandatory component of chiropractic, osteopathic, and naturopathic education because the latter professions utilize manipulative medicine within their therapeutic armamentarium. These diagnostic tools generally include postural analysis, gait analysis, static palpation, motion palpation, and myofascial palpation; within each of these methods are subtypes and nuances that vary by profession and intraprofessional specialization. Specifically, motion palpation assesses multiplanar intersegmental motion and has been validated as a reliable assessment for evaluating spinal motion and the indication for manual spinal manipulation or nonsurgical stabilization.[6,7,8] Clinicians specializing in neuromusculoskeletal disorders may use tools such as tilt tables, myoelectric measurements, or proprioceptive challenges to identify subtle autonomic, neuromuscular, or sensorimotor deficits.

Laboratory Assessment

Laboratory tests are an essential component of the overall evaluation of patients with musculoskeletal pain and inflammation, and functional medicine practitioners employ a wide range of standardized laboratory tests when evaluating and monitoring patients. Such tests can provide for the validation, exclusion, or discovery of underlying disease, quantification of severity, and an objective means for monitoring response to therapy and the need to modify or continue the treatment plan. New patients with musculoskeletal pain should be assessed with these 3 tests at a minimum: complete blood count (CBC), C-reactive protein (CRP), and comprehensive chemistry/metabolic panel. Assessment of serum ferritin, vitamin D, and thyroid status are also highly valuable. The use of these tests on a routine basis helps identify patients with occult diseases and allows for more comprehensive management of the patient's overall health. For patients with chronic inflammatory disease such as an autoimmune condition, comprehensive hormonal evaluation can be performed, and assessment for dysbiosis generally begins with comprehensive stool testing followed by genitourinary swab and culture. A brief description of the most commonly used tests is provided here.

Complete blood count — The CBC can detect hematologic abnormalities and immune response to infection. In the routine evaluation of patients with musculoskeletal pain, this test is primarily used to help exclude anemia, infection, and certain malignancies, particularly myeloproliferative disorders. Anemia in a patient with musculoskeletal pain might be indicative of a functional problem such as nutritional insufficiency (perhaps caused by insufficient intake, malabsorption, or gut dysbiosis) or a more serious pathological lesion such as gastritis or colon cancer. A normal white blood cell count does not exclude acute or chronic musculoskeletal infection; a significant portion of patients with osteomyelitis will have normal CBC and white blood cell indices.

C-reactive protein — CRP is made in the liver following stimulation from interleukin-6 as part of the acute-phase response. CRP thus serves as a sensitive, though nonspecific, marker of inflammation and immune activation, and therefore, it is clinically useful for quantifying the overall level of systemic inflammation. Some patients with major disease will paradoxically have a misleadingly normal CRP value; this is particularly true for some patients with cancer or systemic lupus erythematosus (SLE). Minor limitations acknowledged, CRP or its more sensitive variant, high-sensitivity CRP (hsCRP), should be used for evaluating new patients, assessing complications or new diseases, and monitoring response to treatment. Further, many clinicians use CRP and especially hsCRP as a barometer of health since higher values correlate with increased future risk for diabetes mellitus and cardiovascular disease[9]; this test helps bridge the gap between acute care and wellness promotion. CRP has generally replaced erythrocyte sedimentation rate (ESR) as a laboratory index of inflammation.

Chemistry/metabolic panel — This routine screening panel provides data that correlate with diabetes mellitus, liver disease, kidney failure, bone lesions, electrolyte disturbances, adrenal insufficiency, hyperparathyroidism, and other important clinical conditions. This battery of basic tests is particularly indicated for any patient with nontraumatic musculoskeletal pain, manifestations of systemic disease, hypertension, or diabetes, as well as all patients who use medications that cause hepatotoxicity, nephrotoxicity, or other problems such as electrolyte disturbance. Lipid panels and urinalysis are commonly used with the chemistry panel for initial, follow-up, and annual evaluations.

Serum ferritin — Ferritin is an iron-binding protein, serum levels of which correlate directly with body iron stores. Due to the high population prevalence of iron disorders and the diversity of clinical presentations (including asymptomatic), routine use of serum ferritin to assess iron body iron stores is important in the evaluation of patients with health problems in general and musculoskeletal pain in particular. Hereditary causes of iron overload are among the most common disorders in the human population, and musculoskeletal complications may be the sole clinical manifestation.[10] Secondary forms of iron overload can occur in patients who are not overtreated with supplemental iron or blood transfusions. Virtually any joint may be affected by hemochromatoic (iron overload) arthropathy, and the condition can mimic rheumatoid arthritis, osteoarthritis, ankylosing spondylitis, and other regional and systemic musculoskeletal syndromes.[11]

In the absence of significant inflammation, ferritin values greater than 200 mcg/L in women or greater than 300 mcg/L in men indicate iron overload and the need for treatment with diagnostic and therapeutic phlebotomy regardless of the absence of symptoms or end-stage complications.[12] From a preventive healthcare perspective, research and literature reviews have concluded that in the absence of inflammation, ferritin values greater than 80 mcg/L to 100 mcg/L were associated with increased risk of diseases associated with iron-catalyzed oxidative stress such as cancer and cardiovascular disease; blood donation to safely reduce iron stores is a reasonable and socially beneficial preventive intervention.[13,14,15 16]

Opposite to iron overload on the iron status spectrum, iron deficiency is also common and typically presents with symptoms related to fatigue, increased susceptibility to infection, and various forms of dyscognition, notably including attention-deficit hyperactivity disorder.[17,18] The detection of iron deficiency in adults mandates gastroenterological assessment for pathological causes of blood loss such as gastric ulcer or colon cancer; merely testing for occult fecal blood is inadequate.[19]

Clinical Pearl:

Because ferritin is an acute-phase reactant that increases due to systemic inflammation such as infection or malignancy, an elevated ferritin level may not be indicative of iron overload if systemic inflammation (assessed with CRP or ESR) is also high.

Thyroid assessment — Hypothyroidism, particularly of the autoimmune type (Hashimoto's thyroiditis), is a common problem and is an often overlooked cause of musculoskeletal pain including arthritis, systemic inflammation, myopathy, a fibromyalgia-like clinical presentation, and occasionally carpal tunnel syndrome (CTS) and adhesive capsulitis.[20] Detailed thyroid assessment should include measurements of TSH, free T4, free T3, total T3, reverse T3 (rT3), and antithyroid antibodies (antithyroid peroxidase and antithyroglobulin). TSH levels above 2 µIU/mL[21] or

3.0 µIU/mL[22] warrant consideration for intervention as these indicate subtle thyroid dysfunction and increased risk for future thyroid disease.[ii] Functional medicine clinicians note the importance of the ratio of total T3 to rT3 and consider the optimal range to be between 10 and 14, with lower ratios indicating impaired formation of T3 and/or excess production of rT3.[23] Contrary to the previous view which held that rT3 was simply inactive, we now appreciate that rT3 actually impairs normal thyroid hormone metabolism, thus acting as a "thyrometabolic monkey wrench" or brake on normal metabolism. Elevated rT3 levels predict mortality among critically ill patients.[24]

Aberrancies in thyroid hormone levels may reflect organic disease, psycho-emotional stress, or nutritional deficiency,[25] and therefore, such serological abnormalities warrant consideration of underlying problems and direct treatment when possible. If no underlying cause of the clinically suspected hypothyroidism is apparent, then a trial of thyroid hormones is reasonable in appropriately selected patients.[26,27,28] Beyond stress reduction and nutritional supplementation with iodine, selenium, and zinc (as indicated per patient), correction of overt, subclinical, and functional hypothyroidism generally centers on the administration of natural or synthetic thyroid hormones in the form of T4 and/or T3. Correction of *functional* hypothyroidism (defined here as relatively reduced total T3 and increased rT3 with normal thyroid glandular function; i.e., a mild chronic form of "consumptive hypothyroidism"[29]) is accomplished with either time-released or twice-daily dosing of T3 without T4 to suppress endogenous T4 conversion to T3; this allows temporary downregulation of peripheral transforming enzymes so that rT3 production is reduced following withdrawal of T3 replacement and peripheral thyroid metabolism is normalized following withdrawal of treatment.[30]

Serum 25-hydroxy vitamin D3 (25[OH]D) — Vitamin D deficiency is an epidemic cause of musculoskeletal pain and inflammation,[31] as well as a significant risk factor for cancer, depression, diabetes mellitus, autoimmunity, cardiovascular disease, and other serious health problems.[32,33] Measurement of serum 25(OH)D or empiric treatment with 2000 to 4000 IU of vitamin D3 per day for adults is indicated in patients with chronic musculoskeletal pain and should be the standard of care.[34,35] This author[36,37] initially proposed that optimal vitamin D status correlates with serum 25(OH)D levels of 40 ng/mL to 65 ng/mL (100–160 nmol/L), and in the past few years, evidence and experience have accumulated in favor of allowing even higher serum levels as the upper limit, perhaps up to 100 ng/mL (250 nmol/L). Medicolegal consequences for failure to assess and treat hypovitaminosis D have been proposed.[38] Anyone doubting the importance of vitamin D and its power to alleviate chronic pain and weakness in patients with previously unrecognized deficiency is encouraged to read the case report titled "A woman who left her wheelchair" published in the March 1999 issue of *The Lancet*.[39]

Antinuclear antibodies (ANA) — ANA can be assessed quantitatively and qualitatively for the evaluation of immune function and the detection of autoimmune conditions such as SLE and systemic sclerosis. Occasionally, elevated ANA is seen in patients who do not have autoimmunity, particularly the elderly and patients with infections such as viral hepatitis. ANA titers less than 1:160 should be interpreted cautiously as they may not indicate the presence of *clinical* autoimmunity; titers greater than 1:320 are more strongly correlated with clinically significant autoimmunity. Qualitative assessment of ANA can reveal staining patterns that may refine the

> **Clinical Pearl:**
>
> Measurement of serum 25(OH)D or empiric treatment with 2000 to 4000 IU of vitamin D3 per day for adults is recommended for all patients with chronic musculoskeletal pain.

diagnosis of particular autoimmune diseases. Furthermore, functional medicine clinicians may interpret asymptomatic ANA positivity as an indicator of poor overall health and the need for preventive intervention to restore health and prevent the manifestation of clinically significant autoimmunity. Conversion to ANA negativity can be achieved with nonpharmacological means and can be viewed as a measure of therapeutic efficacy.

---

ii "Until November 2002, doctors had relied on a normal TSH level ranging from 0.5 to 5.0 to diagnose and treat patients with a thyroid disorder who tested outside the boundaries of that range. Now AACE encourages doctors to consider treatment for patients who test outside the boundaries of a narrower margin based on a target TSH level of 0.3 to 3.04. AACE believes the new range will result in proper diagnosis for millions of Americans who suffer from a mild thyroid disorder, but have gone untreated until now." [American Association of Clinical Endocrinologists (AACE). *Over 13 Million Americans with Thyroid Disease Remain Undiagnosed.* January 2003. Available online at http://www.aace.com/newsroom/press/2003/index.php?r=20030118.]

Rheumatoid factor (RF) — Historically, the primary value of this test was in supporting the otherwise unclear diagnosis of rheumatoid arthritis; the specificity and sensitivity of this test are both suboptimal. RF may be positive in normal health and aging, iron overload, chronic infections, hepatitis, sarcoidosis, and bacterial endocarditis. RF has recently been clinically replaced by cyclic citrullinated peptide antibodies as described below.

Cyclic citrullinated protein/peptide (CCP) antibodies — Anti-CCP antibodies have 98% specificity for rheumatoid arthritis,[40] and this test is likely to become the future laboratory standard in the diagnosis and prognosis of rheumatoid arthritis.[41] Anti-CCP antibodies become positive before the clinical onset of rheumatoid arthritis; simultaneous positivity for RF and CCP is termed *conjugate seropositivity*.

Cardiovascular risk assessment — Patients with systemic inflammatory disorders such as rheumatoid arthritis[42] and neuromusculoskeletal pain (including low back pain[43] and migraine with aura[44,45,46]) show an increased prevalence of cardiovascular disease and premature death. Therefore, cardiovascular risk, including traditional and new risk factors, is worthy of assessment. These assessments include total cholesterol, low-density lipoprotein, high-density lipoprotein, triglycerides, homocysteine, CRP and hsCRP, ferritin, lipoprotein(a), apolipoprotein A-1 (protective), apolipoprotein B, fibrinogen, oxidative stress, essential fatty acid levels and ratios (also used for the assessment of inflammatory tendency), thyroid, and vitamin D, among others. Lifestyle risk factors such as diet, stress modulation, smoking cessation, and physical exercise are also important. Drugs used in the treatment of rheumatic disease can exacerbate cardiovascular risk; for example, corticosteroids (e.g., prednisone) worsen dyslipidemia, and methotrexate raises homocysteine.

Hormone assessments — Hormonal imbalances clearly contribute to systemic inflammation and autoimmunity. The classic pattern is that of elevated prolactin and estradiol with lowered dehydroepiandrosterone, testosterone, and cortisol. Most patients with autoimmune-inflammatory disorders will display portions of this pattern; appropriate correction leads to important clinical improvements.[47,48,49,50,51] Routine serological testing for hormones is readily available from standard medical laboratories and, since this is the reference method used in most clinical research studies, allows correlation of clinical intervention with peer-reviewed data. Other methods of hormonal quantification such as random or 24-hour urine collections and saliva testing can also be used clinically, but these methods are not well represented in the research literature in the assessment and treatment of inflammatory disease. This multicomponent approach to the assessment of and intervention with hormones in the treatment of inflammatory disorders has been termed *orthoendocrinology* and is detailed elsewhere.[52]

Lactulose-mannitol assay — The lactulose-mannitol assay became popular among functional medicine clinicians following its validation as an accurate, safe, cost-effective, and noninvasive means for assessing intestinal mucosal integrity in conditions such as Crohn's disease, food allergy, celiac disease, intestinal parasitosis, and other variations of "leaky gut syndrome."[53] The test is often described by other names including *sugar absorption test* and *intestinal permeability test* or *IP test*. Performance of the test is simple: a fasting patient drinks a defined amount of the 2 indigestible sugars, and excreted amounts are measured from a 6-hour urine collection. Elevated lactulose indicates increased paracellular intestinal permeability, whereas reduced mannitol indicates reduced transcellular nutrient absorption. The divergence of these values in cases of mucosal injury is sensitively reflected in an elevated lactulose-to-mannitol ratio and is a nonspecific indicator of intestinal damage,[54] which may be due to one or more of the following six categories[52]:

1. Malnutrition, which may be due to poor intake, catabolism, or malabsorption
2. Enterotoxins, generally high doses of nonsteroidal anti-inflammatory drugs (NSAIDs) or ethanol
3. Food allergies, including celiac disease and type-1 sensitivities
4. Parasites, including protozoa, amebas, helminthes, dysbiotic yeast, and bacteria
5. Systemic inflammation such as tissue hypoxia, trauma, or recent surgery
6. Genetic predisposition toward enteropathy, such as a family history of inflammatory bowel disease or celiac disease

Because an abnormal intestinal permeability result is nonspecific, the clinician must then discover the true identity of the underlying problem(s). In the routine outpatient setting, many of the 6 considerations above can be confirmed or rejected by patient history and rapid clinical assessment; this generally leaves food allergy and intestinal parasitosis and dysbiosis as the holdouts, the former being assessed with serology or the elimination and challenge technique and the latter being assessed with comprehensive stool and parasitology assessments performed by a specialty laboratory as described below.

Microbial analysis of mucosal surfaces and environment — Mucosal colonization or overgrowth of various yeast, bacteria, and other parasites is a major and generally underappreciated contributor to chronic poor health, systemic inflammation, and painful arthritis, despite the substantiating wealth of basic science, molecular, clinical, and epidemiological research. Dysbiosis is the single most efficient and popular term for the different varieties of this phenomenon, which has also been termed autointoxication,[55, 56] bowel-associated dermatosis-arthritis syndrome,[57] intestinal arthritis-dermatitis syndrome,[58] and bypass disease.[59] While a full discussion of dysbiosis is beyond the scope of this monograph, this section provides an overview of the exhaustive reviews published in 2006 and 2007 by this author,[60] which provided the following practical definition of dysbiosis: "a relationship of subacute non-infectious host-microorganism interaction that adversely affects the human host, primarily through metabolic and immunologic disturbances." A defining characteristic of dysbiotic inflammation is that it reflects the uniqueness of the patient's immune response against a particular microbe or combination of microbes; this response is influenced by the patient's nutritional status, genetic background, and hormonal milieu.

The functional medicine understanding of dysbiosis is based on 3 premises:

- Dysbiosis promotes chronic inflammation and autoimmunity by numerous additive and synergistic mechanisms, each of which has been scientifically elucidated in the research literature.
- Dysbiosis can result from a simultaneous multiplicity of microbes at different locations, thus providing for a more comprehensive conceptualization termed *multifocal polydysbiosis*.
- Treatment of dysbiosis without other interventions is often successful at relieving chronic health problems; however, most patients benefit from a more comprehensive approach that corrects associated hormonal, nutritional, and oxidative disorders.

While essentially all mucosal surfaces are subject to colonization, the most common locations are the gastrointestinal tract, genitourinary tract, and oropharynx, and some microbes display location specificity. Subtypes of dysbiosis can be described based on their location and are self-explanatory by name: orodental, sinorespiratory, gastrointestinal, genitourinary, cutaneous, and environmental. The term *environmental dysbiosis* was coined to denote the autoimmune, inflammatory, and painful arthritic syndromes that result from exposure to microbe-infested buildings, particularly water-damaged buildings and those with infested walls, subfloors, and air-conditioning units. Affected patients may display neuronal[61,62] and musculoskeletal[63,64,65,66] autoimmune-type inflammatory reactions resembling multiple sclerosis and rheumatoid arthritis and ankylosing spondylitis, respectively, and respiratory diseases such as asthma[67,68]; these reactions coincide with biotoxin and antigen exposure and remit following either avoidance or remediation of the contaminated building.

Readers should note that the following partial list of arthritogenic microorganisms comprises mostly commensals and microbes generally assumed to be of low pathogenic potential in immunocompetent hosts; because of their intermediate immunoreactivity, these organisms are able to establish chronic mucosal colonization which fails to stimulate the marked immune response that would result in routine antimicrobial treatment or the provocation of an effective immune response. Organisms known to trigger reactive arthritis or dysbiotic arthropathy include:

- *Blastocystis hominis*[69]
- *Endolimax nana*[70]
- *Giardia lamblia*[71,72]

- *Staphylococcus aureus*[73]
- *Staphylococcus epidermidis*[74]
- *Helicobacter pylori*[75]
- *Klebsiella pneumoniae*[76]
- *Streptococcus pyogenes* (Group A streptococci)[77,78,79]
- *Eubacterium aerofaciens*[80]
- *Proteus mirabilis*[81,82]
- *Hafnia alvei*[83]
- *Ureaplasma urealyticum*[84]

Other dysbiotic microbes such as *Candida albicans* may not trigger arthritis directly but can perpetuate other mucosal colorizations through elaboration of mycotoxins and proteases that impair systemic and mucosal defenses, respectively. Commonly found in the gastrointestinal tract of ill and unwell patients, *Pseudomonas aeruginosa* and *Acinetobacter* species may have a role in neurological autoimmunity such as multiple sclerosis and autoimmune peripheral neuropathy.[85,86] *Citrobacter rodentium* (*Citrobacter freundii*) can trigger inflammatory bowel disease in animals and has been a contributing factor to some cases of rheumatoid arthritis and chronic fatigue in this author's practice.

Mechanisms and elements of dysbiosis-induced musculoskeletal pain and inflammation include:

- Molecular mimicry[87]
- Superantigens[88]
- Peptidoglycans[89]
- Endotoxin (lipopolysaccharide)
- Enhanced processing of autoantigens[90]
- Bystander activation
- Immune complexes
- Haptenization and neoantigen formation[91,92]
- Damage to the intestinal mucosa[93]
- Impairment of xenobiotic detoxification[94]
- Immune activation[95]
- Enterohepatic recycling[96] or enterohepatic recirculation[97]
- Various types of immunosuppression mediated by microbial proteases and toxins, such as gliotoxin from *Candida albicans*, which suppresses human neutrophil function[98]

An exhaustive description of the numerous immuno-molecular and biochemical mechanisms involved is beyond the scope of this monograph; interested readers are directed to the primary research of Ebringer[99,100,101] and reviews by Vasquez[52,60] for more details.

Patient assessment for dysbiosis is straightforward using standard analytical and clinical methods. Mucosal surfaces can be swabbed and sampled for analysis by gram stain, Giemsa stain, DNA polymerase chain reaction, and culture. Gastrointestinal dysbiosis is assessed by comprehensive parasitology (including microscopic examination and culture for bacteria and yeast) performed by a specialty laboratory. The genitourinary tract should be swabbed for culture and microbial analysis in patients with inflammatory arthritis, specifically undifferentiated oligoarthritis.[102]

In rare instances, antimicrobial treatment—either with drugs or botanical medicines such as those listed below under *Commonly Employed Therapeutics in Functional Medicine*—is sufficient to effect significant amelioration or resolution of arthritis, systemic inflammation, and other symptoms. More commonly, a multicomponent treatment approach is needed, consisting of dietary modification, allergen avoidance, nutritional supplementation, stress reduction, correction of hormonal imbalances, and, in some patients, xenobiotic depuration. For environmental dysbiosis, the patient's home, work, and recreational environments can be surveyed for microbial contamination, particularly mold. Pier-and-beam homes should be inspected for mold and water in crawl spaces; likewise, attics should be inspected for occult leaks and mold. Mold plates, petri dishes, and filter cartridges can be employed to identify airborne microbes. Contaminated buildings should be repaired, comprehensively remediated, or replaced.

Xenobiotic assessment — Xenobiotics appear to have a primary or contributory role in the induction of inflammation and autoimmunity in humans.[103,104] Researching the effects of xenobiotic exposure is challenging because of the pandemic of xenobiotic exposure,[105,106] as well as the impossibility of finding a xenobiotic-free population to serve as a control group. However, what is known is that xenobiotics have immunotoxic effects that manifest as hyper- and hypofunction, the former promoting the clinical manifestation of allergy, inflammation, and autoimmunity, with the latter increasing the propensity toward infection, which may then reduce immune defenses sufficiently to allow for development of mucosal dysbiosis. Xenobiotics are harmful foreign substances that can generally be classified as metals (e.g., mercury, lead, nickel) and chemicals (e.g., paint fumes, perfume, varnish, new carpet, formaldehyde, food colors, food additives, artificial sweeteners, pesticides, fungicides, herbicides, industrial waste and pollution, pharmaceutical drugs, propellants, synthetic fertilizers, car exhaust, solvents, plastic food/drink containers, polystyrene plastic, trichloroethylene rubber, petroleum fuels, and detergents and other cleaners).

Patients may develop health problems following years of occult exposure to and impaired clearance of numerous xenobiotics or following an acute exposure to a large amount of a single toxin. Chemical xenobiotics and their metabolites can be assayed from blood, urine, and adipose samples. Toxic metals can be measured in blood if the exposure and dose were recent and large, respectively; however, if the exposure and accumulation occurred years ago or have taken place slowly over many years, then chelation-provoked quantitative urinary excretion measurement can be performed[107] (controversy noted[108]).

Imaging

Radiographs, ultrasound imaging, and the various subtypes of magnetic resonance imaging and computed tomography should be utilized as indicated by general standards of care or as approved by institutional review board. A recent development is the potential use of abdominal ultrasound and magnetic resonance imaging in the detection of occult seronegative food allergic reactions,[109] but clinical applicability of this technique, which appears to be specific for patients with gastrointestinal allergy, is still being determined.[110]

Biopsy and Other Tissue and Fluid Sampling

Specialists may perform certain biopsy techniques in their offices on an outpatient basis. Joint aspiration for synovial fluid analysis may be performed for the evaluation and treatment of certain arthropathies and should always be performed if septic arthritis is suspected. Analysis of hair and nail samples can provide some information about nutritional or toxic mineral status when performed and interpreted properly; the utility of these tests is not absolute but is still of sufficient value to support their use, with caveats noted.[111,112] Biopsy acquisition and analysis for functional disorders such as fibromyalgia[113,114] (see *Clinical Focus: Fibromyalgia*) is scientifically valuable but is generally reserved for research purposes and not utilized clinically.

Interventional and Surgical Procedures

Interventional and surgical procedures are generally reserved for conditions outside the scope of outpatient care discussed within this monograph. A noteworthy exception is the surgical closure of patent foramen ovale in the treatment of recalcitrant migraine (see *Clinical Focus: Migraine*).

Commonly Employed Therapeutics in Functional Medicine

Now that we have reviewed fundamental concepts supporting the functional medicine clinical approach (Chapter 1) and patient evaluation (above), in this section we will review commonly employed therapeutics of particular relevance to the treatment of patients with disorders of inflammation and pain. While a generalized schema can be derived from the information presented herein, clinicians must determine the relevance, applicability, and appropriateness of these interventions for each unique patient. Doses listed are for adults without hepatorenal impairment or other contraindication, unless otherwise specified.

Dietary Interventions

Interventional diets are often included in treatment plans for patients with chronically poor health and musculoskeletal pain. The premise that dietary improvement must be implemented and faithfully maintained to allow for the success of other treatments is considered self-evident by clinicians in this field due to the sheer bulk of dietary intake (5.3 pounds per day among Americans[115]) and its manifold qualitative and quantitative effects on gene transcription, inflammatory mediator production, and tissue maintenance and repair.[116,117]

Clinical Pearl:

Between 1970 and 2003 in the United States, total nutrient intake increased 16% and sugar intake increased 19%, resulting in a daily average increase of 523 calories per day; obviously, this is well reflected in the burgeoning epidemics of obesity and diabetes mellitus. Interestingly, at the same time that we note increased food consumption and an increased prevalence of obesity and diabetes, we also note an increase in the prevalence of autoimmune and inflammatory musculoskeletal disorders.[118]

Avoidance of the standard American diet — The standard American diet (SAD) is characterized by overconsumption of simple carbohydrates, sodium chloride, highly fermentable carbohydrates, food additives, *trans*-fatty acids, vegetable oils rich in linoleic acid, animal fats rich in saturated fatty acids and arachidonate, and dietary monotony that promotes allergic sensitization and imbalanced nutrient intake. The SAD is characterized by an insufficiency of fiber, phytonutrients, dietary diversity, vitamins, minerals, high-quality protein, and health-promoting fatty acids such as alpha-linolenic acid (ALA), gamma-linolenic acid (GLA), eicosapentaenoic acid (EPA), docosahexaenoic acid (DHA), and oleic acid. These excesses and insufficiencies synergize to promote a systemic proinflammatory state that promotes the development, perpetuation, and exacerbation of many chronic inflammatory diseases and contributes to therapeutic recalcitrance.[119,120,121] In experimental models, arachidonic acid (but not EPA or oleic acid—see *Fatty Acid Supplements* below) directly promotes inflammation via activation of nuclear transcription factor-kappa B (NF-κB),[122] a major transcription factor for the expression of proinflammatory genes.[123] Self-selected dietary intake should be viewed as self-medication, and clinicians have the responsibility to intervene to prevent self-induced harm and therapeutic subterfuge just as they would if they discovered that a patient was noncompliant with other treatments or was abusing tobacco, drugs, or alcohol.

Paleo-Mediterranean diet, anti-inflammatory diet — The Paleolithic diet[124] and the Mediterranean diet[125,126] are well known for their health-promoting benefits, as described in peer-reviewed journals and the lay press. The Mediterranean diet is characterized by increased proportions of legumes, nuts, seeds, whole-grain products, fruits, vegetables (including potatoes), fish and lean meats, and monounsaturated omega-9 and polyunsaturated omega-3 fatty acids.[127] Consumption of this diet is consistently associated with improvements in insulin sensitivity and reductions in cardiovascular disease, diabetes, cancer, and all-cause mortality.[126] The Paleolithic diet detailed by collaborators Eaton[128] and O'Keefe and Cordain[129] is similar to the Mediterranean diet except for a stronger emphasis on fruits and vegetables (preferably raw or minimally cooked), omega-3-rich lean meats, and reduced consumption of starchy foods such as potatoes and grains, the latter of which promote proinflammatory bacterial overgrowth in the bowel and were not staples in the human diet until the last few millennia. Including the olive oil and red wine per the Mediterranean diet and the absence of grains and potatoes per the Paleolithic diet appears to provide the best of both dietary worlds. The supplemented Paleo-Mediterranean diet extends the benefits of the foundational diet by appropriate use of fatty acid supplementation, multivitamin-multimineral supplementation (including physiological amounts of cholecalciferol), and probiotics. [130]

Biochemical and clinical justification for this type of diet is ample and is well supported by numerous long-term studies in humans wherein both Mediterranean and Paleolithic diets result in dramatic reductions in disease-specific and all-cause mortality.[131,132] Diets rich in fruits and vegetables are sources of more than 5000 phytochemicals, many of which have additive and synergistic nutrigenomic, antioxidant, anti-inflammatory, and anticancer properties.[133] Oleic acid, squalene, and phenolics in olive oil and phenolics and resveratrol in red wine have antioxidant, anti-inflammatory, and anticancer properties.[134] Omega-3 fatty acids have numerous health benefits via multiple mechanisms (see *Fatty Acid Supplements* below). Increased intake of dietary fiber from fruits and vegetables favorably modifies gut flora, promotes xenobiotic elimination (via flora modification, laxation, and overall reductions in enterohepatic recirculation), and is associated with reductions in morbidity and mortality.

Evidence of other benefits includes:

- A Paleolithic diet can lead to urinary alkalinization (average urine pH of ≥ 7.5 according to Sebastian et al[135]), which increases renal retention of minerals for improved musculoskeletal health[136,137,138] and increases urinary elimination of many toxicants and xenobiotics for a reduction in adverse effects from ubiquitous xenobiotic exposure.[139,140] Therapeutic alkalinization, whether by diet or supplementation, appears effective in the alleviation of chronic low back pain as shown in an open trial wherein the use of a low-potency alkalinizing supplement reduced symptoms and disability associated with low back pain in 76 out of 82 patients.[141]
- In obese patients, dietary moderation and the resultant weight loss have been shown to decrease reactive oxygen species generation by leukocytes and oxidative damage to lipids, proteins, and amino acids.[142]
- Implementation of a Mediterranean diet in rheumatoid arthritis patients leads to safe, significant, and cost-effective clinical benefits including reductions in disease activity and improvements in vitality.[143] Another controlled study treating rheumatoid arthritis with a Mediterranean diet showed significant benefit in patient global assessment, pain score, and early morning stiffness.[144] Michalsen et al[145] showed that a poorly designed Mediterranean diet that allowed ad lib overconsumption of highly fermentable carbohydrates provided no benefit in patients with rheumatoid arthritis or fibromyalgia.

Vegan and vegetarian diets — Vegetarian diets generally include grains, fruits, vegetables, nuts, seeds, eggs and milk products (lactoovovegetarian), and occasionally fish (pescovegetarian). Vegan diets are completely void of animal products and emphasize consumption of unprocessed raw foods. Vegan and vegetarian diets have provided benefit to patients with inflammatory and painful musculoskeletal disorders including eczema,[146] fibromyalgia,[147,148] and rheumatoid arthritis.[149] Molecular and physiological mechanisms include exclusion of common allergens and arachidonate, dietary diversity, increased consumption of antioxidant and anti-inflammatory phytonutrients, alkalinization, increased fiber and chlorophyll to promote removal of immunogenic and xenobiotic substances from the bowel, and beneficial qualitative and quantitative modifications of gut flora.

Clinical Pearl:

Rheumatoid arthritis patients who eat a Mediterranean diet have achieved significant benefit in patient global assessment, pain score, and early morning stiffness.

Hypoallergenic and oligoantigenic diets — Consumption of allergenic foods can cause joint pain and inflammation in sensitized patients, and avoidance of allergen consumption alleviates the arthritis.[150,151,152] Mechanisms of food-induced joint inflammation and pain include increased intestinal permeability and the resultant increased absorption of microbial immunogens, as well as food-antibody immune complex deposition in the joints with resultant localized inflammation.[153] Identification of allergenic foods is facilitated by symptomatic correlation with food consumption (including use of diet-symptom diaries) and the elimination and challenge technique (avoidance of the food and then reintroduction and monitoring for exacerbation of symptoms). Laboratory methods for IgE-, IgA- and IgG-mediated allergic reactions are commercially available yet show variable clinical utility. "Rotation diets" are used to avoid the clinically observed progressive sensitization that often occurs in patients with an allergic predisposition or disorders associated with immune activation such as chronic fatigue syndrome and irritable bowel syndrome. Highly sensitive patients may temporarily require elemental nutrition formulas, immunomodulatory interventions, and gastrointestinal repair in order to break the vicious cycles of allergic inflammation and symptomatology.[154]

Hafstrom et al[155] showed that a vegan diet free of gluten improved the signs and symptoms of rheumatoid arthritis, and the clinical benefits correlated with a reduction in IgG antibodies against the food antigens gliadin and beta-lactoglobulin. Hypoallergenic diets also have proven to be beneficial for the treatment of the immune complex disease mixed cryoglobulinemia.[156,157] Migraine headaches are often triggered by consumption and ameliorated by avoidance of food allergens. In a study of migraineurs, Grant[158] found that when an average of 10 triggering foods were avoided, patients experienced a dramatic fall in the number of headaches per month, with 85% of patients becoming headache-free. Hypertensive migraineurs may also experience a normalization of blood pressure following food allergen identification and avoidance.

Fasting — Short-term fasting has numerous health benefits and can be used at the start of dietary and nutritional intervention to expedite change in dietary acclimatization and interrupt pathophysiological vicious cycles.[159] Short-term fasting starves intestinal microbes for a reduction in proinflammatory bacterial overgrowth of the small bowel, temporarily eliminates dietary antigens, stimulates the humoral immune system in the gut to more effectively destroy local microbes,[160,161] and avoids the diet-induced inflammation common to the SAD as cited previously.

Dandona et al[162] showed that a 2-day fast reduced free radical generation, total oxidative load, and oxidative damage to amino acids. Goldhamer et al[163,164,165] have repeatedly proven the safety and effectiveness of supervised fasting in inpatients for the treatment of chronic hypertension, and a similar approach can be used for select patients with musculoskeletal pain and inflammation. Several case reports published by Fuhrman et al[166] showed that water-only fasting provided safe and significant clinical benefits in patients with rheumatoid arthritis (n = 3), fibromyalgia (n = 1), mixed connective tissue disease (n = 1), and SLE (n = 1). Additional evidence on fasting in rheumatoid arthritis includes:

- A systematic review by Muller et al[167] concluded that fasting followed by a vegetarian diet provides statistically and clinically significant long-term benefits in patients with rheumatoid arthritis.
- A controlled clinical trial of fasting followed by a vegetarian diet showed significant improvement in the number of tender joints, Ritchie's articular index, number of swollen joints, pain score, duration of morning stiffness, grip strength, ESR, CRP, white blood cell count, and health assessment questionnaire score in rheumatoid arthritis patients.[168]
- Kjeldsen-Kragh et al[169] showed that fasting followed by a vegetarian diet in patients with rheumatoid arthritis led to clinical improvement and that these clinical improvements are paralleled by reductions in anti-*Proteus* antibodies; this is particularly relevant given the well-described role of *Proteus* urinary tract colonization in the genesis and perpetuation of rheumatoid arthritis. A different study led by the same investigator showed that fasting followed by a vegetarian diet resulted in inhibition of growth of *Proteus mirabilis* and *Escherichia coli* in urine.[170]

Clinical Pearl:

Fasting followed by a vegetarian diet produces safe, effective, long-term subjective and objective benefits in patients with rheumatoid arthritis. Mechanisms of action include avoidance of common food allergens, increased intake of fiber and phytonutrients, qualitative and quantitative modification of gut flora, and increased resistance to urinary tract infection, particularly with *Proteus mirabilis*, which has etiopathological implications.

Fatty Acid Supplements

The fatty acid imbalances inherent in the SAD necessitate the use of precise supplementation in order to restore physiological balance. Patients should be encouraged to change their overall dietary pattern toward one that is more health promoting, such as the Paleo-Mediterranean diet described above, for overall improvement in nutrient intake, as well as food-based improvement in fatty acid balance. However, when supraphysiological effects from nutrients are desired for a "pharmacological" benefit, supplemental fatty acids from liquid or capsule supplements will generally still have to be consumed regardless of dietary optimization. The fatty acids most commonly used in the treatment of painful inflammatory disorders and in preventive medicine are omega-3 ALA, omega-6 GLA, omega-3 EPA, omega-3 DHA, and omega-9 oleic acid. Following brief reviews of the individual fatty acids, research on combination fatty acid supplementation (e.g., ALA+GLA or GLA+EPA+DHA), which more closely resembles the emerging trend in the clinical utilization of fatty acid supplementation, is presented, updated from previous reviews.[171,172]

Alpha-linolenic acid — Flaxseed oil is the most popular supplemental source of ALA, with high-quality expressions providing approximately 57% ALA. ALA has anti-inflammatory benefits, as consistently demonstrated in human studies. The main mechanism of action appears to be downregulation of NF-κB, rather than the direct modulation of eicosanoid biosynthesis. Ren and Chung[173] found that ALA inhibited NF-κB activation and inhibited inducible nitric oxide synthase, cyclooxygenase-2 (COX-2), and tumor necrosis factor-alpha (TNF-α) gene expressions; they also documented "potent antinociceptive effects" in animal models. Antinociceptive benefits of ALA supplementation were also demonstrated in an animal study by Yehuda and Carasso.[174] Moderate intakes of ALA from flaxseed oil have been shown to profoundly reduce production of proinflammatory prostaglandins (e.g., PG-E2, measured by urinary excretion) by 52% to 85% in humans.[175] This level of prostaglandin inhibition is greater than the 42% reduction induced by COX-2 inhibitor rofecoxib.[176] However, because the reduction in prostaglandin formation by ALA is mediated by inhibition of NF-κB rather than specific targeting of the COX-2 enzyme, the anti-inflammatory benefit occurs without adverse cardiovascular effects caused by COX-2 inhibitors, which are well documented.[177,178]

A prospective, randomized, single-blind secondary prevention trial of an ALA-enriched diet among approximately 600 patients (300 per group) who had previously suffered myocardial infarction showed that at 27 months, overall mortality was 20 in the control group but only 8 in the experimental group, providing an adjusted risk ratio of 0.30, clearly favoring the ALA-enriched diet.[179] However due to the dietary (and therefore complex and multicomponent) nature of the intervention, ascription of benefit directly and solely to ALA is not possible from this study. A supplement-based study without dietary intervention by Rallidis et al[180] contrasted results of 15 mL of flaxseed/linseed oil (rich in ALA) per day (n = 50) to those of 15 mL of safflower oil (rich in linoleic acid, 18:2n-6) per day (n = 26) for 3 months and found that ALA resulted in a decrease in CRP of 38% while serum amyloid A dropped by 23.1% and interleukin-6 dropped by 10.5%. This study shows that ALA supplementation reduces several important cardiovascular risk factors, consistent with epidemiological and diet-based studies correlating increased ALA intake with reduced cardiovascular mortality. Similarly, Zhao et al[181] showed that ALA intervention decreased CRP, vascular cell adhesion molecule-1 (-15.6%), E-selectin (-14.6%), and intercellular cell adhesion molecule-1 (-19.1%), leading the authors to conclude, "ALA appears to decrease CVD risk by inhibiting vascular inflammation and endothelial activation beyond its lipid-lowering effects." Thus, research showing safe and effective anti-inflammatory, cardioprotective, and antinociceptive benefits from ALA supplementation justify its use *within comprehensive treatment plans* for patients with neuromusculoskeletal pain and inflammation.

A study using flaxseed oil as a source of ALA to treat rheumatoid arthritis found no clinical or biochemical benefit (i.e., no change in hemoglobin, CRP, or ESR)[182]; however, the poor results of this study may have been due to the inferior quality of the flaxseed oil product, which supplied only 32% ALA compared with the much higher concentration of 57% found in most products.

Gamma-linolenic acid — Unique among omega-6 fatty acids, GLA has predominantly anti-inflammatory effects in contrast to its proinflammatory predecessor (linoleic acid) and successor (arachidonate). GLA is available from seed oils of hemp, evening primrose, blackcurrant, and borage, the latter being the most concentrated source. GLA is efficiently converted to dihomo-GLA and is then preferentially converted to the anti-inflammatory prostaglandin-E1. GLA helps reduce the formation of the arachidonate-derived 2-series prostaglandins, 4-series leukotrienes, and platelet-activating factor.[183] GLA is a ligand for peroxisome proliferator-activated receptor-gamma (PPAR-γ),[184] and activation of PPAR-γ modulates gene transcription and downregulates activation of proinflammatory NF-κB.[185] Thus, GLA has anti-inflammatory effects mediated via biochemical and nutrigenomic mechanisms. Accordingly, GLA has been shown to be clinically effective in reducing inflammation and manifestations of disease activity in patients with rheumatoid arthritis, eczema, respiratory distress syndrome (when used with EPA), breast cancer (when used with tamoxifen), premenstrual syndrome, diabetic neuropathy, and migraine headaches (when used with ALA). Effective adult doses range from 500 mg to 4000 mg with no major adverse effects having been reported, other than the possible exacerbation of temporal lobe epilepsy according to a report on 3 hospitalized schizophrenics.[186]

> **Clinical Pearl:**
>
> GLA is the precursor to arachidonate, and therefore, GLA supplementation can cause a mild increase in arachidonate unless delta-5-desaturase is inhibited by concomitant administration of EPA.[187]

Evidence regarding GLA in rheumatoid arthritis includes:

- In a prospective, 6-month, double-blind, placebo-controlled study of GLA (540 mg/d), 19 patients with rheumatoid arthritis showed a significant reduction in morning stiffness. [188]
- In a randomized, double-blind, placebo-controlled 24-week trial, Leventhal et al[189] used GLA (1400 mg/d) against a placebo of cottonseed oil and found that GLA treatment resulted in clinically important reductions in the signs and symptoms of disease activity in patients with active rheumatoid arthritis: the number of tender joints was reduced by 36%, tender joint score was reduced by 45%, swollen joint count was reduced by 28%, and the swollen joint score was reduced by 41%.
- 56 patients with active rheumatoid arthritis were randomized to treatment groups in a 6-month, double-blind trial of GLA (2800 mg/d) versus placebo, and results showed statistically significant and clinically relevant reductions in the signs and symptoms of disease activity.[190]

Many earlier studies using GLA suffered from methodological errors that led to an underestimation of GLA's anti-inflammatory utility; safety and efficacy have been well documented, but better studies are needed to show GLA's full potential, particularly when used as a component of combination fatty acid therapy and multicomponent intervention.

Eicosapentaenoic acid and docosahexaenoic acid (fish oil) — EPA and DHA generally occur together in dietary sources (cold-water fatty fish) and thus are both present in fatty acid supplements derived from fish oils. From a biochemical perspective, EPA is converted to DHA by the actions of elongase followed by delta-4-desaturase, with the latter being the rate-limiting step. From a practical clinical perspective, however, we see that the interconversion between EPA and DHA is minimal, so that both EPA and DHA need to be provided by the diet or supplementation program in order to obtain the optimal benefits of each. Fatty acids do not substitute for each other; in humans, the biochemical interconversion is slow and subject to genetic and acquired impairments, which are even more common in patients with clinical disease.

Fish oil supplementation has a wide range of applications and a strong history of clinical effectiveness, cost-effectiveness, safety, and collateral benefits that is second to none; no other single treatment is as significantly effective for such a wide range of conditions. Positive results have been documented in clinical trials on hypertension, hypercholesterolemia, cardiovascular disease prevention, depression, stress, bipolar illness, borderline personality disorder, schizophrenia, attention-deficit hyperactivity disorder, multiple sclerosis, psoriasis, ulcerative colitis, Crohn's disease, osteoporosis (when used with GLA), low back pain, SLE, and rheumatoid arthritis. Collateral benefits include reduced risk of the aforementioned conditions in general and depression and cardiovascular disease in particular. Rather than showing specificity for any one disease, the provision of EPA and DHA via diet and/or supplementation improves overall health by supplying the long-chain omega-3 fatty acids that are necessary for proper cell membrane structure and function, eicosanoid elaboration, and gene transcription. Significant cardioprotective benefit is seen even with the use of low doses; administration of less than 900 mg/d of combined EPA and DHA from fish oil resulted in a 45% decrease in risk of sudden cardiac death and a 20% reduction in all-cause mortality in a study of more than 11 000 patients.[191,192] For the assertive treatment of inflammatory disease, higher doses are used, generally 3000 mg/d of combined EPA and DHA.

For hundreds of thousands of years, premodern humans who consumed diets obtained from hunting and foraging had omega-3 fatty acid intake of approximately 7000 mg/d.[193] Supplemental EPA and DHA have been used in relatively high doses with little or no evidence of important adverse effects. In a Phase 1 dose-escalation trial to determine the maximum tolerated dose of fish oil in cachexia cancer patients, dosages reached up to 13 100 mg/d of EPA+DHA for 2 months without generalizable adverse effects other than diarrhea and abdominal discomfort due to lipid excess.[194] Due to its anti-inflammatory and antithrombotic effects, high-dose fish oil may potentate anticoagulant medication such as warfarin, and thus, caution should be employed in presurgical and anticoagulated patients. Some, but not all, fish oil supplements contain variable amounts of vitamin D3 and vitamin A, but the amounts of these vitamins are not high enough to cause toxicity except in the most extreme circumstances of high-dose, long-term supplementation. A quarter-cup of cod liver oil can provide 6000 IU of vitamin D and 15 000 IU to 23 000 IU of vitamin A; such doses would be safe for most adults, but the vitamin A dose is clearly above the 10 000 IU/d limit for pregnant women. The potential and largely theoretical problems of hypervitaminoses D and A are avoided by keeping the routine daily dose at approximately 3000 mg of EPA+DHA, which is consistent with the amounts used in the research literature to provide clinical benefit in the treatment of inflammatory disease.[195]

Standard medical training generally does not include dietetics and basic nutrition, let alone interventional nutrition and therapeutic diets. The lack of patentability of most nutritional products keeps prices low for consumers but also keeps motivation low for nutrition companies to promote a concept or product that could be usurped by a competitor. Cleland et al[196] described this situation accurately in a 2003 review of fatty acid therapy for rheumatoid arthritis: "Since fish oils do not provide industry with the opportunities for substantial profit associated with patented prescription items, they have not received the marketing inputs that underpin the adoption of usual pharmacotherapies. Accordingly, many prescribers remain ignorant of their biochemistry, therapeutic effects, formulations, principles of application and complementary dietary modifications."

The safety and effectiveness of fish oil, EPA, and DHA in the treatment of painful neuromusculoskeletal disorders are generally well established in the research literature. Mechanisms of action relevant to the treatment of pain include:

- Increased formation of anti-inflammatory prostaglandins, leukotrienes, resolvins, and docosatrienes
- Increased central serotonergic activity and reduced adrenergic activity, which culminate in the alleviation of depression, pain, and the experience of stress
- Modulation of gene transcription via the aforementioned resolvins and activation of PPAR-α for suppression of NF-κB
- Stimulation of chondrogenesis for the repair and preservation of articular structures
- Increased mineral (calcium) absorption from the gut
- Reductions in intracellular calcium, high levels of which promote inflammation and pathogenic patterns of gene expression

Representative clinical studies and reviews include:

- In a randomized, double-blind crossover study of 23 adolescent migraineurs, Harel et al[197] compared fish oil (756 mg EPA, 498 mg DHA) against a "placebo" of olive oil (1382 mg oleic acid) and found that both treatments were effective but that fish oil was more effective than olive oil.
- In a recent open trial with data from 125 patients with discogenic low back pain seen by a neurosurgeon, a daily dose of 1200 mg to 2400 mg EPA and DHA was shown to alleviate low back pain. Further, 59% of

patients were able to discontinue NSAID use thanks to pain relief from fish oil supplementation; 80% of patients were satisfied with their improvement, and 88% chose to continue treatment.[198]

- Long-term fish oil supplementation reduces cardiovascular risk in patients with rheumatoid arthritis as demonstrated by a study showing 30% to 40% reductions in cell membrane arachidonate, 35% reduction in serum thromboxane B2, 41% reduction in lipopolysaccharide-stimulated whole-blood prostaglandin E2, and 38% greater reduction in NSAID use compared with placebo results; disease remission occurred in 72% of patients receiving fish oil compared with only 31% of patients taking placebo.[199]

- A nonrandomized, double-blind, placebo-controlled crossover trial with 14-week treatment periods and 4-week washout periods among 32 patients with active rheumatoid arthritis used 2700 mg EPA and 1800 mg DHA with no dietary change; patients benefited from increased time to onset of fatigue (increased by 156 minutes) and fewer tender joints (average reduction 3.5 affected joints) while biochemical studies showed reductions in leukotriene B4 production.[200]

- In a placebo-controlled, double-blind crossover study contrasting the benefits of fish oil therapy in rheumatoid arthritis patients with or without dietary modification (an anti-inflammatory diet providing an arachidonic acid intake of less than 90 mg/d), Adam et al[201] showed a 14% reduction in tender and swollen joints with the anti-inflammatory diet alone (with placebo). While both fish oil supplementation and the low-arachidonate diet were safe and effective, clinical and biochemical efficacy increased significantly by the combination of the two.

- Shapiro[202] reviewed evidence showing that an important mechanism of action of omega-3 fatty acids is their central neurological effects, such as inhibiting eicosanoid production in glial cells, blocking voltage-gated sodium channels, inhibiting neuronal protein kinases, increasing serotonergic activity, and modulating gene expression, which helps contribute to the observed mood-stabilizing, analgesic, and sympatholytic effects.

- A meta-analysis of the analgesic effects of omega-3 fatty acid supplementation for inflammatory joint pain published by Goldberg and Katz[203] in 2007 concluded that supplementation with omega-3 fatty acids for 3 to 4 months reduces patient-reported joint pain intensity, duration of morning stiffness, and number of painful and/or tender joints but that effects on physician-assessed pain or Ritchie articular index were not significant. These latter findings were refuted by Kremer et al[204] who found significant physician-observed improvements and noted that many rheumatoid arthritis patients receive so much benefit from the simple use of fish oil supplementation that they are able to discontinue NSAIDs without experiencing a disease flare.

Overall, the research shows the safety and clinical benefit of fish oil supplementation for the alleviation of musculoskeletal pain and inflammation, and many of the biochemical and neurophysiological mechanisms have been elucidated. The biggest problems noted in most fatty acid studies are insufficient duration of treatment (i.e., less than 3 to 4 months), inappropriate selection of placebo (e.g., olive oil), concomitant use of drugs that impair eicosanoid production, product impurity, inadequate dosing, and failure to implement dietary restriction of arachidonate. The latter 2 factors are critically important because a basic premise of fatty acid therapy is ensuring the appropriate ratio of omega-3 to omega-6 fatty acids; a high-arachidonate diet can practically nullify the benefits of omega-3 supplementation, especially if the omega-3 dose is low or modest.

Oleic acid (olive oil) — The predominant fatty acid in olive oil, oleic acid is also found in borage seed and flaxseed oils, among others. Oleic acid has anti-inflammatory and cardioprotective effects via inhibition of NF-κB.[205] Olive oil is a complex mixture of fatty acids such as squalene and phytonutrients such as oleocanthal, which have highly potent anti-inflammatory and antioxidant actions of clinical significance. Earlier researchers erroneously believed olive oil to be clinically inert and were therefore surprised when their "placebo" showed clinical benefits. Olive oil consumption has consistently proven to be cardioprotective, and for this reason, it is an essential component of the Mediterranean diet strategy for reducing cardiovascular mortality. Fresh olive oil contains oleocanthal, which is "a natural anti-inflammatory compound that has a potency and profile strikingly similar to that of ibuprofen" and is the phytonutrient whose pungency induces the characteristic stinging sensation in the throat.[206]

Combination fatty acid supplementation — Because fatty acids compete for space within cell membranes and the active sites of converting enzymes, overconsumption of one fatty acid can cause relative and absolute depletions of fatty acids. This is used advantageously to reduce the adverse effects of arachidonate; however, beneficial fatty acids can also be compromised if they are "outnumbered and overpowered" by overzealous monotherapy with another fatty acid. For example:

- Monotherapy with GLA causes unfavorable reductions in oleic acid and EPA while raising proinflammatory arachidonate.[207]
- EPA/fish oil monotherapy reduces oleic acid[208] and dihomo-GLA.[209]
- ALA monotherapy reduces oleic acid.[210]

Further, with the recognition of the slow and unreliable interconversion of fatty acids in patients with clinical disease, researchers and clinicians have clearly begun transitioning away from fatty acid monotherapy and have begun using fatty acids in combination. This approach has provided superior results in animal models and available human studies wherein comparisons were performed with different ratios of various omega-3 (ALA, EPA, DHA) and omega-6 (GLA) fatty acids. Clinical trials that have used combination fatty acid therapy in the treatment of neuro-musculoskeletal disorders include the following:

- With an interventional design that resembled the functional medicine practice of therapeutic synergism, Wagner et al[211] treated 168 migraineurs in an open prospective study with the combination of 1800 mg GLA and ALA, multivitamins, progressive relaxation, encouragement to limit reliance on drugs, and a low-arachidonate diet. Of the 129 patients who completed the study, 82 were improved and 29 became migraine-free (total improved: 86%); overall migraine severity dropped from 88 points to 25 points (1-100 scale), and average time to the onset of therapeutic effectiveness was 3.2 months (such a delay in therapeutic onset makes placebo effect unlikely and is consistent with fatty acid exchange time frames). Given the high efficacy and safety, the authors stated that administration of a placebo would have been unethical.
- In a double-blind, placebo-controlled study, Belch et al[212] treated 3 rheumatoid arthritis groups (540 mg GLA, n = 16; 240 mg EPA and 450 mg GLA, n = 15; placebo, n = 18) for 12 months. By the end of the study, patients receiving GLA and GLA/fish oil had significantly replaced their NSAIDs in favor of fatty acids with no loss in disease control; 3 months of placebo treatment caused disease relapse.
- Berbert et al[213] added olive oil (9.6 mL) to the treatment plan of 43 rheumatoid arthritis patients already taking fish oil (3000 mg/d) in a placebo-controlled, randomized study; fish oil alone provided significant benefit on several parameters of disease activity, and the addition of olive oil further reduced morning stiffness and improved patient global assessment and ability to turn faucets. An important and unique finding in this study was a significant drop in serum levels of RF, used as a prognostic marker and believed to have a pathogenic role in rheumatoid arthritis.
- A double-blind, placebo-controlled, parallel group study by Remans et al[214] used combination fatty acid therapy "with micronutrients" (1400 mg EPA, 211 mg DHA, 500 mg GLA) in patients with active RA and found no benefit of therapy, which they ascribed to the subtherapeutic dosing; note that previous studies established that the minimum dose for EPA+DHA is 3000 mg in patients with inflammatory disease. Additional reasons for inefficacy may be that the supplement also contained linoleic acid (440 mg) and iron (9 mg), both of which are known to have proinflammatory and pro-oxidant effects; in addition, researchers co-administered bovine whey protein to which the patients may have been allergic, no dietary changes were implemented, and patients suffered from severe disease (selection bias) for which achieving improvement is difficult by any means.

Clinical Pearl:

While the therapeutic use of individual fatty acids is justified on biochemical, clinical, cardioprotective, and ethical bases, improved efficacy is obtained with combination fatty acid therapy, particularly in conjunction with a low-arachidonate diet and preferably with supplemental vitamin use.

Vitamin and Mineral Supplements

Reviewed in this section are specific vitamin and mineral interventions that are particularly noteworthy for their relevance to the treatment of chronic neuromusculoskeletal pain. Clinicians should ensure that their patients are taking an appropriately dosed basic multivitamin-multimineral supplement for chronic disease prevention.[215,216,217] When needed, supraphysiological doses of specific nutrients are not used in isolation, but are rather used atop a foundational program that includes dietary optimization and basic nutritional supplementation (multivitamin-multimineral, combination fatty acids [low dose for prevention, higher doses for intervention], and probiotics/synbiotics). As is well known, an important purpose of high-dose nutritional supplementation is to compensate for genotropic enzyme defects resultant from single nucleotide polymorphisms that cause decreased binding affinity for the corresponding vitamin coenzyme.[218] Because vitamins and minerals function cohesively and synergistically, isolated megadose supplementation is less rational, safe, and efficacious than combination supplementation.

Vitamin D3 (cholecalciferol) — Vitamin D deficiency is a prevalent international health problem that affects all strata of society and occurs in many sunlight-rich geographic regions. The finding by Heaney et al[219] that the adult physiological requirement for vitamin D3 is in the range of 3000 to 5000 IU/d is consistent with data showing that endogenous production from less than 1 hour of full-body sun exposure can easily range from 4000 IU to 20 000 IU. In the United States, the FDA's Recommended Daily Intake for vitamin D (200–600 IU/d for adults) was based on flawed logic and the observation that rickets could be prevented and treated in infants with administration of 1 teaspoon of cod liver oil, which contains 400 IU of vitamin D.

Vitamin D deficiency causes dull, achy musculoskeletal pain that is not appropriately treated by pharmacological, surgical, or manual interventions. The mechanism by which this pain is produced has been clearly elucidated by Holick[220]:

- Vitamin D deficiency causes a reduction in calcium absorption.
- Production of parathyroid hormone is increased to maintain blood calcium levels.
- Parathyroid hormone results in increased urinary excretion of phosphorus, which leads to hypophosphatemia.
- Insufficient calcium phosphate results in deposition of unmineralized collagen matrix on the endosteum (inside) and periosteum (outside) of bones.
- When the collagen matrix hydrates and swells, it compresses the sensory-innervated periosteum, resulting in pain.

Furthermore, vitamin D deficiency produces a systemic pro-inflammatory state, reversible with vitamin D supplementation,[221] that adversely affects central nervous system serotonergic transmission (and perhaps adrenergic transmission) to contribute to central hyperalgesia and depression.[222] Accordingly, vitamin D supplementation at 4000 IU/d improves mood and enhances well-being.[223]

Clinical Pearl:

Pain caused by vitamin D deficiency may be widespread or confined to a particular area, most commonly the lumbar spine.

Several clinical investigations have shown that vitamin D deficiency is particularly common among people with musculoskeletal pain and that vitamin D repletion alleviates pain.[224,225] In a landmark study by Plotnikoff and Quigley,[226] of 150 patients with persistent, nonspecific musculoskeletal pain syndromes refractory to standard therapies, 93% were found to have severe vitamin D deficiency, leading these researchers to conclude, "All patients with persistent, nonspecific musculoskeletal pain are at high risk for the consequences of unrecognized and untreated severe hypovitaminosis D … Because osteomalacia is a known cause of persistent, nonspecific musculoskeletal pain, screening all outpatients with such pain for hypovitaminosis D should be standard practice in clinical care." In a more recent study, hypovitaminosis D was found in 49 of 60 female patients with chronic low back pain.[227]

Proof of the cause-and-effect relationship between vitamin D deficiency and chronic musculoskeletal pain comes from clinical trials among deficient patients showing that vitamin D monotherapy alleviates pain. The exemplary study by Al Faraj and Al Mutairi[35] showed that among patients with "idiopathic chronic low back pain," 83% (n = 299) were vitamin D deficient, and supplementation with 5000 to 10 000 IU/d of cholecalciferol for 3 months alleviated or cured the low back pain in more than 95% of patients. The authors concluded that, in the evaluation of chronic musculoskeletal pain among populations with a sufficiently high prevalence of vitamin D deficiency, "Screening for vitamin D deficiency and treatment with supplements should be mandatory in this setting."

Vitamin D has a wide range of safety according to an extensive review of the literature performed by Vieth.[228] Doses of 2000 IU/d of vitamin D3 have been given to children starting at 1 year of age and were not associated with toxicity but led to a reduction in the incidence of type 1 diabetes by 80%, consistent with the vitamin's anti-infective and immunomodulatory roles.[229] A 2004 review[36] on the clinical importance of vitamin D proposed that optimal vitamin D status is defined as 40 ng/mL to 65 ng/mL (100–160 nmol/L) and that "until proven otherwise, the balance of the research indicates that oral supplementation in the range of 1000 IU per day for infants, 2000 IU per day for children and 4000 IU per day for adults is safe and reasonable to meet physiological requirements, to promote optimal health, and to reduce the risk of several serious diseases. Safety and effectiveness of supplementation are assured by periodic monitoring of serum 25(OH)D and serum calcium." Current data and laboratory reference ranges support a higher top limit for serum 25(OH)D of approximately 100 ng/mL (250 nmol/L). Vitamin D hypersensitivity is seen with primary hyperparathyroidism, granulomatous diseases (such as sarcoidosis, Crohn's disease, and tuberculosis), adrenal insufficiency, hyperthyroidism, hypothyroidism, and various forms of cancer, as well as adverse drug effects, particularly with thiazide diuretics. Thiazide diuretics are known to potentiate hypercalcemia.

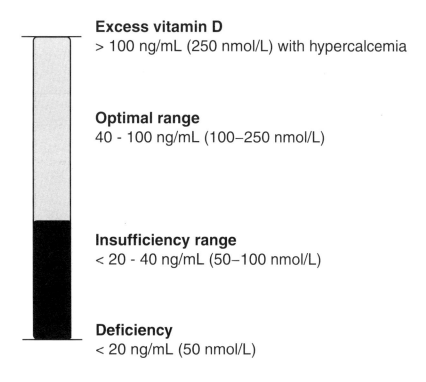

Excess vitamin D
> 100 ng/mL (250 nmol/L) with hypercalcemia

Optimal range
40 - 100 ng/mL (100–250 nmol/L)

Insufficiency range
< 20 - 40 ng/mL (50–100 nmol/L)

Deficiency
< 20 ng/mL (50 nmol/L)

Figure 2.1—Interpretation of Serum 25(OH)D Levels
Adapted from Vasquez A, Manso G, Cannell J. *Altern Ther Health Med.* 2004;10:28-37.36

Riboflavin (vitamin B2) — The neuromusculoskeletal applications for riboflavin include migraine headaches and CTS. Flavin adenine dinucleotide is required at Complex 2 of the mitochondrial electron transport chain (ETC), and high-dose riboflavin (400 mg/d) showed high efficacy, excellent tolerability, and low cost in the prevention of recurrent migraine attacks, according to a randomized controlled trial by Schoenen et al[230]; this study confirmed the safety and efficacy data from 2 open trials.[231,232] In small comparative groups of 11 and 15 patients, Sandor et al[233] showed that riboflavin has comparable effectiveness to beta-blocker drugs in the prophylaxis of migraine and suggested that these 2 treatments can be used together. In the treatment of CTS, Folkers et al[234] described a patient with a 3-year history of CTS and marked reductions in the activities of erythrocyte glutamic-oxaloacetic transaminase (EGOT) and erythrocyte glutathione reductase; riboflavin supplemented at 50 mg/d for 5 months normalized erythrocyte glutathione reductase and nearly resolved the CTS, which completely resolved (along with normalization of EGOT activity) following addition of pyridoxine (500 mg/d). By virtue of the safety and effectiveness of vitamin therapy for the treatment of migraine and CTS, some patients are able to avoid the need for expensive and potentially risky drugs and surgery.

Pyridoxine (vitamin B6) — Pyridoxine has been used in neuromuscular conditions including generalized pain with a "central" component, as well as CTS. Use of pyridoxine for the treatment of CTS has been advocated by individual practitioners[235] and by standard medical textbooks such as *The Merck Manual*, which advocates a trial of 50 mg twice daily.[236] In a small double-blind, placebo-controlled trial of pyridoxine (100–150 mg/d), Ellis and Folkers et al[237] found that most patients with CTS had deficient activity of pyridoxine-dependent EGOT and that clinical improvement in CTS paralleled biochemical improvements in EGOT over 10 to 12 weeks; the authors concluded, "Clinical improvement of the syndrome with pyridoxine therapy may frequently obviate hand surgery." Another case report published by the same authors[238] was that of a patient with CTS who had partial clinical (CTS) and biochemical (EGOT) response to pyridoxine at 2 mg/d; progressing to 100 mg/d maximized EGOT function and eliminated CTS symptoms.

Pain-relieving mechanisms of vitamin B6 include:

- Amelioration of previously undiagnosed pyridoxine-deficient peripheral neuropathy
- Enhanced conversion of tryptophan to serotonin for its analgesic effects
- Reduced plasma and brain levels of glutamate, an excitatory neurotransmitter that augments pain perception; increased levels of glutamate are seen in migraine and fibromyalgia[239]
- A diuretic effect in some patients, particularly women, due to reduced estrogen, increased progesterone, and suppression of aldosterone[240]

High levels of glutamate are noted peripherally and centrally in patients with chronic pain and some seizure disorders, while reduced levels of gamma-amino butyric acid (GABA), an inhibitory neurotransmitter, are seen in these disorders. The conversion of glutamate to GABA directly influences the tendency toward pain hypersensitivity and seizures; this glutamate-to-GABA enzymatic conversion in nerve terminals requires pyridoxine-dependent glutamic acid decarboxylase.[241] High-dose pyridoxine supplementation therefore promotes conversion of glutamate to GABA and thus promotes normalization of neurocortical excitation and alleviation of pain; importantly, the ratio of these "adversarial" neurotransmitters is favorably altered to a greater extent than the relative amounts of either one. Conversion of pyridoxine hydrochloride to the active intracellular form of the vitamin requires magnesium, zinc, and riboflavin, underscoring the importance of optimizing the diet and nutritional program to enhance therapeutic effectiveness.

Niacinamide (nicotinamide) — The general term *vitamin B3* can include niacin and its derivatives niacinamide (nicotinamide), niacinamide adenine dinucleotide (NADH), time-released or sustained-release niacin, prescription extended-release niacin, and inositol hexaniacinate. Each has its unique form, function, clinical applications, risk, and safety; time- or sustained-release niacin is notoriously hepatotoxic.[242] Of these forms, only the amide form— niacinamide—is useful for osteoarthritis-type degenerative joint disease. The credit for discovering the effectiveness of niacinamide in the treatment of painful arthritis goes to Kaufman,[243] who documented its safety and efficacy in hundreds of patients with rheumatoid arthritis and osteoarthritis. A generalized rejuvenative effect of vitamin therapy was also noted by Kaufman,[244] and this is consistent with experimental research showing that niacinamide induces "rapid reversion of aging phenotypes" through modulation of histone acetylation.[245] Reduced formation of joint-destroying nitric oxide appears to be an important mechanism of action,[246] and the reversal of aging phenotypes may counteract chondrocyte senescence. Further, as an endogenous ligand for and modulator of benzodiazepine receptors, niacinamide in supraphysiological doses might alleviate pain, exert anxiolytic benefits, and enhance well-being by acting centrally.

A recent double-blind, placebo-controlled study found that niacinamide therapy improved joint mobility, reduced objective inflammation as assessed by ESR, reduced the impact of arthritis on the activities of daily living, and allowed a reduction in medication use.[247] Given that a small risk for liver damage exists, liver enzymes should be assessed before and after the first month of treatment and periodically thereafter in patients receiving more than 2000 mg/d. Patients are advised to discontinue treatment with the onset of abdominal pain, jaundice, or nausea. Administration in divided doses is essential for efficacy; 500 mg given 4 to 6 times per day is a common dosing regimen, and the same daily dose could be achieved with more frequent use of 250 mg. As Gaby and Wright[248] pointed out, "500 mg taken 3 times a day is about half as effective as 250 mg taken every 3 hours for 6 doses, even though the total daily dose is the same." Treatment must be maintained for a minimum of 4 weeks before beneficial subjective and objective improvements can be expected. The general trend is rapid improvement in joint mobility and a reduction in pain in the first 1 to 2 months, followed by slower improvement which may continue for the next 1 to 3 years.

Niacin — NADH is an essential component of the first stage (Complex 1) of the mitochondrial ETC, a step that is commonly defective in patients with migraine. In addition to its tryptophan-sparing and vasodilatory roles, high-dose niacin facilitates mitochondrial energy production and thereby alleviates and reduces recurrence of migraine headaches.[249,250]

Cobalamins (vitamin B12) — Clinicians should be aware that routine laboratory assessment for vitamin B12 status is not reliable for the assurance of B12 sufficiency and that normal results on such tests do not preclude therapeutic efficacy of B12 administration.[251] Vitamin B12 is clinically available as cyanocobalamin, hydroxocobalamin (hydroxycobalamin), methylcobalamin, and adenosylocobalamin. Arguments against cyanocobalamin have been made due to its content of cyanide, a known mitochondrial toxin, whereas hydroxocobalamin actually promotes removal of cyanide from the human body.[252] Thus, the preferred forms are hydroxocobalamin, methylcobalamin, and adenosylocobalamin, and some patients may prefer or respond to one form over another.

Clinical trials using vitamin B12 in the treatment of pain include:

- A systematic review of 7 controlled clinical trials (4 used methylcobalamin, and 3 used vitamin B complex) using vitamin B12 to treat painful diabetic neuropathy indicated that vitamin B12's benefits include symptomatic relief of pain and paresthesia improvement in autonomic symptoms; effects on vibration perception and electrophysiological measures were not consistent and were generally of less magnitude than the symptomatic relief. [253]
- Methylcobalamin (500 mcg, intravenously three times weekly for 6 months) was used to treat patients receiving maintenance hemodialysis, and efficacy was evaluated using neuropathic pain grading and a nerve conduction study. Researchers found that patients' pain or paresthesia had lessened, and the ulnar motor and median sensory nerve conduction velocities showed significant improvement with no adverse effects of treatment.[254]
- Administration of hydroxocobalamin (1000 mcg, intranasal application daily for 3 months) in an open trial of patients with migraine headaches was shown to impressively lower the migraine attack frequency by 42% and to lower the duration, total number of migraine days per month, and the number of medication doses for acute treatment used per month.[255] The authors attributed the efficacy to the known ability of hydroxocobalamin to scavenge nitric oxide.
- Mauro et al[256] conducted a randomized, double-blind, placebo-controlled study using intramuscular vitamin B12 in 60 patients with chronic low back pain. Patients showed significant improvements in the visual

analog scale for pain and in a standardized disability questionnaire; acetaminophen use was also reduced by the nutritional therapy.

Thus, vitamin B12, which can be administered at 2000 mcg/d orally with results comparable or superior to parenteral administration,[257,258] appears to have a role in the treatment and adjunctive treatment of painful neuromusculoskeletal disorders.

Tocopherols (vitamin E) — Vitamin E is a general term that includes various tocopherols (alpha, beta, gamma, and delta, as well as tocopherol succinate), tocotrienols (alpha, beta, gamma, and delta), and tocopheryl congeners, each of which differs in nuances of pharmacokinetics and pharmacodynamics and therefore clinical effect. Clinicians and the public have been confused and misled by overzealous misinterpretations of flawed research that used synthetic and isolated forms of vitamin E without the context of balanced antioxidant supplementation and requisite dietary improvement.[259] Supplementation with synthetic forms of vitamin E should be avoided,[260] and the synthetic dl-tocopherol has been noted by some clinicians to trigger transient hypertension and headache. Most research in the use of vitamin E for the treatment of neuromusculoskeletal conditions has used alpha-tocopherol (inexpensive and widely available) or an unspecified "vitamin E."

Anti-inflammatory and analgesic mechanisms, particularly but not exclusively attributable to alpha- and gamma-tocopherols, include:

- Favorable modulation of eicosanoid production and reduction in isoprostane and CRP levels[261,262]
- Reduced transcription or direct inhibition of enzymes with proinflammatory effects (e.g., 5-lipoxygenase, phospholipase A2, COX-2)[263,264]
- Enhanced xenobiotic clearance secondary to induction of drug metabolizing (cytochrome P450) enzymes induced by the pregnane X receptor[265,266]
- Activation of PPAR-γ, which inhibits NF-κB activation to reduce transcription of proinflammatory genes[267]

Further, by virtue of its antioxidant and membrane-stabilizing effects, vitamin E may suppress development and perpetuation of certain autoimmune conditions by reducing oxidative modification of cellular and nuclear constituents that can become neoantigens and (auto)immunogens.

Ayres and Mihan[268] reported "successful control" of various autoimmune diseases by vitamin E including scleroderma, discoid lupus erythematosus, porphyria cutanea tarda, several types of vasculitis, and polymyositis; they offered that "since vitamin E is a physiological stabilizer of cellular and lysosomal membranes, and since some autoimmune diseases respond to vitamin E, we suggest that a relative deficiency of vitamin E damages lysosomal membranes, thus initiating the autoimmune process." A double-blind, placebo-controlled, randomized study used alpha-tocopherol (600 mg twice daily) in 42 medicated rheumatoid arthritis patients for 12 weeks and found a "small but significant analgesic activity," but no objective change in laboratory or clinical parameters.[269] Researchers in Egypt described a controlled trial using adjunctive vitamin E to produce improved subjective responses and objective control of rheumatoid arthritis.[270]

Vitamin E treatment studies in patients with osteoarthritis are conflicting, with results showing "good tocopherol analgesic effect"[271] or "no benefit for the management of symptomatic knee osteoarthritis."[272] Large-scale trials with modern research methods using isolated and mixed forms of vitamin E with and without additional diet and drug therapy need to be conducted in order to supplement, confirm, or refute the previously reports of successful vitamin E use in inflammatory conditions.[273,274] In dialysis patients who suffer from leg cramps, vitamin E is just as effective but less toxic and less expensive than quinine.[275]

Although vitamin E shows no short-term toxicity in doses up to 3200 IU/d,[276] most clinicians utilize lower doses (800–2400 IU/d) of mixed (not isolated) tocopherols in combination with diet optimization and additional supplementation when treating inflammatory musculoskeletal disorders.

Magnesium — Required for hundreds of biochemical reactions in the body, magnesium modulates pain perception by partially blocking (with zinc) N-methyl-D-aspartate receptors, which appear to be overstimulated in pain syndromes such as fibromyalgia, migraine, and most other types of headaches. Magnesium insufficiency is therefore associated with widespread, nonspecific biochemical derangements (i.e., "medically unexplained symptoms") and idiopathic drug-recalcitrant pain syndromes. The term *magnesium insufficiency* will be used here to include overt deficiency (deficiency of serum or ionized Mg) and functional disturbances (deficiency of intracellular Mg or a reduced ionized-to-serum ratio); not all research articles distinguish between these types of magnesium derangement. Magnesium insufficiency is common in American patients and the general population and can be assessed clinically (e.g., history, response to supplementation) and with laboratory tests (e.g., leukocyte intracellular Mg, urinary excretion following oral Mg administration).[277]

Support for the use of magnesium for preventive medicine and therapeutic analgesia are provided by the following reports:

- Magnesium insufficiency is seen in approximately 20% to 34% of the general population,[278,279] and the incidence is increased (43%) in trauma patients.[280] Insufficiency correlates with an increased risk of diabetes mellitus and cardiovascular disease.
- Overt magnesium insufficiency or response to magnesium supplementation characterizes migraine, tension headaches,[281] menstrual migraine,[282] post-traumatic headaches,[283] and nearly all other subtypes of headache due to the almost universal disturbances in magnesium ion homeostasis which appear to contribute to brain cortex hyperexcitability.[284]
- A prospective, multicenter, placebo-controlled, double-blind, randomized study evaluated the use of oral magnesium (600 mg/d) for 12 weeks and found that after 9 to 12 weeks of treatment, migraine attack frequency was reduced by 42% in the magnesium group and by 16% in the placebo group. In addition, the number of days with migraine and the drug consumption for symptomatic treatment per patient also decreased significantly in the magnesium group. The researchers concluded, "High-dose oral magnesium appears to be effective in migraine prophylaxis."[285]
- A randomized, double-blind, placebo-controlled trial of oral magnesium oxide prophylaxis of frequent migrainous headache in children (Mg oxide, n = 42; placebo, n = 44) found a statistically significant decrease over time in headache frequency in the magnesium oxide group but not in the placebo group. The group treated with magnesium oxide also had significantly lower headache severity relative to the placebo group.[286]
- In a case-control comparison at an outpatient headache clinic, Mauskop et al[287] sought to determine the efficacy of intravenous magnesium sulfate (1 g) in the treatment of various headaches (n = 40; patients included 11 with chronic migrainous headaches, 16 with migraines without aura, 9 with cluster headaches, and 4 with chronic tension-type headaches). Results showed complete elimination of pain in 80% of the patients within 15 minutes of infusion of magnesium sulfate. Further, no recurrence or worsening of pain was observed within 24 hours in 56% of the patients; patients treated with magnesium sulfate observed complete elimination of photophobia, phonophobia, and nausea. A brief, transient "flushed feeling" was the only side effect observed.
- The incidence of painful diabetic neuropathy among type 1 diabetics was reduced over 5 years among patients orally supplemented with 300 mg of magnesium per day (39% improved, 49% no change, 12% worse) compared with placebo (8% improved, 31% no change, 61% worse).[288]

Future studies should evaluate the efficacy of different forms of magnesium (e.g., Mg oxide, Mg citrate, Mg malate) and the roles of concomitant alkalinization, dietary optimization, and supplementation with pyridoxine, vitamin D, and omega-3 fatty acids.

Coenzyme Q10 (CoQ10) — CoQ10 is an endogenously produced and dietarily available antioxidant and an essential component of the mitochondrial ETC. Originally procured from bovine myocardium (i.e., raw cow hearts), its biosynthetic manufacture has made CoQ10 affordable, widely available, and one of the most popular nutritional supplements on the market. Its supplementation is supported by an abundance of safety and efficacy data. Reviewed here are the considerations relevant to the treatment of pain disorders.

An important component of migraines and certain other headaches is reduced energy production due to mitochondrial impairment, which can be either genotropic or secondary to nutritional deficiency or toxic insult. Painful migraine headaches can be successfully, safely, and cost-effectively prevented by supplementation with CoQ10 as demonstrated in an open trial in adults (150 mg/d),[289] an open trial among adolescent migraineurs deficient in CoQ10 (1–3 mg/kg/d),[290] and a double-blind, randomized, placebo-controlled trial (300 mg/d).[291]

A major adverse effect of statin drugs (3-hydroxy-3-methylglutaryl coenzyme A [HMG-CoA] reductase inhibitors) used for the treatment of hyperlipidemias and dyslipidemias and the prevention of cardiovascular disease is the painful myopathy and occasional sensorimotor neuropathy that often force discontinuation of the drug. HMG-CoA is necessary for the endogenous production of CoQ10; pharmacological inhibition of HMG-CoA reduces CoQ10 levels and results in iatrogenic mitochondrial myopathy, which is often painful. Statin-treated patients with symptoms of myopathy were treated in a double-blind protocol with CoQ10 (100 mg/d, n = 18) or vitamin E (400 IU/d, n = 14) for 30 days; pain severity decreased by 40% and pain interference with daily activities decreased by 38% in the CoQ10 group compared with no statistically significant improvement in the group treated with vitamin E.[292]

An underappreciated effect of CoQ10 is that of antiallergic immunomodulation, which was first described by Ye and Folkers et al,[293] who found that 40% of allergic patients had severe CoQ10 deficiency similar to that seen in dying class IV cardiac patients. Folkers et al[294] showed that CoQ10 increases T4/T8 ratios of lymphocytes in healthy subjects. Patients with bronchial asthma have significantly lower than normal CoQ10 levels,[295] and this finding was confirmed and extended by Gvozdjakova et al,[296] who showed that daily CoQ10 supplementation (120 mg, with 400 mg alpha-tocopherol and 250 mg ascorbate) reduced corticosteroid dosage in patients with bronchial asthma, a benefit possibly mediated through immunomodulation; the latter trial should be repeated without the additional vitamins E and C. Despite their imperfections, these studies have shown an association between CoQ10, immune function, and allergy, and combination antioxidant therapy with CoQ10 appears to have an antiallergic effect in patients with bronchial asthma. This raises the possibility that the benefit of CoQ10 in migraine, a condition known to be strongly associated with food allergies, might occur in part via antiallergic immunomodulation rather than completely via mitochondrial support. This would be in accord with the popular use of CoQ10 by integrative clinicians and the lay public for the treatment of various allergic diatheses. Furthermore, beneficial immunomodulation by CoQ10 might have relevance in the treatment of other immune disorders, autoimmunity in particular.

This author has used CoQ10 (100–250 mg/d, with other nutritional supplements such as cholecalciferol, EPA, and DHA) in a few patients with SLE to achieve complete normalization of high titers of ANA. Normalization of ANA occurred with CoQ10+nutrient supplementation, became elevated at ≥ 1:320 with treatment discontinuation, and again reduced to negative (normal) with reinstitution of CoQ10+nutrient supplementation. This technique of using over-the-counter nutritional supplements for *orthomolecular immunomodulation* has been detailed elsewhere[52,154] and deserves further study in the treatment of allergy and neuromusculoskeletal and systemic autoimmunity.

Protein and Amino Acids

Dietary protein intake, digestion, absorption, assimilation, and utilization must be adequate for the healing of injuries (including daily microtrauma) and the maintenance of muscle mass, immune function, neurotransmitter synthesis, and other functions. Dietary protein quality, determined by how well the amino acid profile matches the needs of human physiology, must also receive attention and can generally be ensured by consumption of a variety of protein sources and avoidance of dietary monotony. Excellent sources of high-quality protein include soy, whey, and rice protein isolates, eggs, milk(s), poultry, lamb, bison, seafood, and other animals; these can be selected by patients based on affordability, availability, palatability, allergenicity, and socioreligious considerations.

Individual patients can vary significantly in their efficiency of protein utilization and their need for particular amino acids; these factors can change over time and with the onset or regression of disease. For complete metabolism, interconversion, and utilization, nutritional cofactors (e.g., vitamins and minerals) must also be present, and therefore, any discussion of protein and amino acid nutriture or intervention must also consider the cofactors necessary for biochemical and therapeutic optimization. While any patient may have a unique need for and may derive benefit from one or more specific amino acids, we will concentrate here on amino acids that are particularly relevant to and researched in the treatment of chronic musculoskeletal pain, namely 5-hydroxytryptophan (5-HTP), DL-phenylalanine, L-arginine, and S-adenosylmethionine (SAMe).

> **Clinical Pearl:**
> Patients with recalcitrant fatigue, depression, pain, and other neuro-psychiatric conditions often respond to individual amino acid therapy or customized supplementation of amino acid blends based on correction of imbalances identified by measurement of urine or plasma amino acid levels.

5-hydroxytryptophan — 5-HTP is the hydroxylated form of L-tryptophan and occurs naturally in the human body as a normal intermediate in the conversion of L-tryptophan into serotonin. 5-HTP is available as a nutritional supplement isolated from a woody climbing shrub (*Bandeiraea simplicifolia*) native to West and Central Africa. Clinically, 5-HTP is administered orally, with 50 to 300 mg/d given either in divided doses or as a single dose. The therapeutic benefits of 5-HTP supplementation are derived from its conversion to serotonin, a portion of which is ultimately converted to melatonin. The supplement is used for its neurotransmitter and neuroendocrine effects in the treatment of anxiety, depression, hyperphagia, fibromyalgia, migraine, pain, and insomnia.[297] Interestingly, the analgesic and antinociceptive benefits of 5-HTP may be partly or largely mediated by beta-endorphin, in addition to serotonin; administration of 5-HTP (particularly with coadministration of carbidopa) significantly increases plasma levels of beta-endorphin.[298] Patients with disorders of both pain and mitochondrial dysfunction such as migraine and fibromyalgia derive dual benefit from 5-HTP because serotonin downregulates pain reception and sustains adrenal secretion of cortisol while melatonin functions as a powerful antioxidant and helps sustain mitochondrial function.

Research conducted on 5-HTP includes:

- An open 90-day study showed significant improvement in all measured parameters (number of tender points, anxiety, pain intensity, quality of sleep, fatigue) among 50 fibromyalgia patients treated with 5-HTP; global clinical improvement assessed by the patients and the investigator indicated a "good" or "fair" response in nearly 50% of the patients during the treatment period.[299]
- A double-blind, placebo-controlled study using 5-HTP in 50 patients with fibromyalgia showed significant improvement in all measured parameters with minimal adverse effects.[300]
- 5-HTP has a better safety and efficacy profile than the drug methysergide in the treatment of migraine, according to a study of 124 adults and children with migraine.[301]
- A randomized, double-blind, placebo-controlled trial of 65 patients with chronic tension-type headaches using 5-HTP (300 mg/d) showed a significant reduction in the use of pharmaceutical analgesics in patients treated with 5-HTP, but overall headache frequency and intensity remained constant[302]; in other words, patients replaced their analgesics with 5-HTP. The 300 mg/d dose was probably higher than necessary and higher than desirable; this contention is supported by the finding in this study that headache frequency declined and subjective opinion favored 5-HTP during the 2 weeks after termination of treatment.
- A double-blind, placebo-controlled crossover study in 31 patients with chronic primary headache used 5-HTP (400 mg/d) for 2 months to achieve "moderate efficacy and remarkable safety" in reducing frequency and severity of headaches.[303]

DL-phenylalanine — Supplementation with DL-phenylalanine has long been used in the treatment of pain and for the enhancement of opiate analgesia as reviewed by Russell and McCarty.[304] The nutritional L-isomer is converted from phenylalanine to tyrosine to L-dopa to dopamine to norepinephrine to epinephrine; augmentation of this pathway promotes resistance to fatigue, depression, and pain. The synthetic D-isomer inhibits the endorphin-degrading enzyme enkephalinase and thereby preserves endogenous opioids and augments their pain-relieving, mood-elevating function. Some chronic pain conditions are associated with reduced endogenous production of endorphins, which is thought to promote hypersensitivity to pain. Endorphins can be measured in plasma and mononuclear cells; in one study, patients with migraine and tension headaches had significantly lower plasma beta-endorphin compared with healthy controls (migraine 16.2 pmol/L, tension headache 14.5 pmol/L, controls 21.3 pmol/L) and lower beta-endorphin in mononuclear cells compared with controls (migraine 110.5 units, tension headache 142.3 units, controls 359.3 units).[305] While benefit has been shown in controlled trials in the treatment of depression, new high-quality clinical studies are needed in large groups to reaffirm empiric use and previous trials for the treatment of pain.[306,307] Attention to dosing is important, as some studies have used as little as 400 mg whereas doctors in clinical practice commonly use up to 1500 mg/d; one study in particular used bolus doses of 4000 mg of D-phenylalanine to augment acupuncture anesthesia in patients with low back pain and those undergoing tooth extraction.[308] Amino acid therapy is generally given between meals to avoid problems with competitive absorption.

L-arginine — Chronic and subacute pain can result from delayed healing of macrotrauma or recurrent micro-trauma, and therefore, facilitation of healing by the use of supplemental arginine can alleviate pain, promote optimal healing, and lessen reliance upon analgesic pharmaceutical drugs. Lack of dietary arginine impairs experimental wound healing, whereas arginine supplementation promotes formation of nitric oxide (necessary for wound healing), L-proline (substrate for collagen synthesis), and polyamines (stimulate cellular proliferation).[309,310]

Clinical studies in humans have shown qualitative and chronological improvements in wound healing following administration of arginine.

- A randomized, double-blind, placebo-controlled study of oral arginine supplementation (15 g/d) in elderly patients (>65 years) showed significantly enhanced wound hydroxyproline accumulation and total protein content; peripheral blood lymphocyte responses to mitogenic and allogenic stimulation were greater in the arginine-supplemented group, and serum insulin-like growth factor-1 levels were significantly elevated in the arginine group.[311]
- In a placebo-controlled study of 36 healthy volunteers, oral arginine supplementation (17 or 25 g/d) doubled the amount of collagen deposition into a standardized wound as assessed by the amount of hydroxyproline present (controls: 10.1 nmol/cm; 17 g arginine daily: 17.57 nmol/cm; 25 g arginine daily: 23.85 nmol/cm); immunostimulatory activity was evidenced by increased lymphocyte mitogenesis in response to phytohemagglutinin and concanavalin A.[312]
- Pressure ulcers can cause severe pain and disability and are correlated with increased risk for mortality; in a randomized controlled trial among 16 hospitalized patients with a stage 2, 3, or 4 pressure ulcer, patients receiving additional arginine (9 g), vitamin C (500 mg), and zinc (30 mg) demonstrated clinically significant improvement in pressure ulcer healing.[313]

Patients who are slow to recover from acute or chronic injury should be counseled on the importance of sufficient protein intake, screened for digestive problems that impair proteolysis and absorption, assessed for the anabolic-catabolic balance of their hormonal milieu, and supplemented with arginine (and perhaps other amino acids and nutrients) in order to expedite healing and alleviate pain.

S-adenosylmethionine — A critically important molecule present in every cell of the body, SAMe is involved in numerous biochemical pathways. Supplementation with SAMe has shown benefit in numerous and divergent conditions including osteoarthritis, depression, and liver injury. In the treatment of depression, SAMe at doses of 200 to 1600 mg/d has been shown to be superior to placebo, "relatively free of adverse effects," and as effective as tricyclic antidepressants in alleviating depression with a faster onset of action.[314] In the treatment of painful neuromusculoskeletal disorders, SAMe has shown consistent benefit in osteoarthritis. Although some of the clinical benefits of SAMe are certainly due to its modulation of neurotransmitter status (serotonergic and adrenergic effects), what makes SAMe unique in the treatment of osteoarthritis is its ability to promote cartilage regeneration.

Evidence of the benefits of SAMe in neuromusculoskeletal disorders includes:

- Experimental studies have shown that intermediate doses of SAMe promote sulfate incorporation and protein synthesis by chondrocytes.[315] Animal studies (rabbits) with experimental osteoarthritis showed improved cartilage regeneration following SAMe administration.[316]
- A 4-week randomized, double-blind study of 36 patients with osteoarthritis (knee, hip, and/or spine) showed that SAMe (1200 mg/d) was safer and at least as effective as drug treatment with indomethacin (150 mg/d).[317]
- A 12-week, randomized, double-blind, controlled clinical trial with 56-day post-treatment follow-up compared SAMe (1200 mg/d) with oral piroxicam (20 mg/d) in 45 patients with unilateral knee osteoarthritis; efficacy and tolerability were similar, but SAMe provided sustained clinical improvement following the discontinuation of treatment that was not demonstrated by piroxicam.[318]
- A 2-year multicenter open trial involving 108 patients with osteoarthritis of the knee, hip, and spine used 400 to 600 mg of SAMe daily; benefits (alleviation of musculoskeletal pain and associated depression) began at 2 weeks and continued for the entire 24 months, with only mild and self-limiting adverse effects such as mild nausea.[319]
- In a placebo-controlled crossover trial in which 34 patients with fibromyalgia received daily intravenous SAMe (600 mg) for 10 days, no change in tender point score was recorded, but results favored SAMe on subjective perception of pain at rest, pain on movement, overall well-being, fatigue, quality of sleep, and morning stiffness, as well as on the Fibromyalgia Impact Questionnaire for pain[320]; the dose of SAMe and the short duration of this study may have precluded any opportunity for more meaningful benefits.
- In a double-blind, placebo-controlled study among 44 fibromyalgia patients, Jacobsen et al[321] administered 800 mg of SAMe orally for 6 weeks and found improvements in clinical disease activity, pain during the last week, fatigue, and morning stiffness; tender point score and muscle strength did not change.
- Tavoni et al[322] also showed modest benefit of SAMe in the treatment of fibromyalgia, while Gatto et al[323] showed anti-migraine benefit in an open trial.

Clinical doses range from 400 to 1600 mg/d and can be tailored to patient response and body weight. Conversion to mania in patients with bipolar disorder has been reported.[324] SAMe should be stored away from light, air, and heat.

Botanical Medicines

Botanical medicines have been used for thousands of years for the preservation, maintenance, and restoration of health. As massive as it is, the sum total use of pharmacological drugs, the vast majority of which have been developed only within the past 50 years, is miniscule compared to the collective use of botanical medicines across all populations. Reviewed in this section are those botanical medicines that are commonly employed in the comprehensive management of painful and inflammatory neuromusculoskeletal disorders. The botanical medicines discussed below will be categorized either as anti-inflammatory/analgesic or antimicrobial/anti-dysbiotic, although some botanicals such as ginger and *Uncaria* species are simultaneously anti-inflammatory and antimicrobial.

Clinical Pearl:

Therapeutics discussed here may be employed indirectly or directly depending on the perspective employed. For example, if a patient presents with joint pain secondary to gastrointestinal dysbiosis, which is the proper treatment—one that targets the joint pain and inflammation or one that eradicates the dysbiosis? Solely treating the consequence of dysbiosis by targeting the joint pain condemns the patient to suffer endlessly as the underlying cause of disease remains untouched, whereas direct and effective eradication of the causative dysbiosis removes the stimulus for inflammation and thereby eliminates both the cause and its secondary manifestation of joint pain.

Anti-inflammatory and analgesic botanical medicines

Willow bark, *Salix* **species** — Salicylates are widely present in fruits, vegetables, herbs, and spices and are partly responsible for the anticancer, anti-inflammatory, and health-promoting benefits of plant consumption.[325,326] As a source of salicylates and related components such as salicin, willow bark has a positive history of safety and efficacy in the clinical treatment of musculoskeletal pain. Because willow bark's salicylates were the original source for the chemical manufacture of acetylsalicylic acid (aspirin), researchers and clinicians have erroneously described willow bark as synonymous with aspirin; however, this is inaccurate, and clarification of willow's pharmacodynamics will be provided here.

Aspirin has 2 primary effects via 3 primary mechanisms of action: (1) anticoagulant effects mediated by the acetylation and permanent inactivation of thromboxane-A synthase (the enzyme that makes the powerful proaggregatory thromboxane-A2), (2) antiprostaglandin action via acetylation of both isoforms of cyclooxygenase (COX-1 inhibition 25 to 166 times greater than COX-2 inhibition), and (3) antiprostaglandin formation via "retroconversion" of acetylsalicylate into salicylic acid, which then inhibits COX-2 gene transcription.[327] It is important to note that the acetylation reactions are specific to aspirin (*acetyl*salicylic acid), and thus, mechanisms #1 and #2 are not seen with willow bark; in contrast, mechanism #3—inhibition of COX-2 gene transcription—appears to be the major mechanism of action of willow bark extract. Proof of this principle is supported by the lack of adverse effects associated with willow bark in the research literature. If willow bark were pharmacodynamically synonymous with aspirin, then we would expect case reports of gastric ulceration, hemorrhage, and Reye's syndrome; this is not the case, and therefore—with the exception of possible allergic reactions in patients previously allergic to aspirin and salicylates—extensive warnings on willow bark products[328] are unnecessary.[329] A single case report of serious anaphylaxis following use of willow bark in a patient previously sensitized to aspirin suggests that willow bark extract may be contraindicated in aspirin-allergic patients.[330] The daily dose should not exceed 240 mg of salicin, and products should include other components of the whole plant (especially polyphenols).[331]

In a double-blind, placebo-controlled study of 210 patients with moderate/severe low back pain (20% of patients had positive straight-leg raising test), extract of willow bark showed a dose-dependent analgesic effect, with benefits beginning in the first week of treatment.[332] In a head-to-head study of 228 patients comparing willow bark (standardized for 240 mg salicin) with rofecoxib (12.5 mg), both treatments were equally effective, yet willow bark was safer and 40% less expensive.[333]

Boswellia serrata, frankincense, salai guggal — The *Boswellia serrata* tree is commonly found in India and has been used for hundreds of years for its anti-inflammatory, antiarthritic, and analgesic activity. Boswellia's mechanisms of action include inhibition of 5-lipoxygenase with no apparent effect on cyclooxygenase[334]; a recent discovery has shown that it also inhibits NF-κB.[335,336] Evidence of boswellia's efficacy includes:

- A randomized, double-blind, placebo-controlled crossover study evaluated the efficacy, safety, and tolerability of boswellia for 8 weeks in 30 patients with knee osteoarthritis; patients receiving boswellia reported decreased knee pain and swelling, with increased knee flexion and walking distance.[337]
- A controlled trial found that boswellia provided a higher response rate (82%) than sulfasalazine (75%) in the treatment of ulcerative colitis.[338,339]
- In a double-blind, placebo-controlled study, 40 asthmatic patients were treated with boswellia gum resin (300 mg three times daily) for 6 weeks, with 70% of patients showing reduction in disease severity contrasted with only 27% response rate in the placebo group.

Products are commonly standardized to contain 37.5% to 65% boswellic acids, which have generally been considered the active constituents with clinical benefit. The daily dose is generally 450 mg of boswellic acids (e.g., 150 mg three times daily), with lower doses needed when treatment is multifaceted. Minor gastrointestinal upset has been reported. The recent discovery that incensole acetate from boswellia resin inhibits NF-κB activation[340] will probably lead to a reformulation of boswellia products, favoring standardization of both the boswellic acid and incensole derivatives.

***Harpagophytum procumbens*, devil's claw** — *Harpagophytum*'s mechanisms appear to include a central analgesic action localized at the periaqueductal gray[341] and a peripheral anti-inflammatory effect mediated by inhibition of inflammatory gene transcription via suppression of NF-κB.[342] Accordingly, administration of *Harpagophytum* to healthy volunteers does not alter eicosanoid production.[343] The literature includes these studies on *Harpagophytum*:

- In short-term, open, and head-to-head studies against pharmaceutical drugs, *Harpagophytum* has demonstrated safety and clinically relevant efficacy in the alleviation of hip pain, low back pain, and knee pain.[344]
- A double-blind, randomized, multicenter clinical study compared daily treatment with 435 mg of cryo-ground powder *Harpagophytum procumbens* against 100 mg of the NSAID diacerein for 4 months in patients with osteoarthritis of the knee and hip; the results of this study showed that *Harpagophytum* is comparable in efficacy and superior in safety to diacerhein.[345]
- Another randomized, double-blind trial compared 60 mg harpagoside (an active ingredient in *Harpagophytum procumbens*) against 12.5 mg of rofecoxib among 88 patients with low back pain; the botanical medicine provided greater patient retention, fewer adverse effects, and comparable efficacy.[346]
- In a randomized, double-blind study among 197 patients with chronic low back pain who were experiencing an acute exacerbation (some patients demonstrating radicular pain and neurological deficit), *Harpagophytum procumbens* extract containing 50 and 100 mg harpagoside showed superiority over placebo and significant clinical efficacy.[347]

Therefore, *Harpagophytum procumbens* appears to be a safe and moderately effective botanical analgesic with defined mechanisms of action that are appropriate for clinical use in patients with acute and chronic musculoskeletal pain. Side effects are rare and are generally less common with *Harpagophytum* than with NSAIDs in comparison studies; mild gastrointestinal upset, dizziness, and allergic reactions have been reported.[348] Treatment should be continued for at least 4 weeks, and many patients will continue to improve after several weeks of treatment. Products are generally standardized for the content of harpagoside, with a target dose of 60 mg/d. However, the whole plant is considered to contain effective constituents, not only the iridoid glycosides. The results of one laboratory study suggest that the some of the active components are degraded following exposure to acid,[349] and so the product might be consumed between meals, perhaps with sodium bicarbonate, to theoretically increase bioavailablity and efficacy.

***Zingiber officinale*, ginger** — Ginger is a well-known spice and food with a long history of use as an anti-inflammatory, antinausea, and gastroprotective agent. Components of ginger reduce production of the leukotriene LTB4 (by inhibiting 5-lipoxygenase) and of the prostaglandin PG-E2 (by inhibiting cyclooxygenase). Thus, as a safe and effective dual inhibitor of inflammatory eicosanoid production, ginger has been advocated as a clinically applicable therapy against musculoskeletal pain.[350,351] A randomized, double-blind, placebo-controlled, multicenter trial using a standardized concentrated extract of 2 ginger species (*Zingiber officinale* and *Alpinia galanga*) for 6 weeks in 261 patients with knee osteoarthritis showed that the ginger group had a higher rate of response, greater improvement in global status, greater reduction in knee pain on standing, greater reduction in knee pain after walking 50 feet, greater reduction in standardized osteoarthritis indexes, and greater reduction in intake of rescue medication.[352] A placebo-controlled, drug-controlled, double-blind crossover study ranked effectiveness as ibuprofen > ginger > placebo as assessed by a visual analogue scale of pain and the Lequesne index[353]; given ginger's slow onset of action compared to pharmaceutical drugs, a short-term (3-week) trial such as this is not an appropriate reflection of long-term treatment or dietary intake. In addition, doses of up to 1 g of ginger per day have been safely used during pregnancy to reduce nausea, vomiting, and the more severe hyperemesis gravidarum.[354,355] The pungent principles of ginger often create a warm or burning sensation in the stomach that is mild, reducible with food consumption, and not indicative of tissue irritation. Ginger can be consumed as a root or in capsule or powder form; most products designed for clinical used arc standardized for the concentration of gingerols.

***Uncaria tomentosa, Uncaria guianensis*, cat's claw, una de gato** — *Uncaria tomentosa* and *Uncaria guianensis* are flowering tropical vines native to Asia, Africa, and South America with similar *in vitro* activities. Extracts from *Uncaria* inhibit NF-κB, TNF-α, nitric oxide, and PGE-2 production *in vivo*, and clinical benefits correspond to these anti-inflammatory mechanisms.[356] A placebo-controlled trial using freeze-dried aqueous extraction of *Uncaria guianensis*

(100 mg daily) for 4 weeks among 45 patients with knee osteoarthritis revealed no major adverse effects and showed significant reductions in pain and subjective and objective measures of disease severity within the first week of therapy.[357] In a placebo-controlled, 2-phase, 52-week trial among 40 patients with rheumatoid arthritis using sulfasalazine or hydroxychloroquine, treatment with *Uncaria tomentosa* reduced the number of painful and swollen joints and the Ritchie Index; researchers concluded that the botanical showed "relative safety and modest benefit."[358]

Adverse effects are generally nonexistent or limited to mild headache and dizziness. Use during contraception or pregnancy is probably contraindicated based on the historical use of *Uncaria* as a contraceptive. High-quality extractions from reputable manufacturers used according to directions are recommended.

***Capsicum annuum, Capsicum frutescens,* cayenne pepper, capsaicin (topical)** — Controlled clinical trials have demonstrated the ability of topically applied capsaicin (8-methyl-N-vanillyl-6-nonenamide) to safely reduce pain, mostly via depletion, blocked transport, and reduced *de novo* synthesis of the neuropeptide substance P in sensory fibers. To the extent that capsaicin alleviates pain without improving underlying dysfunction, its use is not consistent with the functional medicine model, which aims to improve overall health by addressing underlying dysfunction. However, functional medicine clinicians appreciate the need for pain relief, especially if it helps avoid the cost and adverse effects of potentially addicting narcotic analgesics, and therefore, capsaicin has a role in functional medicine practice.

Evidence of capsaicin's efficacy includes:

- 200 patients with chronic neuropathic pain were treated with topical 0.025% capsaicin, 3.3% doxepin (analgesic, anesthetic), both, or placebo; doxepin, capsaicin, and doxepin-capsaicin were similar in their pain-reliving effect, while capsaicin significantly reduced sensitivity and shooting pain.[359]
- An 8-week, double-blind, multicenter parallel study compared the safety and efficacy of topical capsaicin and oral amitriptyline in 235 patients with painful diabetic neuropathy involving the feet; pain relief and reduction in disability were comparable, but topical capsaicin was much safer and avoided the costs and adverse effects of amitriptyline (somnolence [46%], neuromuscular [23%] and cardiovascular [9%] effects). The authors concluded, "Topically applied capsaicin is an equally effective but considerably safer alternative to amitriptyline for relief of the pain of diabetic neuropathy."[360]
- A very assertive intervention study by Robbins et al[361] used high-concentration (5%–10%) capsaicin administered with regional anesthesia in patients with intractable pain, complex regional pain syndromes, and neuropathic pain; the effectiveness of this approach led the authors to conclude, "The intermittent application of large-dose topical capsaicin may provide significant pain relief, decrease chronic analgesic dependence, and decrease aggregate health care expenditures."
- A double-blind, placebo-controlled study among 108 children undergoing pediatric hernia repair showed that acupoint capsaicin application provided pain relief and allowed for reduced dependence on meperidine (opioid analgesic).[362]
- A double-blind, placebo-controlled study among 90 women undergoing abdominal hysterectomy showed that topical capsaicin reduced the need for morphine and postoperative antiemetics.[363]
- A double-blind, randomized, placebo-controlled, multicenter parallel study with 320 patients with chronic low back pain used topical capsicum to obtain clinically relevant and statistically significant reductions in pain and disability without systemic adverse effects.[364]
- Treatment of active cluster headache with intranasal capsaicin (compared with placebo) reduced severity after 7 days of treatment.[365]
- In a small controlled clinical trial, patients stated that intranasal application of capsaicin alleviated chronic migraine suffering by 50% to 80%.[366]

Patients must be instructed to not get capsaicin in the eyes and to wash hands thoroughly after application. Transient (10 minutes) burning, sneezing, and coughing are common following intranasal application. Topical application of capsaicin during pregnancy has not been evaluated but is thought to be safe since the therapeutic mechanism of action is local. Over-the-counter capsaicin creams are available at strengths ranging from 0.025% to 0.1%. The stronger creams have a more powerful analgesic effect but result in more initial burning, which abates with continued use. The cream is generally not applied to areas of skin that are broken or bleeding. Since topical capsaicin reduces sensitivity to pain, patients should use increased vigilance and good judgment to avoid burns or freeze injuries if using heating pads or cryotherapy, respectively.

Antimicrobial and anti-dysbiotic botanicals

***Origanum vulgare*, Mediterranean oregano** — An *in vitro* study[367] and clinical experience support the use of emulsified oregano against *Candida albicans*. In an open clinical trial among 14 gastrosymptomatic patients infected with *Blastocystis hominis*, *Entamoeba hartmanni*, and/or *Endolimax nana*, administration of time-released, emulsified oil of oregano in tablets (600 mg/d in divided doses) for 6 weeks resulted in symptomatic improvement and complete disappearance of *Entamoeba hartmanni* (4 cases), *Endolimax nana* (1 case), and *Blastocystis hominis* (8 cases).[368] Gastro-intestinal colonization with *Blastocystis hominis* or *Endolimax nana* can cause an inflammatory reactive arthritis that mimics rheumatoid arthritis and remits following eradication of the parasite.

Berberine — Berberine is an alkaloid extracted from plant such as *Berberis vulgaris* and *Hydrastis canadensis*, and it shows effectiveness against *Giardia*, *Candida*, and *Streptococcus* in addition to its direct anti-inflammatory and antidi-arrheal actions. An oral divided dose of 400 mg/d is common for antimicrobial purposes in adults,[369] while a recent study using oral berberine to successfully lower low-density lipoprotein employed 1000 mg/d for 3 months.[370] Topical *Mahonia/Berberis aquifolium* is effective for dermal psoriasis via its combined anti-inflammatory and antimicrobial mechanisms.[371]

***Artemisia annua*, sweet wormwood** — Artemisinin consumed as a tea made from the dried leaves of *Artemisia annua* has been safely used for centuries in Asia in the treatment of malaria. Modern studies have used *Artemisia* tea, standardized preparations of artemisinin, or synthetic derivatives.[372,373] Beyond its proven effectiveness against malaria, artemisinin is also effective against anaerobic bacteria due to its pro-oxidative sesquiterpene endoperoxide. In a recent study of malaria patients, the adult artemisinin dose was 500 mg while children younger than age 15 received 10 mg/kg per dose.[374] Although research studies have used up to 1000 mg/d of artemisinin, such a high dose is generally not necessary in clinical practice when treating non-malarial infections or dysbiosis. For the treatment of gastrointestinal dysbiosis in this author's practice, a common dosing scheme for adults is 60 mg/d of artemisinin twice daily orally, and this is commonly combined with other antimicrobial botanicals such as berberine. Rectal administration of artemisinin extracts and derivatives is safe and highly efficacious for the treatment of malaria.[375] While it is effective in the gut, an additional benefit of artemisinin is its systemic bioavailability.

***Vaccinium macrocarpon*, cranberry** — Cranberry juice is effective for the prevention and treatment of mild urinary tract infections, mostly due to proanthocyanidin-mediated inhibition of *Escherichia coli* adherence to epithelial cells.[376] Evidence clearly implicates occult urinary tract infections (urogenital dysbiosis) as an important causative factor in rheumatoid arthritis, and therefore, dietary modification and nutritional supplementation including cranberry should be pursued.[377,378] Cranberry is available as juice (500 mL/d) and as standardized extracts in tablet and capsule form (400 mg twice daily).

Other anti-dysbiotic botanical medicines — In addition to those listed above, botanical medicines and plant-derived extracts employed against clinical and subclinical infections in humans include *Hypericum perforatum* (St. John's wort), *Commiphora myrrha* (myrrh), *Mentha x piperita* (peppermint), *Arctostaphylos uva-ursi* (bearberry), *Thymus vulgaris* (thyme), *Syzygium aromaticum* (clove), *Pimpinella anisum* (anise), buchu/betulina, caprylic acid and undecy-lenic acid, *Anethum graveolens* (dill), *Brucea javanica*, and *Acacia catechu*. Each of these is supported by historical use and modern experimental validation of its antimicrobial effects *in vitro*; clinical trials in infected humans exist for a few of these treatments. *Commiphora myrrha* is remarkably effective against the parasitic infection schistosomiasis[379]; researchers commented, "The parasitological cure rate after 3 months was 97.4% and 96.2% for *S. haematobium* and

S. mansoni cases with the marvelous clinical cure without any side effects."[380] *Arctostaphylos uva-ursi* has been used for the treatment and prevention of urinary tract infections and requires an alkaline urine for optimal effectiveness[381]; it shows some ocular and neurological toxicity and should be used with professional supervision for low-dose and/or short-term administration only.[382]

Antimicrobial pharmaceuticals — Drug treatments (e.g., ciprofloxacin, metronidazole, nystatin, amphoteri-cin B, vancomycin, the tetracyclines) can be used for the eradication of dysbiosis and subclinical infections and are chosen per microbe sensitivity, patient tolerance, and systemic bioavailablity or locational specificity. Antimicrobial treatments may need to be maintained for many months, as recently demonstrated in a trial of 2 years' duration which showed clinical improvement in psoriasis only after the initial 12 weeks of treatment with penicillin.[383]

Accessory Supplements

Glucosamine sulfate and chondroitin sulfate — From its precursor glucose, fructose-6-phosphate combines with glutamine to form glucosamine-6-phosphate, which is eventually converted to UDP-N-acetylglucosamine, then to UDP-N-acetylgalactosamine, which alternates with glucuronic acid to form the glycosaminoglycan chondroitin sulfate, a critical component of the hyaline cartilage matrix of articular surfaces.[384] Oral supplementation with glu-cosamine sulfate or chondroitin sulfate is used to prevent and alleviate degenerative arthritis pain by promoting the preservation and restoration of articular cartilage. Oral dosages of glucosamine and chondroitin sulfates are each in the range of 1000 to 2000 mg/d. Despite the safety and biochemical logic of supplementing with glucosamine and chondroitin sulfates for the treatment of osteoarthritis, controversy exists regarding the clinical efficacy of this ap-proach. In order to achieve a more advanced comprehension of the appropriate clinical use of these therapeutics, a review of the following considerations is necessary: (1) safety, (2) efficacy of monotherapy, (3) efficacy of multicom-ponent therapy, and (4) extra-articular benefits, namely cardioprotection. The first and last of these considerations will be grouped together for the sake of efficiency.

Chondroitin sulfate was first widely documented to be cardioprotective in several landmark studies by Morrison and colleagues,[385,386,387,388] beginning in 1968 with a clinical trial published in *Journal of the American Geriatric Society* and later in *Experimental Medicine and Surgery* and *Angiology*. In sum, these studies documented the consistent ability of chondroitin sulfate-A to reverse atherosclerosis and its consequences *in vitro* (cell/tissue culture), *in vivo* (animal stud-ies with spontaneously atherosclerotic primates), and *in clinico* (human patients with pre-existing atherosclerosis and clinically apparent cardiovascular disease). The reduction in morbidity and mortality in these clinical studies, when contrasted to the results of conventional therapy (control group), lends credence to the view that chondroitin is safe for human use. Glucosamine's safety was called into question based on the assumption that glucosamine contains glucose and would therefore be harmful for patients with diabetes mellitus[389]; this er-roneous presupposition has been thoroughly disproved by studies showing that daily supplementation with 1500 mg of glucosamine hydrochloride with 1200 mg of chondroitin does not appreciably alter hemoglobin-A1c levels nor adversely affect diabetes manage-ment.[390,391] Further, the application of simple mathematics to this conundrum is resolutory since glucosamine sulfate is administered therapeutically at doses of 1500 mg/d and an equivalent weight of pure glucose would contain only 6 dietary calories (carbohydrate = 4 kilocalories per gram). When sourced from shellfish (rather than bovine, porcine, or synthetic sources), supplemental glucosamine and chondroitin may possibly incite an allergic response in patients previously sensitized to shellfish; a case report describes an exacer-bation of asthma in a patient so treated.[392] Such allergic and idio-

---

Clinical Pearl:

While both glucosamine sulfate and glucosamine hydrochloride are 90% absorbed following oral administration, glucosamine hydrochloride is better tolerated by sulfur-sensitive patients (clinical observation); however, gluco-samine sulfate is therapeutically superior and is the preferred form for alleviating osteoarthritis pain and preserving articular cartilage.[396]

---

syncratic responses are extremely rare and are miniscule in comparison with the 17,000 annual deaths due to NSAID-induced hemorrhagic gastropathy and the tens of thousands of deaths attributed to coxibs such as valdecoxib and rofecoxib (both have been removed from the U.S. market).[177,393,394,395]

Glucosamine sulfate, glucosamine hydrochloride, and/or chondroitin sulfate can be described as chondroanabolic monotherapy when used in isolation (without appropriate supportive nutrients) for the preservation and rebuilding of articular cartilage. While glucosamine sulfate and chondroitin sulfate have some anti-inflammatory effects that can promote resolution of symptoms within 2 weeks, the full power of these interventions is realized only with long-term, multiyear consumption. Therefore, contrasting these slow-acting, sustained-benefit nutraceuticals against a rapidly acting anti-inflammatory pharmaceutical drug would be an inappropriate comparison.

The literature on these supplements includes the following osteoarthritis studies:

- A systematic quality assessment and meta-analysis by McAlindon et al[397] that included published and unpublished data found "moderate to large effects" of glucosamine and chondroitin preparations in the treatment of osteoarthritis, but the inclusion of studies of less than 6-months' duration and with abnormally low dosages clearly underpowered the demonstrable effects.
- A comprehensive meta-analysis by Richy et al[398] based on "an exhaustive systematic research of randomized, placebo-controlled clinical trials" found "highly significant efficacy of glucosamine on all outcomes, including joint space narrowing and Western Ontario and MacMaster Universities Osteoarthritis Index (WOMAC™). Chondroitin was found to be effective on Lequesne index, visual analog scale pain, mobility, and responding status." The authors noted excellent safety and "indistinguishable symptomatic efficacies for both compounds."
- A 3-year, randomized, double-blind, placebo-controlled trial among 212 patients with knee osteoarthritis used 1500 mg/d of glucosamine sulfate and showed preservation of joint space (contrasted with joint-space loss among the placebo-treated patients) and alleviation of pain (contrasted with exacerbation of pain among the placebo-treated patients).[399]
- A randomized, double-blind, parallel-group study of glucosamine sulfate (1500 mg/d) versus ibuprofen (1200 mg/d) orally for 4 weeks among 200 hospitalized patients showed more rapid symptomatic relief among patients treated with ibuprofen (48% responders versus 28% after the first treatment week) but no difference from the second week onward; success rates were comparable, but adverse effects were noted in 35% of patients taking ibuprofen compared to only 6% among patients taking glucosamine sulfate.[400]
- In a 3-year, randomized, placebo-controlled trial among 202 patients with knee osteoarthritis, placebo-treated patients showed progressive joint space (-0.19 mm) whereas glucosamine sulfate-treated patients (1500 mg/d) maintained or increased cartilage thickness (+0.04 mm), with a significant difference between groups. Standardized assessments and pain, function, and stiffness subscales significantly favored glucosamine sulfate, while safety was similar between glucosamine sulfate and placebo.[401]
- A combination of 2 randomized, placebo-controlled, prospective 3-year studies evaluated glucosamine sulfate among 414 knee osteoarthritis patients containing a subset of 319 postmenopausal women; joint space thickness decreased (-0.33 mm) and pain increased in the placebo group, while the glucosamine group maintained joint space (+0.003 mm) and achieved significant symptomatic benefit.[402]
- In a 6-month, randomized, acetaminophen-controlled (3 g/d), placebo-controlled, double-blind trial, 318 osteoarthritis patients used a prescription formulation of glucosamine sulfate (1500 mg/d). More patients responded to glucosamine sulfate (39.6%) than acetaminophen (33.3%) and placebo (21.2%).[403] Such a high acetaminophen dose would almost certainly result in hepatorenal complications (potentially serious, lethal, and expensive) if used long term.
- A 6-month, randomized, placebo-controlled trial of modest dose chondroitin sulfate (1000 mg/d) among 307 patients with knee osteoarthritis found that pain was reduced and function was improved in the chondroitin group compared with placebo; the chondroitin group also had a higher percentage of responders than the placebo group.[404]

- A short-term, multicenter study using glucosamine hydrochloride (less effective than glucosamine sulfate[405]) and chondroitin in which several of the authors (11 of 25) received payment from or have equity interests in the competing drug company (Pfizer, maker of celecoxib) may suggest that glucosamine and chondroitin are insufficiently therapeutic, despite the authors' own data to the contrary.[406]

By utilizing monotherapeutic interventions, clinical studies have failed to accurately reflect the practices and benefits seen in clinical practice, wherein a comprehensive protocol for treating osteoarthritis[407] would also include diet modification, basic vitamin and mineral supplementation, and supplementation with vitamin D, fish oil, and olive oil to retard chrondrolysis and promote chondrogenesis. Additionally, glucosamine and chondroitin sulfates can be used with the aforementioned nutrients such as niacinamide and botanicals such as *Uncaria* for additive and synergistic enhancement of clinical efficacy.[408]

Proteolytic and pancreatic enzymes — The clinical use of orally administered pancreatic and proteolytic enzymes, including pancreatin, bromelain, papain, trypsin, and alpha-chymotrypsin, began with the experimental work of Beard in 1906 in the *British Medical Journal*[409] and was soon followed by human data by Cutfield[410] and numerous reports in the *Journal of the American Medical Association*.[411,412,413] Orally administered proteolytic enzymes are well absorbed from the gastrointestinal tract into the systemic circulation by the body's intrinsic system for conserving such enzymes.[414,415] The antitumor, anti-metastatic, anti-infectious, anti-inflammatory, analgesic, and anti-edematous actions result from synergism between a variety of mechanisms of action, including the dose-dependent stimulation of reactive oxygen species production and anticancer cytotoxicity in human neutrophils, a pro-differentiative effect, reduction in PG-E2 production, reduction in substance P production, modulation of adhesion molecules and cytokine levels, fibrinolytic effects, and a antithrombotic effect mediated at least in part by a reduction in 2-series thromboxanes.

Enzymes must be consumed between meals so that they are absorbed systemically without being partly or completely exhausted or destroyed, as they might be if consumed with food. Therapeutic potency is determined by amount and enzyme activity, with the latter being rarely quantified or standardized in most research studies, making comparisons very difficult. Although bromelain may be used in isolation, enzyme therapy is generally delivered in the form of polyenzyme preparations containing pancreatin, bromelain, papain, amylase, lipase, trypsin, and alpha-chymotrypsin. Dosage is determined per product and tailored somewhat to patient and the severity and intensity of the situation. The therapeutic margin is very wide, and therefore, overdose/toxicity is unlikely with any reasonable dosage regimen.

Research data on these enzymes include:

- In a double-blind, placebo-controlled trial with 59 patients, Taub[416] documented that oral administration of bromelain significantly promoted the resolution of congestion, inflammation, and edema in patients with acute and chronic refractory sinusitis; no adverse effects were seen in any patient.
- In an open trial report of clinical experience, Trickett[417] reported that a papain-containing preparation benefited 40 patients with various injuries (e.g., contusions, sprains, lacerations, strains, fracture, surgical repair, muscle tears); no adverse effects were seen.
- In a randomized open trial of 77 adults with subchronic (less than 3 months' duration) mild acute knee pain, bromelain at either 200 or 400 mg/d provided dose-dependent reductions in the WOMAC symptom score of 41% and 59%, respectively, along with improvements in stiffness, physical function, and overall psychological well-being.[418]
- A randomized, double-blind, placebo-controlled trial among 47 patients with confirmed moderate to severe knee osteoarthritis used bromelain (800 mg/d) for 12 weeks but found no significant difference in outcomes between placebo and treatment groups[419]; negative peculiarities of this study are the once daily dosing and no mention that patients were advised to consume the proteolytic enzyme away from food.
- In a phase 3 randomized, double-blind, drug-controlled parallel group trial, 90 patients with painful hip osteoarthritis were treated for 6 weeks with either combination proteolytic enzymes or the NSAID diclofenac

(100 mg/d); proteolytic enzyme therapy was superior to diclofenac for WOMAC subscales of pain, joint stiff-ness, physical function, Lequesne index, and higher response rate (71.1% versus 61.4%).[420]

- A randomized, double-blind trial contrasted an oral bromelain-trypsin-rutosid combination (n = 52) with diclofenac (n = 51) in the treatment of knee osteoarthritis; researchers found that the Lequesne index improved from 13.0 to 9.4 (-3.6 change) in the enzyme group and from 12.5 to 9.4 (-3.1 change) in the diclofenac group, while physicians' global judgment of efficacy favored enzyme therapy (51.4% responders) over diclofenac (37.2% responders).[421]

- Rutosid, bromelain, and trypsin (in various combinations) were contrasted against placebo in a multinational, multicenter, double-blind, randomized parallel group trial in orthopedic surgery and emergency departments in 27 European hospitals. Among 721 patients, ages 16 to 53, presenting with acute unilateral sprain of the lateral ankle joint, the greatest reduction in pain (at the primary end point after 7 days) was in the bromelain/trypsin group (73.7%), which was marginally superior to that seen with rutoside-bromelain-trypsin (60.3%) and placebo (73.3%); the largest increase in range of motion was in the placebo group (60% increase from baseline) contrasted to the rutosid-bromelain-trypsin group (42.9%). Decreases in swelling were -3.9% for trypsin, -2.3% for rutoside-bromelain-trypsin, and -2.9% for placebo.[422]

- In a 3-week, prospective, randomized, drug-controlled, single-blind study, 50 patients ages 40-75 with knee osteoarthritis received diclofenac sodium (100 mg/d) or a combination of rutoside, bromelain, and trypsin (enzyme group); both groups benefited but the enzyme group showed better improvements in joint tenderness and range of motion.[423]

Overall, the results for enzyme therapy in the treatment of chronic pain and post-traumatic pain are modest but clinically significant, and the wide therapeutic index makes enzyme therapy a very reasonable consideration for patients with pain, particularly when pain does not respond to other treatments.[424,425] In the future, properly designed clinical trials should emphasize dose escalation so that published research reflects dosages used by nutritionally knowledgeable clinicians.

Physical Medicine: Spinal and Myofascial Manipulative Therapy

As mentioned above, many functional medicine practitioners extend their general physical examination to include the more detailed techniques of postural assessment, motion palpation, and static palpation to allow detection and assessment of subtle biomechanical faults and articular and myofascial aberrancies, which significantly contribute to chronic pain. Naturopathic, chiropractic, and osteopathic physicians receive classroom and practical hands-on training in physical medicine during their formal college training and must display cognitive and practical competence in this area on national and state licensing examinations. The additional training in somatic assessment and physical treatment provides these clinicians with safe and effective nonpharmacological and nonsurgical means for addressing acute and chronic musculoskeletal pain. Relatively exhaustive evidence-based reviews of physical medicine have been compiled by Leach,[426] Hammer,[427] Bergman, Peterson, and Lawrence,[428] and Vasquez.[407] The physical medicine paradigm is clinically synergistic with, yet conceptually divergent from, the biochemical paradigm that underlies the use of pharmacological, nutritional, and botanical medicines; the latter is based on biochemistry and pharmacology, while the former is primarily based on mechanical physics and neurophysiology. Below is a short survey of mechanisms and clinical results. (Also see discussion relevant to low back pain in Chapter 4, *Clinical Focus: Low Back Pain*.)

Spinal manipulation — Briefly, mechanisms of manipulative therapy[429,430] include:

- Releasing entrapped intraarticular menisci and synovial folds
- Acutely reducing intradiscal pressure, thus promoting replacement of decentralized disc material
- Stretching of deep periarticular muscles to break the cycle of chronic autonomous muscle contraction by lengthening the muscles and thereby releasing excessive actin-myosin binding
- Promoting restoration of proper kinesthesia and proprioception
- Modulating central neuronal pathways involved in pain perception

The clinical benefits and cost-effectiveness of manipulative management of musculoskeletal conditions are extensively documented, and it is well established that spinal manipulation generally shows superior safety to drug and surgical treatment of back and neck pain.[431,432,433,434,435] In a randomized trial involving 741 patients, Meade et al[436] showed: "Chiropractic treatment was more effective than hospital outpatient management, mainly for patients with chronic or severe back pain. … The benefit of chiropractic treatment became more evident throughout the follow up period. Secondary outcome measures also showed that chiropractic was more beneficial." A 3-year follow-up study by these same authors[437] in 1995 confirmed that "when chiropractic or hospital therapists treat patients with low-back pain as they would in day to day practice, those treated by chiropractic derive more benefit and long term satisfaction than those treated by hospitals."

Spinal manipulation provides benefits that extend beyond the spinal column and musculoskeletal system.[438] Such benefits include improved pulmonary function and/or quality of life in patients with asthma[439,440,441,442,443] and improvement or restoration of vision in patients with post-traumatic visual loss.[444,445,446,447,448,449,450,451] More research is required to quantify the potential benefits of spinal manipulation in patients with wide-ranging conditions such as epilepsy,[452,453] attention-deficit hyperactivity disorder,[454,455] and Parkinson's disease.[456] Modulation of immune function has been documented following spinal manipulation[457,458]; however, the clinical relevance of this effect has not been fully demonstrated. Upper cervical spine manipulation using a specific chiropractic technique is as effective as two-drug pharmacotherapy for the treatment of essential hypertension.[459]

Soft tissue manipulation — Adjunctive therapies such as post-isometric relaxation[460] and correction of myofascial dysfunction[461] can lead to tremendous and rapid reductions in musculoskeletal pain without the hazards and expense associated with pharmaceutical drugs. Soft tissue therapeutics such as massage can reduce adolescent aggression,[462] improve outcome in preterm infants,[463] alleviate premenstrual syndrome,[464] and increase serotonin and dopamine levels in patients with low back pain.[465]

Manipulative therapy can also be applied with clinical benefit to problems of the appendicular skeleton, including the shoulder,[466,467] wrist,[468] and ankle.[469] Manipulative therapy also appears to provide therapeutic benefit in the treatment of depression,[470] geriatric pneumonia,[471] and carpal tunnel syndrome,[472] as well as in recovery from cardiac bypass surgery.[473]

Conclusion

This chapter has reviewed assessments and interventions commonly utilized in the practice of integrative and functional medicine and has provided the scientific basis for each. When applied by skilled clinicians to appropriate patients, these interventions can generally be used in combination to maximize and expedite the clinical benefits while also minimizing adverse effects and overall costs. In the following chapters, the monograph will illustrate the application of these interventions in four clinical focus sections: migraine, low back pain, fibromyalgia, and rheumatoid arthritis.

References

1. Bickley LS, Szilagyi PG. *Bates' Guide to Physical Examination and History Taking*. 9th ed. Lippincott Williams & Wilkins; 2007.
2. Girard C, Dereure O, Blatière V, Guillot B, Bessis D. Vitamin a deficiency phrynoderma associated with chronic giardiasis. *Pediatr Dermatol*. 2006;23:346-349.
3. Khurana AK, Sinha RS, Ghorai BK, Bihari N. Ankle reflex photomotogram in thyroid dysfunctions. *J Assoc Physicians India*. 1990;38:201-203.
4. Celik S, Erdoğan T, Gedikli O, Kiriş A, Erem C. Diagonal ear-lobe crease is associated with carotid intima-media thickness in subjects free of clinical cardiovascular disease. *Atherosclerosis*. 2007;192:428-431.
5. Edston E. The earlobe crease, coronary artery disease, and sudden cardiac death: an autopsy study of 520 individuals. *Am J Forensic Med Pathol*. 2006;27:129-133.
6. Humphreys BK, Delahaye M, Peterson CK. An investigation into the validity of cervical spine motion palpation using subjects with congenital block vertebrae as a "gold standard." *BMC Musculoskelet Disord*. 2004;5:19.

7. Haas M, Panzer D, Peterson D, Raphael R. Short-term responsiveness of manual thoracic end-play assessment to spinal manipulation: a randomized controlled trial of construct validity. *J Manipulative Physiol Ther*. 1995;18:582-589.

8. Fritz JM, Whitman JM, Childs JD. Lumbar spine segmental mobility assessment: an examination of validity for determining intervention strategies in patients with low back pain. *Arch Phys Med Rehabil*. 2005;86:1745-1752.

9. Ridker PM. C-reactive protein and the prediction of cardiovascular events among those at intermediate risk: moving an inflammatory hypothesis toward consensus. *J Am Coll Cardiol*. 2007;49:2129-2138.

10. M'Seffar A, Fornasier VL, Fox IH. Arthropathy as the major clinical indicator of occult iron storage disease. *JAMA*. 1977;238:1825-8.

11. Vasquez A. Musculoskeletal disorders and iron overload disease: comment on the American College of Rheumatology guidelines for the initial evaluation of the adult patient with acute musculoskeletal symptoms. *Arthritis Rheum* 1996;39:1767-1768.

12. Barton JC, McDonnell SM, Adams PC, et al. Management of hemochromatosis. Hemochromatosis Management Working Group. *Ann Intern Med*. 1998;129:932-939.

13. Lauffer RB. *Iron and Your Heart*. New York, NY: St. Martin's Press; 1991.

14. Sullivan JL. Iron and the sex difference in heart disease risk. *Lancet*. 1981;1(8233):1293-1294.

15. Vasquez A. High body iron stores: causes, effects, diagnosis, and treatment. *Nutritional Perspectives*. 1994;17:13, 15-17, 19, 21, 28.

16. Vasquez A. Iron in men: why men store this nutrient in their bodies and the harm that it does. *M.E.N. Magazine*. January 1997: 11, 21-23. Available online at: http://www.menweb.org/alexiron.htm.

17. Konofal E, Lecendreux M, Deron J, et al. Effects of iron supplementation on attention deficit hyperactivity disorder in children. *Pediatr Neurol*. 2008;38:20-26.

18. Konofal E, Lecendreux M, Arnulf I, Mouren MC. Iron deficiency in children with attention-deficit/hyperactivity disorder. *Arch Pediatr Adolesc Med*. 2004;158:1113-1115.

19. Rockey DC, Cello JP. Evaluation of the gastrointestinal tract in patients with iron-deficiency anemia. *N Engl J Med*. 1993;329:1691-1695.

20. Punzi L, Betterle C. Chronic autoimmune thyroiditis and rheumatic manifestations. *Joint Bone Spine*. 2004;71:275-283.

21. Weetman AP. Hypothyroidism: screening and subclinical disease. *BMJ*. 1997;314:1175.

22. American Association of Clinical Endocrinologists Medical Guidelines for Clinical Practice for the Evaluation and Treatment of Hyperthyroidism and Hypothyroidism. Endocr Pract. 2002;8:457-469.

23. McDaniel AB. Thyroid assessment: Controversies and conundrums. Presented at: The 14th International Symposium on Functional Medicine; May 23-26, 2007; Tucson, Ariz.

24. Peeters RP, Wouters PJ, van Toor H, Kaptein E, Visser TJ, Van den Berghe G. Serum 3,3',5'-triiodothyronine (rT3) and 3,5,3'-triiodothyronine/rT3 are prognostic markers in critically ill patients and are associated with postmortem tissue deiodinase activities. *J Clin Endocrinol Metab*. 2005;90:4559-4565.

25. Kelly GS. Peripheral metabolism of thyroid hormones: a review. *Altern Med Rev*. 2000;5:306-333.

26. Gaby AR. Sub-laboratory hypothyroidism and the empirical use of Armour thyroid. *Altern Med Rev*. 2004;9:157-179.

27. Weetman AP. Hypothyroidism: screening and subclinical disease. *BMJ*. 1997;314(7088):1175-1178.

28. Skinner GR, Thomas R, Taylor M, et al. Thyroxine should be tried in clinically hypothyroid but biochemically euthyroid patients. *BMJ*. 1997;314(7096):1764.

29. Peeters RP, Wouters PJ, Kaptein E, van Toor H, Visser TJ, Van den Berghe G. Reduced activation and increased inactivation of thyroid hormone in tissues of critically ill patients. *J Clin Endocrinol Metab*. 2003;88:3202-3211.

30. Friedman M, Miranda-Massari JR, Gonzalez MJ. Supraphysiological cyclic dosing of sustained release T3 in order to reset low basal body temperature. *P R Health Sci J*. 2006;25:23-29.

31. Holick MF. Vitamin D deficiency: what a pain it is. *Mayo Clin Proc*. 2003;78:1457-1459.

32. Zittermannn A. Vitamin D in preventive medicine: are we ignoring the evidence? *Br J Nutr*. 2003;89:552-572.

33. Holick MF. Vitamin D: importance in the prevention of cancers, type 1 diabetes, heart disease, and osteoporosis. *Am J Clin Nutr*. 2004;79:362-371.

34. Plotnikoff GA, Quigley JM. Prevalence of severe hypovitaminosis D in patients with persistent, nonspecific musculoskeletal pain. *Mayo Clin Proc*. 2003;78:1463-1470.

35. Al Faraj S, Al Mutairi K. Vitamin D deficiency and chronic low back pain in Saudi Arabia. *Spine*. 2003;28:177-179.

36. Vasquez A, Manso G, Cannell J. The clinical importance of vitamin D (cholecalciferol): A paradigm shift with implications for all healthcare providers. *Altern Ther Health Med*. 2004;10:28-37.

37. Vasquez A, Cannell J. Calcium and vitamin D in preventing fractures: data are not sufficient to show inefficacy [letter]. *BMJ*. 2005;331:108-109.

38. Heaney RP. Vitamin D, nutritional deficiency, and the medical paradigm. *J Clin Endocrinol Metab*. 2003;88:5107-5108.

39. Mingrone G, Greco AV, Castagneto M, Gasbarrini G. A woman who left her wheelchair. *Lancet*. 1999;353(9155):806.

40. Hill J, Cairns E, Bell DA. The joy of citrulline: new insights into the diagnosis, pathogenesis, and treatment of rheumatoid arthritis. *J Rheumatol*. 2004;31:1471-1473.

41. van Boekel MA, Vossenaar ER, van den Hoogen FH, van Venrooij WJ. Autoantibody systems in rheumatoid arthritis: specificity, sensitivity and diagnostic value. *Arthritis Res*. 2002;4:87-93.

42. Frostegard J. Atherosclerosis in patients with autoimmune disorders. *Arterioscler Thromb Vasc Biol*. 2005;25:1776-1785.

43. Zhu K, Devine A, Dick IM, Prince RL. Association of back pain frequency with mortality, coronary heart events, mobility, and quality of life in elderly women. *Spine*. 2007;32:2012-2018.

44. Kurth T, Gaziano JM, Cook NR, Logroscino G, Diener HC, Buring JE. Migraine and risk of cardiovascular disease in women. *JAMA*. 2006;296:283-291.

45. Wingerchuk DM, Spencer B, Dodick DW, Demaerschalk BM. Migraine with aura is a risk factor for cardiovascular and cerebrovascular disease: a critically appraised topic. *Neurologist*. 2007;13:231-233.

46. Kurth T, Gaziano JM, Cook NR, et al. Migraine and risk of cardiovascular disease in men. *Arch Intern Med*. 2007;167:795-801.

47. McMurray RW. Bromocriptine in rheumatic and autoimmune diseases. *Semin Arthritis Rheum*. 2001;31:21-32.

48. Sereda D, Werth VP. Improvement in dermatomyositis rash associated with the use of antiestrogen medication. *Arch Dermatol*. 2006;142:70-72.

49. Jefferies WM. Mild adrenocortical deficiency, chronic allergies, autoimmune disorders and the chronic fatigue syndrome: a continuation of the cortisone story. *Med Hypotheses*. 1994;42:183-189.

50. Chang DM, Lan JL, Lin HY, Luo SF. Dehydroepiandrosterone treatment of women with mild-to-moderate systemic lupus erythematosus: a multicenter randomized, double-blind, placebo-controlled trial. *Arthritis Rheum.* 2002;46:2924-2927.

51. Booji A, Biewenga-Booji CM, Huber-Bruning O, Cornelis C, Jacobs JW, Bijlsma JW. Androgens as adjuvant treatment in postmenopausal female patients with rheumatoid arthritis. *Ann Rheum Dis.* 1996;55:811-815.

52. Vasquez A. *Integrative Rheumatology.* 2nd ed. Fort Worth, Tex: Integrative and Biological Medicine Research and Consulting; 2007.

53. Miller A. The pathogenesis, clinical implications, and treatment of intestinal hyperpermeability. *Alt Med Rev.* 1997:2:330-345.

54. Dastych M, Dastych M Jr, Novotná H, Cíhalová J. Lactulose/mannitol test and specificity, sensitivity, and area under curve of intestinal permeability parameters in patients with liver cirrhosis and Crohn's disease. *Dig Dis Sci.* 2008 Mar 5 [Epub ahead of print].

55. Person JR, Bernhard JD. Autointoxication revisited. *J Am Acad Dermatol.* 1986;15:559-563.

56. Snyder RG. The value of colonic irrigations in countering auto-intoxication of intestinal origin. *Med Clin North Am.* May 1939:781-788.

57. Jorizzo JL, Apisarnthanarax P, Subrt P, et al. Bowel-bypass syndrome without bowel bypass. Bowel-associated dermatosis-arthritis syndrome. *Arch Intern Med.* 1983;143:457-461.

58. Stein HB, Schlappner OL, Boyko W, Gourlay RH, Reeve CE. The intestinal bypass: arthritis-dermatitis syndrome. *Arthritis Rheum.* 1981;24:684-690.

59. Utsinger PD. Systemic immune complex disease following intestinal bypass surgery: bypass disease. *J Am Acad Dermatol.* 1980;2:488-495.

60. Vasquez A. Reducing pain and inflammation naturally, part 6: Nutritional and botanical treatments against "silent infections" and gastrointestinal dysbiosis, commonly overlooked causes of neuromusculoskeletal inflammation and chronic health problems. *Nutritional Perspectives.* January 2006: 5-21.

61. Campbell AW, Thrasher JD, Madison RA, Vojdani A, Gray MR, Johnson A. Neural autoantibodies and neurophysiologic abnormalities in patients exposed to molds in water-damaged buildings. *Arch Environ Health.* 2003;58:464-474.

62. Gray MR, Thrasher JD, Crago R, et al. Mixed mold mycotoxicosis: immunological changes in humans following exposure in water-damaged buildings. *Arch Environ Health.* 2003;58:410-420.

63. Luosujärvi RA, Husman TM, Seuri M, et al. Joint symptoms and diseases associated with moisture damage in a health center. *Clin Rheumatol.* 2003;22:381-385.

64. Myllykangas-Luosujärvi R, Seuri M, Husman T, Korhonen R, Pakkala K, Aho K. A cluster of inflammatory rheumatic diseases in a moisture-damaged office. *Clin Exp Rheumatol.* 2002;20:833-836.

65. Roponen M, Kiviranta J, Seuri M, et al. Inflammatory mediators in nasal lavage, induced sputum and serum of employees with rheumatic and respiratory disorders. *Eur Respir J.* 200;18:542-548.

66. Seuri M, Paldanius M, Leinonen M, Roponen M, Hirvonen MR, Saikku P. Chlamydophila pneumoniae antibodies in office workers with and without inflammatory rheumatic diseases in a moisture-damaged building. *Eur J Clin Microbiol Infect Dis.* 2005;24:236-237.

67. Tuomainen A, Seuri M, Sieppi A. Indoor air quality and health problems associated with damp floor coverings. *Int Arch Occup Environ Health.* 2004;77:222-226.

68. Hirvonen MR, Ruotsalainen M, Roponen M, et al. Nitric oxide and proinflammatory cytokines in nasal lavage fluid associated with symptoms and exposure to moldy building microbes. *Am J Respir Crit Care Med.* 1999;160:1943-1946.

69. Lakhanpal S, Cohen SB, Fleischmann RM. Reactive arthritis from Blastocystis hominis. Arthritis Rheum. 1991 Feb;34(2):251-3

70. "Endolimax nana grew on stool culture. Both the patient's diarrhea and arthritis responded effectively to therapy with metronidazole. The diagnosis of parasitic rheumatism was made in retrospect." Burnstein SL, Liakos S. Parasitic rheumatism presenting as rheumatoid arthritis. *J Rheumatol.* 1983 Jun;10(3):514-5

71. Meza-Ortíz F. Giardiasis-associated arthralgia in children. Arch Med Res. 2001 May-Jun;32(3):248-50

72. Layton MA, Dziedzic K, Dawes PT. Sacroiliitis in an HLA B27-negative patient following giardiasis. *Br J Rheumatol.* 1998 May;37(5):581-3

73. Siam AR, Hammoudeh M. Staphylococcus aureus triggered reactive arthritis. *Ann Rheum Dis.* 1995 Feb;54(2):131-3

74. Mondillo S, Giordano N, Senesi M, Battisti E, Palazzuoli V, Gennari C. An unusual case of restrictive cardiomyopathy in a patient with reactive arthritis caused by Staphylococcus epidermidis. Eur Heart J. 1996 Jan;17(1):152-3

75. Melby KK, Kvien TK, Glennas A. Helicobacter pylori--a trigger of reactive arthritis? *Infection.* 1999;27(4-5):252-5

76. Ahmadi K, Wilson C, Tiwana H, Binder A, Ebringer A. Antibodies to Klebsiella pneumoniae lipopolysaccharide in patients with ankylosing spondylitis. *Br J Rheumatol.* 1998 Dec;37(12):1330-3

77. Ely PH. The bowel bypass syndrome: a response to bacterial peptidoglycans. *J Am Acad Dermatol.* 1980 Jun;2(6):473-87

78. Shulman ST, Ayoub EM. Poststreptococcal reactive arthritis. Curr Opin Rheumatol. 2002 Sep;14(5):562-5

79. Howell EE, Bathon J. A case of post-streptococcal reactive arthritis. *Md Med J.* 1999 Nov-Dec;48(6):292-4

80. Severijnen AJ, Kool J, Swaak AJ, Hazenberg MP. Intestinal flora of patients with rheumatoid arthritis: induction of chronic arthritis in rats by cell wall fragments from isolated Eubacterium aerofaciens strains. Br J Rheumatol. 1990 Dec;29(6):433-9

81. Rashid T, Darlington G, Kjeldsen-Kragh J, Forre O, Collado A, Ebringer A. Proteus IgG antibodies and C-reactive protein in English, Norwegian and Spanish patients with rheumatoid arthritis. *Clin Rheumatol* 1999;18(3):190-5

82. Tiwana H, Wilson C, Alvarez A, Abuknesha R, Bansal S, Ebringer A. Cross-reactivity between the rheumatoid arthritis-associated motif EQKRAA and structurally related sequences found in Proteus mirabilis. Infect Immun. 1999 Jun;67(6):2769-75

83. Newmark JJ, Hobbs WN, Wilson BE. Reactive arthritis associated with Hafnia alvei enteritis. Arthritis Rheum. 1994 Jun;37(6):960

84. Toivanen P, Toivanen A. Two forms of reactive arthritis? *Ann Rheum Dis.* 1999 Dec;58(12):737-41

85. Hughes LE, Bonell S, Natt RS, Wilson C, Tiwana H, Ebringer A, Cunningham P, Chamoun V, Thompson EJ, Croker J, Vowles J. Antibody responses to Acinetobacter spp. and Pseudomonas aeruginosa in multiple sclerosis: prospects for diagnosis using the myelin-acinetobacter-neurofilament antibody index. *Clin Diagn Lab Immunol.* 2001 Nov;8(6):1181-8

86. Ebringer A, Hughes L, Rashid T, Wilson C. Acinetobacter immune responses in multiple sclerosis: etiopathogenetic role and its possible use as a diagnostic marker. Arch Neurol. 2005 Jan;62(1):33-6

87. Wucherpfennig KW. Mechanisms for the induction of autoimmunity by infectious agents. *J Clin Invest.* 2001;108:1097-1104.

88. Hemalatha V, Srikanth P, Mallika M. Superantigens: Concepts, clinical disease and therapy. *Indian J Med Microbiol.* 2004;22:204-211.

89. Ely PH. The bowel bypass syndrome: a response to bacterial peptidoglycans. *J Am Acad Dermatol.* 1980;2:473-487.

90. Harel M, Aron-Maor A, Sherer Y, Blank M, Shoenfeld Y. The infectious etiology of the antiphospholipid syndrome: links between infection and autoimmunity. *Immunobiology.* 2005;210:743-747.

91. Van Ghelue M, Moens U, Bendiksen S, Rekvig OP. Autoimmunity to nucleosomes related to viral infection: a focus on hapten-carrier complex formation. *J Autoimmun.* 2003;20:171-182.

92. Brons RH, Bakker HI, Van Wijk RT, et al. Staphylococcal acid phosphatase binds to endothelial cells via charge interaction; a pathogenic role in Wegener's granulomatosis? *Clin Exp Immunol.* 2000;119:566-573.

93. Picco P, Gattorno M, Marchese N, et al Increased gut permeability in juvenile chronic arthritides. A multivariate analysis of the diagnostic parameters. *Clin Exp Rheumatol.* 2000;18:773-778.

94. Shedlofsky SI, Israel BC, McClain CJ, Hill DB, Blouin RA. Endotoxin administration to humans inhibits hepatic cytochrome P450-mediated drug metabolism. *J Clin Invest.* 1994;94:2209-2214.

95. Lin HC. Small intestinal bacterial overgrowth: a framework for understanding irritable bowel syndrome. *JAMA.* 2004;292:852-858.

96. Roberts MS, Magnusson BM, Burczynski FJ, Weiss M. Enterohepatic circulation: physiological, pharmacokinetic and clinical implications. *Clin Pharmacokinet.* 2002;41:751-790.

97. Liska DJ. The detoxification enzyme systems. *Altern Med Rev.* 1998;3:187-198.

98. Shah DT, Jackman S, Engle J, Larsen B. Effect of gliotoxin on human polymorphonuclear neutrophils. *Infect Dis Obstet Gynecol.* 1998;6:168-175.

99. Ebringer A, Rashid T, Wilson C. Rheumatoid arthritis: proposal for the use of anti-microbial therapy in early cases. *Scand J Rheumatol* 2003;32(1):2-11

100. Rashid T, Darlington G, Kjeldsen-Kragh J, Forre O, Collado A, Ebringer A. Proteus IgG antibodies and C-reactive protein in English, Norwegian and Spanish patients with rheumatoid arthritis. *Clin Rheumatol* 1999;18(3):190-5

101. Ebringer A, Wilson C. The use of a low starch diet in the treatment of patients suffering from ankylosing spondylitis. Clin Rheumatol. 1996 Jan;15 Suppl 1:62-66

102. Erlacher L, Wintersberger W, Menschik M, et al. Reactive arthritis: urogenital swab culture is the only useful diagnostic method for the detection of the arthritogenic infection in extra-articularly asymptomatic patients with undifferentiated oligoarthritis. *Br J Rheumatol.* 1995;34:838-842.

103. Cooper GS, Parks CG, Treadwell EL, St Clair EW, Gilkeson GS, Dooley MA. Occupational risk factors for the development of systemic lupus erythematosus. *J Rheumatol.* 2004;31:1928-1933.

104. Vojdani A, Pangborn JB, Vojdani E, Cooper EL. Infections, toxic chemicals and dietary peptides binding to lymphocyte receptors and tissue enzymes are major instigators of autoimmunity in autism. *Int J Immunopathol Pharmacol.* 2003;16:189-199.

105. Schafer KS, Reeves M, Spitzer S, Kegley SE. *Chemical Trespass: Pesticides in Our Bodies and Corporate Accountability.* Pesticide Action Network North America. May 2004. Available online at: http://www.panna.org/docsTrespass/chemicalTrespass2004.dv.html.

106. Human Toxome Project. Available online at: http://www.ewg.org/sites/humantoxome.

107. Bradstreet J, Geier DA, Kartzinel J, Adams JB, Geier MR. A case-control study of mercury burden in children with autistic spectrum disorders. *Journal of American Physicians and Surgeons.* 2003;8:76-79.

108. Frumkin H, Manning CC, Williams PL, et al. Diagnostic chelation challenge with DMSA: a biomarker of long-term mercury exposure? *Environ Health Perspect.* 2001;109:167-171.

109. Arslan G, Lillestol K, Mulahasanovic A, Florvaag E, Berstad A. Food hypersensitivity reactions visualised by ultrasonography and magnetic resonance imaging in a patient lacking systemic food-specific IgE. *Digestion.* 2006;73(2-3):111-115.

110. Arslan G, Gilja OH, Lind R, Florvaag E, Berstad A. Response to intestinal provocation monitored by transabdominal ultrasound in patients with food hypersensitivity. *Scand J Gastroenterol.* 2005;40:386-394.

111. Shamberger RJ. Validity of hair mineral testing. *Biol Trace Elem Res.* 2002;87(1-3):1-28.

112. Bass DA, Hickock D, Quig D, Urek K. Trace element analysis in hair: factors determining accuracy, precision, and reliability. *Altern Med Rev.* 2001;6:472-481.

113. Olsen NJ, Park JH. Skeletal muscle abnormalities in patients with fibromyalgia. *Am J Med Sci.* 1998;315:351-358.

114. Sprott H, Salemi S, Gay RE, et al. Increased DNA fragmentation and ultrastructural changes in fibromyalgic muscle fibres. *Ann Rheum Dis.* 2004;63:245-251.

115. Farah H, Buzby J. U.S. food consumption up 16 percent since 1970. *Amber Waves.* November 2005. Available online at: http://www.ers.usda.gov/AmberWaves/November05/Findings/USFoodConsumption.htm.

116. Seaman D. The dietary pursuit of disease overwhelms the power of nutritional supplements. *Nutritional Wellness.* August 2007. Available online at: http://www.nutritionalwellness.com/archives/2007/aug/08_seaman.php.

117. Vasquez A. Common oversights and shortcomings in the study and implementation of nutritional supplementation. *Naturopathy Digest.* June 2007. Available online at: http://www.naturopathydigest.com/archives/2007/jun/vasquez.php.

118. Bach JF. The effect of infections on susceptibility to autoimmune and allergic diseases. *N Engl J Med.* 2002;347:911-920.

119. Seaman DR. The diet-induced proinflammatory state: a cause of chronic pain and other degenerative diseases? *J Manipulative Physiol Ther.* 2002;25:168-179.

120. Aljada A, Mohanty P, Ghanim H, et al. Increase in intranuclear nuclear factor kappaB and decrease in inhibitor kappaB in mononuclear cells after a mixed meal: evidence for a proinflammatory effect. *Am J Clin Nutr.* 2004;79:682-690.

121. Mohanty P, Hamouda W, Garg R, Aljada A, Ghanim H, Dandona P. Glucose challenge stimulates reactive oxygen species (ROS) generation by leucocytes. *J Clin Endocrinol Metab.* 2000;85:2970-2973.

122. Ramakers JD, Mensink RP, Schaart G, Plat J. Arachidonic acid but not eicosapentaenoic acid (EPA) and oleic acid activates NF-kappaB and elevates ICAM-1 expression in Caco-2 cells. *Lipids.* 2007;42:687-698.

123. Tak PP, Firestein GS. NF-kappaB: a key role in inflammatory diseases. *J Clin Invest.* 2001;107:7-11.

124. Cordain L. *The Paleo Diet: Lose Weight and Get Healthy by Eating the Food You Were Designed to Eat.* Indianapolis, Ind: John Wiley and Sons; 2002.

125. de Lorgeril M, Salen P, Martin JL, Monjaud I, Boucher P, Mamelle N. Mediterranean dietary pattern in a randomized trial: prolonged survival and possible reduced cancer rate. *Arch Intern Med.* 1998;158:1181-1187.

126. Knoops KT, de Groot LC, Kromhout D, et al. Mediterranean diet, lifestyle factors, and 10-year mortality in elderly European men and women: the HALE project. *JAMA.* 2004;292:1433-1439.

127. Curtis BM, O'Keefe JH Jr. Understanding the Mediterranean diet. Could this be the new "gold standard" for heart disease prevention? *Postgrad Med.* 2002;112:35-38, 41-45.

128. Eaton SB, Shostak M, Konner M. *The Paleolithic Prescription: A program of Diet and Exercise and a Design for Living,* New York, NY: Harper & Row; 1988.

129. O'Keefe JH Jr, Cordain L. Cardiovascular disease resulting from a diet and lifestyle at odds with our Paleolithic genome: how to become a 21st-century hunter-gatherer. *Mayo Clin Proc.* 2004;79:101-108.

130. Vasquez A. A five-part nutritional protocol that produces consistently positive results. *Nutritional Wellness*. September 2005. Available online at: http://nutritionalwellness.com/archives/2005/sep/09_vasquez.php.

131. Lindeberg S, Cordain L, Eaton SB. Biological and clinical potential of a Paleolithic diet. *J Nutri Environ Med*. 2003;13:149-160.

132. O'Keefe JH Jr, Cordain L, Harris WH, Moe RM, Vogel R. Optimal low-density lipoprotein is 50 to 70 mg/dl: lower is better and physiologically normal. *J Am Coll Cardiol*. 2004;43:2142-2146.

133. Liu RH. Health benefits of fruit and vegetables are from additive and synergistic combinations of phytochemicals. *Am J Clin Nutr*. 2003;78(Suppl 3):517S-520S.

134. Alarcon de la Lastra C, Barranco MD, Motilva V, Herrerias JM. Mediterranean diet and health: biological importance of olive oil. *Curr Pharm Des*. 2001;7:933-950.

135. Sebastian A, Frassetto LA, Sellmeyer DE, Merriam RL, Morris RC Jr. Estimation of the net acid load of the diet of ancestral preagricultural Homo sapiens and their hominid ancestors. *Am J Clin Nutr*. 2002;76:1308-1316.

136. Sebastian A, Harris ST, Ottaway JH, Todd KM, Morris RC Jr. Improved mineral balance and skeletal metabolism in postmenopausal women treated with potassium bicarbonate. *N Engl J Med*. 1994;330:1776-1781.

137. Tucker KL, Hannan MT, Chen H, Cupples LA, Wilson PW, Kiel DP. Potassium, magnesium, and fruit and vegetable intakes are associated with greater bone mineral density in elderly men and women. *Am J Clin Nutr*. 1999;69:727-736.

138. Whiting SJ, Boyle JL, Thompson A, Mirwald RL, Faulkner RA. Dietary protein, phosphorus and potassium are beneficial to bone mineral density in adult men consuming adequate dietary calcium. *J Am Coll Nutr*. 2002;21:402-409.

139. Proudfoot AT, Krenzelok EP, Vale JA. Position Paper on urine alkalinization. *J Toxicol Clin Toxicol*. 2004;42:1-26.

140. Minich DM, Bland JS. Acid-alkaline balance: role in chronic disease and detoxification. *Altern Ther Health Med*. 2007;13:62-65.

141. Vormann J, Worlitschek M, Goedecke T, Silver B. Supplementation with alkaline minerals reduces symptoms in patients with chronic low back pain. *J Trace Elem Med Biol*. 2001;15(2-3):179-183.

142. Dandona P, Mohanty P, Ghanim H, et al. The suppressive effect of dietary restriction and weight loss in the obese on the generation of reactive oxygen species by leukocytes, lipid peroxidation, and protein carbonylation. *J Clin Endocrinol Metab*. 2001;86:355-362.

143. Sköldstam L, Hagfors L, Johansson G. An experimental study of a Mediterranean diet intervention for patients with rheumatoid arthritis. *Ann Rheum Dis*. 2003;62:208-214.

144. McKellar G, Morrison E, McEntegart A, et al. A pilot study of a Mediterranean-type diet intervention in female patients with rheumatoid arthritis living in areas of social deprivation in Glasgow. *Ann Rheum Dis*. 2007;66:1239-1243.

145. Michalsen A, Riegert M, Lüdtke R, et al. Mediterranean diet or extended fasting's influence on changing the intestinal microflora, immunoglobulin A secretion and clinical outcome in patients with rheumatoid arthritis and fibromyalgia: an observational study. *BMC Complement Altern Med*. 2005;5:22.

146. Tanaka T, Kouda K, Kotani M, et al. Vegetarian diet ameliorates symptoms of atopic dermatitis through reduction of the number of peripheral eosinophils and of PGE2 synthesis by monocytes. *J Physiol Anthropol Appl Human Sci*. 2001;20:353-361.

147. Donaldson MS, Speight N, Loomis S. Fibromyalgia syndrome improved using a mostly raw vegetarian diet: an observational study. *BMC Complement Altern Med*. 2001;1:7.

148. Kaartinen K, Lammi K, Hypen M, Nenonen M, Hanninen O, Rauma AL. Vegan diet alleviates fibromyalgia symptoms. *Scand J Rheumatol*. 2000;29:308-313.

149. Peltonen R, Nenonen M, Helve T, Hänninen O, Toivanen P, Eerola E. Faecal microbial flora and disease activity in rheumatoid arthritis during a vegan diet. *Br J Rheumatol*. 1997;36:64-68.

150. van de Laar MA, Aalbers M, Bruins FG, van Dinther-Janssen AC, van der Korst JK, Meijer CJ. Food intolerance in rheumatoid arthritis. II. Clinical and histological aspects. *Ann Rheum Dis*. 1992;51:303-306.

151. Golding DN. Is there an allergic synovitis? *J R Soc Med*. 1990;83:312-314.

152. Hvatum M, Kanerud L, Hällgren R, Brandtzaeg P. The gut-joint axis: cross reactive food antibodies in rheumatoid arthritis. *Gut*. 2006;55:1240-1247.

153. Inman RD. Antigens, the gastrointestinal tract, and arthritis. *Rheum Dis Clin North Am*. 1991;17:309-321.

154. Vasquez A. Improving neuromusculoskeletal health by optimizing immune function and reducing allergic reactions: a review of 16 treatments and a three-step clinical approach. *Nutritional Perspectives*. October 2005: 27-35, 40.

155. Hafström I, Ringertz B, Spångberg A, et al. A vegan diet free of gluten improves the signs and symptoms of rheumatoid arthritis: the effects on arthritis correlate with a reduction in antibodies to food antigens. *Rheumatology (Oxford)*. 2001;40:1175-1179.

156. Ferri C, Pietrogrande M, Cecchetti R, et al. Low-antigen-content diet in the treatment of patients with mixed cryoglobulinemia. *Am J Med*. 1989;87:519-524.

157. Pietrogrande M, Cefalo A, Nicora F, Marchesini D. Dietetic treatment of essential mixed cryoglobulinemia. *Ric Clin Lab*. 1986;16:413-416.

158. Grant EC. Food allergies and migraine. *Lancet* 1979;1(8123):966-969.

159. McCarty MF. A preliminary fast may potentiate response to a subsequent low-salt, low-fat vegan diet in the management of hypertension: fasting as a strategy for breaking metabolic vicious cycles. *Med Hypotheses*. 2003;60:624-633.

160. Trollmo C, Verdrengh M, Tarkowski A. Fasting enhances mucosal antigen specific B cell responses in rheumatoid arthritis. *Ann Rheum Dis*. 1997;56:130-134.

161. Ramakrishnan T, Stokes P. Beneficial effects of fasting and low carbohydrate diet in D-lactic acidosis associated with short-bowel syndrome. *JPEN J Parenter Enteral Nutr*. 1985;9:361-363.

162. Dandona P, Mohanty P, Hamouda W, et al. Inhibitory effect of a two day fast on reactive oxygen species (ROS) generation by leucocytes and plasma ortho-tyrosine and meta-tyrosine concentrations. *J Clin Endocrinol Metab*. 2001;86:2899-2902.

163. Goldhamer A, Lisle D, Parpia B, Anderson SV, Campbell TC. Medically supervised water-only fasting in the treatment of hypertension. *J Manipulative Physiol Ther*. 2001;24:335-339.

164. Goldhamer AC, Lisle DJ, Sultana P, et al. Medically supervised water-only fasting in the treatment of borderline hypertension. *J Altern Complement Med*. 2002;8:643-650.

165. Goldhamer AC. Initial cost of care results in medically supervised water-only fasting for treating high blood pressure and diabetes. *J Altern Complement Med*. 2002;8:696-897.

166. Fuhrman J, Sarter B, Calabro DJ. Brief case reports of medically supervised, water-only fasting associated with remission of autoimmune disease. *Altern Ther Health Med*. 2002;8:112, 110-111.

167. Müller H, de Toledo FW, Resch KL. Fasting followed by vegetarian diet in patients with rheumatoid arthritis: a systematic review. *Scand J Rheumatol*. 2001;30:1-10.

168. Kjeldsen-Kragh J, Haugen M, Borchgrevink CF, et al. Controlled trial of fasting and one-year vegetarian diet in rheumatoid arthritis. *Lancet*. 1991;338(8772):899-902.

169. Kjeldsen-Kragh J, Rashid T, Dybwad A, et al. Decrease in anti-Proteus mirabilis but not anti-Escherichia coli antibody levels in rheumatoid arthritis patients treated with fasting and a one year vegetarian diet. *Ann Rheum Dis*. 1995;54:221-224.

170. Kjeldsen-Kragh J, Kvaavik E, Bottolfs M, Lingaas E. Inhibition of growth of Proteus mirabilis and Escherichia coli in urine in response to fasting and vegetarian diet. *APMIS*. 1995;103:818-822.

171. Vasquez A. Reducing pain and inflammation naturally, part 1: New insights into fatty acid biochemistry and the influence of diet. *Nutritional Perspectives*. October 2004:5, 7-10, 12, 14.

172. Vasquez A. Reducing pain and inflammation naturally, part 2: New insights into fatty acid supplementation and its effect on eicosanoid production and genetic expression. *Nutritional Perspectives*. January 2005: 5-16.

173. Ren J, Chung SH. Anti-inflammatory effect of alpha-linolenic acid and its mode of action through the inhibition of nitric oxide production and inducible nitric oxide synthase gene expression via NF-kappaB and mitogen-activated protein kinase pathways. *J Agric Food Chem*. 2007;55:5073-5080.

174. Yehuda S, Carasso RL. Modulation of learning, pain thresholds, and thermoregulation in the rat by preparations of free purified alpha-linolenic and linoleic acids: determination of the optimal omega 3-to-omega 6 ratio. *Proc Natl Acad Sci U S A*. 1993;90:10345-10349.

175. Adam O, Wolfram G, Zollner N. Effect of alpha-linolenic acid in the human diet on linoleic acid metabolism and prostaglandin biosynthesis. *J Lipid Res*. 1986;27:421-426.

176. Van Hecken A, Schwartz JI, Depre M, et al. Comparative inhibitory activity of rofecoxib, meloxicam, diclofenac, ibuprofen, and naproxen on COX-2 versus COX-1 in healthy volunteers. *J Clin Pharmacol*. 2000;40:1109-1120.

177. Topol EJ. Failing the public health: rofecoxib, Merck, and the FDA. *N Engl J Med*. 2004;351:1707-1709.

178. Sooriakumaran P. COX-2 inhibitors and the heart: are all coxibs the same? *Postgrad Med J*. 2006;82:242-245.

179. de Lorgeril M, Renaud S, Mamelle N, et al. Mediterranean alpha-linolenic acid-rich diet in secondary prevention of coronary heart disease. *Lancet*. 1994;343(8911):1454-1459.

180. Rallidis LS, Paschos G, Liakos GK, Velissaridou AH, Anastasiadis G, Zampelas A. Dietary alpha-linolenic acid decreases C-reactive protein, serum amyloid A and interleukin-6 in dyslipidaemic patients. *Atherosclerosis*. 2003;167:237-242.

181. Zhao G, Etherton TD, Martin KR, West SG, Gillies PJ, Kris-Etherton PM. Dietary alpha-linolenic acid reduces inflammatory and lipid cardiovascular risk factors in hypercholesterolemic men and women. *J Nutr*. 2004;134:2991-2997.

182. Nordstrom DC, Honkanen VE, Nasu Y, Antila E, Friman C, Konttinen YT. Alpha-linolenic acid in the treatment of rheumatoid arthritis. A double-blind, placebo-controlled and randomized study: flaxseed vs. safflower seed. *Rheumatol Int*. 1995;14:231-234.

183. Fan YY, Chapkin RS. Importance of dietary gamma-linolenic acid in human health and nutrition. *J Nutr*. 1998;128:1411-1414.

184. Jiang WG, Redfern A, Bryce RP, Mansel RE. Peroxisome proliferator activated receptor-gamma (PPAR-gamma) mediates the action of gamma linolenic acid in breast cancer cells. *Prostaglandins Leukot Essent Fatty Acids*. 2000;62:119-127.

185. De Bosscher K, Vanden Berghe W, Haegeman G. Cross-talk between nuclear receptors and nuclear factor kappaB. *Oncogene*. 2006;25:6868-6886.

186. Vaddadi KS. The use of gamma-linolenic acid and linoleic acid to differentiate between temporal lobe epilepsy and schizophrenia. *Prostaglandins Med*. 1981;6:375-379.

187. Barham JB, Edens MB, Fonteh AN, Johnson MM, Easter L, Chilton FH. Addition of eicosapentaenoic acid to gamma-linolenic acid-supplemented diets prevents serum arachidonic acid accumulation in humans. *J Nutr*. 2000;130:1925-1931.

188. Brzeski M, Madhok R, Capell HA. Evening primrose oil in patients with rheumatoid arthritis and side-effects of non-steroidal anti-inflammatory drugs. *Br J Rheumatol*. 1991;30:370-372.

189. Leventhal LJ, Boyce EG, Zurier RB. Treatment of rheumatoid arthritis with gammalinolenic acid. *Ann Intern Med*. 1993;119:867-873.

190. Zurier RB, Rossetti RG, Jacobson EW, et al. gamma-Linolenic acid treatment of rheumatoid arthritis. A randomized, placebo-controlled trial. *Arthritis Rheum*. 1996;39:1808-1817.

191. Dietary supplementation with n-3 polyunsaturated fatty acids and vitamin E after myocardial infarction: results of the GISSI-Prevenzione trial. Gruppo Italiano per lo Studio della Sopravvivenza nell'Infarto miocardico. *Lancet*. 1999;354(9177):447-455.

192. Marchioli R, Barzi F, Bomba E, et al. Early protection against sudden death by n-3 polyunsaturated fatty acids after myocardial infarction: time-course analysis of the results of the Gruppo Italiano per lo Studio della Sopravvivenza nell'Infarto Miocardico (GISSI)-Prevenzione. *Circulation*. 2002;105:1897-1903.

193. Cordain L. *The Paleo Diet: Lose Weight and Get Healthy by Eating the Food You Were Designed to Eat*. Indianapolis, Ind: John Wiley and Sons; 2002

194. Burns CP, Halabi S, Clamon GH, et al. Phase I clinical study of fish oil fatty acid capsules for patients with cancer cachexia: cancer and leukemia group B study 9473. *Clin Cancer Res*. 1999;5:3942-3947.

195. Kremer JM. n-3 fatty acid supplements in rheumatoid arthritis. *Am J Clin Nutr*. 2000;71(Suppl 1):349S-351S.

196. Cleland LG, James MJ, Proudman SM. The role of fish oils in the treatment of rheumatoid arthritis. *Drugs*. 2003;63:845-853.

197. Harel Z, Gascon G, Riggs S, Vaz R, Brown W, Exil G. Supplementation with omega-3 polyunsaturated fatty acids in the management of recurrent migraines in adolescents. *J Adolesc Health*. 2002;31:154-161.

198. Maroon JC, Bost JW. Omega-3 fatty acids (fish oil) as an anti-inflammatory: an alternative to nonsteroidal anti-inflammatory drugs for discogenic pain. *Surg Neurol*. 2006;65:326-331.

199. Cleland LG, Caughey GE, James MJ, Proudman SM. Reduction of cardiovascular risk factors with longterm fish oil treatment in early rheumatoid arthritis. *J Rheumatol*. 2006;33:1973-1979.

200. Kremer JM, Jubiz W, Michalek A, et al. Fish-oil fatty acid supplementation in active rheumatoid arthritis. A double-blinded, controlled, crossover study. *Ann Intern Med*. 1987;106:497-503.

201. Adam O, Beringer C, Kless T, et al. Anti-inflammatory effects of a low arachidonic acid diet and fish oil in patients with rheumatoid arthritis. *Rheumatol Int*. 2003;23:27-36.

202. Shapiro H. Could n-3 polyunsaturated fatty acids reduce pathological pain by direct actions on the nervous system? *Prostaglandins Leukot Essent Fatty Acids*. 2003;68:219-224.

203. Goldberg RJ, Katz J. A meta-analysis of the analgesic effects of omega-3 polyunsaturated fatty acid supplementation for inflammatory joint pain. *Pain*. 2007;129(1-2):210-223.

204. Kremer JM, Lawrence DA, Petrillo GF, et al. Effects of high-dose fish oil on rheumatoid arthritis after stopping nonsteroidal antiinflammatory drugs. Clinical and immune correlates. *Arthritis Rheum*. 1995;38:1107-1114.

205. Carluccio MA, Massaro M, Bonfrate C, et al. Oleic acid inhibits endothelial activation: A direct vascular antiatherogenic mechanism of a nutritional component in the mediterranean diet. *Arterioscler Thromb Vasc Biol*. 1999;19:220-228.

206. Beauchamp GK, Keast RS, Morel D, et al. Phytochemistry: ibuprofen-like activity in extra-virgin olive oil. *Nature*. 2005;437(7055):45-46.

207. Jäntti J, Nikkari T, Solakivi T, Vapaatalo H, Isomäki H. Evening primrose oil in rheumatoid arthritis: changes in serum lipids and fatty acids. *Ann Rheum Dis*. 1989;48:124-127.

208. Haban P, Zidekova E, Klvanova J. Supplementation with long-chain n-3 fatty acids in non-insulin-dependent diabetes mellitus (NIDDM) patients leads to the lowering of oleic acid content in serum phospholipids. Eur J Nutr. 2000;39:201-206.

209. Cleland LG, Gibson RA, Neumann M, French JK. The effect of dietary fish oil supplement upon the content of dihomo-gammalinolenic acid in human plasma phospholipids. *Prostaglandins Leukot Essent Fatty Acids*. 1990;40:9-12.

210. Adam O, Wolfram G, Zöllner N. Effect of alpha-linolenic acid in the human diet on linoleic acid metabolism and prostaglandin biosynthesis. *J Lipid Res*. 1986;27:421-426.

211. Wagner W, Nootbaar-Wagner U. Prophylactic treatment of migraine with gamma-linolenic and alpha-linolenic acids. *Cephalalgia*. 1997;17:127-130.

212. Belch JJ, Ansell D, Madhok R, O'Dowd A, Sturrock RD. Effects of altering dietary essential fatty acids on requirements for non-steroidal anti-inflammatory drugs in patients with rheumatoid arthritis: a double blind placebo controlled study. *Ann Rheum Dis*. 1988;47:96-104.

213. Berbert AA, Kondo CR, Almendra CL, Matsuo T, Dichi I. Supplementation of fish oil and olive oil in patients with rheumatoid arthritis. *Nutrition*. 2005;21:131-136.

214. Remans PH, Sont JK, Wagenaar LW, et al. Nutrient supplementation with polyunsaturated fatty acids and micronutrients in rheumatoid arthritis: clinical and biochemical effects. *Eur J Clin Nutr*. 2004;58:839-845.

215. Fletcher RH, Fairfield KM. Vitamins for chronic disease prevention in adults: clinical applications. *JAMA*. 2002;287:3127-3129.

216. Heaney RP. Long-latency deficiency disease: insights from calcium and vitamin D. *Am J Clin Nutr*. 2003;78:912-919.

217. Ames BN. Low micronutrient intake may accelerate the degenerative diseases of aging through allocation of scarce micronutrients by triage. *Proc Natl Acad Sci U S A*. 2006;103:17589-17594.

218. Ames BN, Elson-Schwab I, Silver EA. High-dose vitamin therapy stimulates variant enzymes with decreased coenzyme binding affinity (increased K(m)): relevance to genetic disease and polymorphisms. Am J Clin Nutr. 2002 Apr;75(4):616-58

219. Heaney RP, Davies KM, Chen TC, Holick MF, Barger-Lux MJ. Human serum 25-hydroxycholecalciferol response to extended oral dosing with cholecalciferol. *Am J Clin Nutr*. 2003;77:204-210.

220. Holick MF. Vitamin D deficiency: what a pain it is. *Mayo Clin Proc*. 2003;78:1457-1459.

221. Timms PM, Mannan N, Hitman GA, et al. Circulating MMP9, vitamin D and variation in the TIMP-1 response with VDR genotype: mechanisms for inflammatory damage in chronic disorders? *QJM*. 2002;95:787-796.

222. Lansdowne AT, Provost SC. Vitamin D3 enhances mood in healthy subjects during winter. *Psychopharmacology (Berl)*. 1998;135:319-323.

223. Vieth R, Kimball S, Hu A, Walfish PG. Randomized comparison of the effects of the vitamin D3 adequate intake versus 100 mcg (4000 IU) per day on biochemical responses and the wellbeing of patients. *Nutr J*. 2004;3:8.

224. Masood H, Narang AP, Bhat IA, Shah GN. Persistent limb pain and raised serum alkaline phosphatase the earliest markers of subclinical hypovitaminosis D in Kashmir. *Indian J Physiol Pharmacol*. 1989;33:259-261.

225. Heath KM, Elovic EP. Vitamin D deficiency: implications in the rehabilitation setting. *Am J Phys Med Rehabil*. 2006;85:916-923.

226. Plotnikoff GA, Quigley JM. Prevalence of severe hypovitaminosis D in patients with persistent, nonspecific musculoskeletal pain. *Mayo Clin Proc*. 2003;78:1463-1470.

227. Lotfi A, Abdel-Nasser AM, Hamdy A, Omran AA, El-Rehany MA. Hypovitaminosis D in female patients with chronic low back pain. *Clin Rheumatol*. 2007;26:1895-1901.

228. Vieth R. Vitamin D supplementation, 25-hydroxyvitamin D concentrations, and safety. *Am J Clin Nutr*. 1999;69:842-856.

229. Hypponen E, Laara E, Reunanen A, Jarvelin MR, Virtanen SM. Intake of vitamin D and risk of type 1 diabetes: a birth-cohort study. *Lancet*. 2001;358(9292):1500-1503.

230. Schoenen J, Jacquy J, Lenaerts M. Effectiveness of high-dose riboflavin in migraine prophylaxis. A randomized controlled trial. *Neurology* 1998;50:466-470.

231. Schoenen J, Lenaerts M, Bastings E. High-dose riboflavin as a prophylactic treatment of migraine: results of an open pilot study. *Cephalalgia*. 1994;14:328-329.

232. Boehnke C, Reuter U, Flach U, Schuh-Hofer S, Einhäupl KM, Arnold G. High-dose riboflavin treatment is efficacious in migraine prophylaxis: an open study in a tertiary care centre. *Eur J Neurol*. 2004;11:475-477.

233. Sándor PS, Afra J, Ambrosini A, Schoenen J. Prophylactic treatment of migraine with beta-blockers and riboflavin: differential effects on the intensity dependence of auditory evoked cortical potentials. *Headache*. 2000;40:30-35.

234. Folkers K, Wolaniuk A, Vadhanavikit S. Enzymology of the response of the carpal tunnel syndrome to riboflavin and to combined riboflavin and pyridoxine. *Proc Natl Acad Sci U S A*. 1984;81:7076-7078.

235. Ellis JM. Treatment of carpal tunnel syndrome with vitamin B6. *South Med J*. 1987;80:882-884.

236. Beers MH, Berkow R, eds. *The Merck Manual of Diagnosis and Therapy*. 17th ed. Whitehouse Station: Merck Research Laboratories; 1999: 492

237. Ellis JM, Folkers K, Levy M, et al. Response of vitamin B-6 deficiency and the carpal tunnel syndrome to pyridoxine. *Proc Natl Acad Sci U S A*. 1982;79:7494-7498.

238. Folkers K, Ellis J, Watanabe T, Saji S, Kaji M. Biochemical evidence for a deficiency of vitamin B6 in the carpal tunnel syndrome based on a crossover clinical study. *Proc Natl Acad Sci U S A*. 1978;75:3410-3412.

239. Sarchielli P, Di Filippo M, Nardi K, Calabresi P. Sensitization, glutamate, and the link between migraine and fibromyalgia. *Curr Pain Headache Rep*. 2007;11:343-351.

240. Abraham GE. Nutritional factors in the etiology of the premenstrual tension syndromes. *J Reprod Med*. 1983;28:446-464.

241. Kelly A, Stanley CA. Disorders of glutamate metabolism. *Ment Retard Dev Disabil Res Rev*. 2001;7:287-295.

242. Rader JI, Calvert RJ, Hathcock JN. Hepatic toxicity of unmodified and time-release preparations of niacin. *Am J Med*. 1992;92:77-81.

243. Kaufman W. Niacinamide therapy for joint mobility; therapeutic reversal of a common clinical manifestation of the normal aging process. *Conn Med*. 1953;17:584-589.

244. Kaufman W. The use of vitamin therapy to reverse certain concomitants of aging. *J Am Geriatr Soc*. 1955;3:927-936.

245. Matuoka K, Chen KY, Takenawa T. Rapid reversion of aging phenotypes by nicotinamide through possible modulation of histone acetylation. *Cell Mol Life Sci*. 2001;58:2108-2116.

246. McCarty MF, Russell AL. Niacinamide therapy for osteoarthritis: does it inhibit nitric oxide synthase induction by interleukin 1 in chondrocytes? *Med Hypotheses*. 1999;53:350-360.

247. Jonas WB, Rapoza CP, Blair WF. The effect of niacinamide on osteoarthritis: a pilot study. *Inflamm Res*. 1996;45:330-334.

248. Gaby AR, Wright JV. *Nutritional Therapy in Medical Practice. Reference Manual and Study Guide*. 1996 ed. Wright/Gaby Seminars; 1996: 102.

249. Velling DA, Dodick DW, Muir JJ. Sustained-release niacin for prevention of migraine headache. *Mayo Clin Proc*. 2003;78:770-771.

250. Prousky J, Seely D. The treatment of migraines and tension-type headaches with intravenous and oral niacin (nicotinic acid): systematic review of the literature. *Nutr J*. 2005;4:3.

251. Solomon LR. Cobalamin-responsive disorders in the ambulatory care setting: unreliability of cobalamin, methylmalonic acid, and homocysteine testing. *Blood*. 2005;105:978-985.

252. Freeman AG. Cyanocobalamin-a case for withdrawal: discussion paper. *J R Soc Med*. 1992;85:686-687.

253. Sun Y, Lai MS, Lu CJ. Effectiveness of vitamin B12 on diabetic neuropathy: systematic review of clinical controlled trials. *Acta Neurol Taiwan*. 2005;14:48-54.

254. Kuwabara S, Nakazawa R, Azuma N, et al. Intravenous methylcobalamin treatment for uremic and diabetic neuropathy in chronic hemodialysis patients. *Intern Med*. 1999;38:472-475.

255. van der Kuy PH, Merkus FW, Lohman JJ, ter Berg JW, Hooymans PM. Hydroxocobalamin, a nitric oxide scavenger, in the prophylaxis of migraine: an open, pilot study. *Cephalalgia*. 2002;22:513-519.

256. Mauro GL, Martorana U, Cataldo P, Brancato G, Letizia G. Vitamin B12 in low back pain: a randomised, double-blind, placebo-controlled study. *Eur Rev Med Pharmacol Sci*. 2000;4:53-58.

257. Kaltenbach G, Noblet-Dick M, Barnier-Figue G, Berthel M, Kuntzmann F, Andres E. Early normalization of low vitamin B12 levels by oral cobalamin therapy in three older patients with pernicious anemia. *J Am Geriatr Soc*. 2002;50:1914-1915.

258. Butler CC, Vidal-Alaball J, Cannings-John R, et al. Oral vitamin B12 versus intramuscular vitamin B12 for vitamin B12 deficiency: a systematic review of randomized controlled trials. *Fam Pract*. 2006;23:279-285.

259. Hyman M, Pizzorno J, Weil A. A rational approach to antioxidant therapy and vitamin E. *Altern Ther Health Med*. 2005;11:14-17.

260. Neustadt J, Pizzorno J. Vitamin E and all-cause mortality. *Integrative Med*. 2005;4:14-17.

261. Devaraj S, Tang R, Adams-Huet B, et al. Effect of high-dose alpha-tocopherol supplementation on biomarkers of oxidative stress and inflammation and carotid atherosclerosis in patients with coronary artery disease. *Am J Clin Nutr*. 2007;86:1392-1398.

262. Sutherland WH, Manning PJ, Walker RJ, de Jong SA, Ryalls AR, Berry EA. Vitamin E supplementation and plasma 8-isoprostane and adiponectin in overweight subjects. *Obesity (Silver Spring)*. 2007;15:386-391.

263. Zingg JM, Azzi A. Non-antioxidant activities of vitamin E. *Curr Med Chem*. 2004;11:1113-1133.

264. Jiang Q, Christen S, Shigenaga MK, Ames BN. Gamma-tocopherol, the major form of vitamin E in the US diet, deserves more attention. *Am J Clin Nutr*. 2001;74:714-722.

265. Brigelius-Flohé R. Vitamin E and drug metabolism. *Biochem Biophys Res Commun*. 2003;305:737-740.

266. Landes N, Pfluger P, Kluth D, et al. Vitamin E activates gene expression via the pregnane X receptor. *Biochem Pharmacol*. 2003;65:269-273.

267. Azzi A, Gysin R, Kempná P, et al. Regulation of gene expression by alpha-tocopherol. *Biol Chem*. 2004;385:585-591.

268. Ayres S Jr, Mihan R. Is vitamin E involved in the autoimmune mechanism? *Cutis*. 1978;21:321-325

269. Edmonds SE, Winyard PG, Guo R, et al. Putative analgesic activity of repeated oral doses of vitamin E in the treatment of rheumatoid arthritis. Results of a prospective placebo controlled double blind trial. *Ann Rheum Dis*. 1997;56:649-655.

270. Helmy M, Shohayeb M, Helmy MH, el-Bassiouni EA. Antioxidants as adjuvant therapy in rheumatoid disease. A preliminary study. *Arzneimittelforschung*. 2001;51:293-298.

271. Machtey I, Ouaknine L. Tocopherol in osteoarthritis: a controlled pilot study. *J Am Geriatr Soc*. 1978;26:328-330,

272. Brand C, Snaddon J, Bailey M, Cicuttini F. Vitamin E is ineffective for symptomatic relief of knee osteoarthritis: a six month double blind, randomised, placebo controlled study. *Ann Rheum Dis*. 2001;60:946-949.

273. Yell JA, Burge S, Wojnarowska F. Vitamin E and discoid lupus erythematosus. *Lupus*. 1992;1:303-305.

274. Ayres S Jr, Mihan R. Lupus erythematosus and vitamin E: an effective and nontoxic therapy. *Cutis*. 1979;23:49-52, 54.

275. Roca AO, Jarjoura D, Blend D, et al. Dialysis leg cramps. Efficacy of quinine versus vitamin E. *ASAIO J*. 1992;38:M481-485.

276. Meydani M. Vitamin E. *Lancet*. 1995;345(8943):170-175.

277. Innerarity S. Hypomagnesemia in acute and chronic illness. *Crit Care Nurs Q*. 2000;23:1-19.

278. Fox CH, Ramsoomair D, Mahoney MC, Carter C, Young B, Graham R. An investigation of hypomagnesemia among ambulatory urban African Americans. *J Fam Pract*. 1999;48(8):636-639.

279. Schimatschek HF, Rempis R. Prevalence of hypomagnesemia in an unselected German population of 16,000 individuals. *Magnes Res*. 2001;14:283-290.

280. Frankel H, Haskell R, Lee SY, Miller D, Rotondo M, Schwab CW. Hypomagnesemia in trauma patients. *World J Surg*. 1999;23:966-969.

281. Mishima K, Takeshima T, Shimomura T, et al. Platelet ionized magnesium, cyclic AMP, and cyclic GMP levels in migraine and tension-type headache. *Headache*. 1997;37:561-564.

282. Mauskop A, Altura BT, Altura BM. Serum ionized magnesium levels and serum ionized calcium/ionized magnesium ratios in women with menstrual migraine. *Headache*. 2002;42:242-248.

283. Marcus JC, Altura BT, Altura BM. Serum ionized magnesium in post-traumatic headaches. *J Pediatr*. 2001;139:459-462.

284. Boska MD, Welch KM, Barker PB, Nelson JA, Schultz L. Contrasts in cortical magnesium, phospholipid and energy metabolism between migraine syndromes. *Neurology*. 2002;58:1227-1233.

285. Peikert A, Wilimzig C, Kohne-Volland R. Prophylaxis of migraine with oral magnesium: results from a prospective, multi-center, placebo-controlled and double-blind randomized study. *Cephalalgia*. 1996;16:257-263.

286. Wang F, Van Den Eeden SK, Ackerson LM, Salk SE, Reince RH, Elin RJ. Oral magnesium oxide prophylaxis of frequent migrainous headache in children: a randomized, double-blind, placebo-controlled trial. *Headache*. 2003;43:601-610.

287. Mauskop A, Altura BT, Cracco RQ, Altura BM. Intravenous magnesium sulfate rapidly alleviates headaches of various types. *Headache* 1996;36:154-160.

288. De Leeuw I, Engelen W, De Block C, Van Gaal L. Long term magnesium supplementation influences favourably the natural evolution of neuropathy in Mg-depleted type 1 diabetic patients (T1dm). *Magnes Res*. 2004;17:109-114.

289. Rozen TD, Oshinsky ML, Gebeline CA, et al. Open label trial of coenzyme Q10 as a migraine preventive. *Cephalalgia*. 2002;22:137-141.

290. Hershey AD, Powers SW, Vockell AL, et al. Coenzyme Q10 deficiency and response to supplementation in pediatric and adolescent migraine. *Headache*. 2007;47:73-80.

291. Sándor PS, Di Clemente L, Coppola G, et al. Efficacy of coenzyme Q10 in migraine prophylaxis: a randomized controlled trial. *Neurology*. 2005;64:713-715.

292. Caso G, Kelly P, McNurlan MA, Lawson WE. Effect of coenzyme q10 on myopathic symptoms in patients treated with statins. *Am J Cardiol*. 2007;99:1409-1412.

293. Ye CQ, Folkers K, Tamagawa H, Pfeiffer C. A modified determination of coenzyme Q10 in human blood and CoQ10 blood levels in diverse patients with allergies. *Biofactors*. 1988;1:303-306.

294. Folkers K, Hanioka T, Xia LJ, McRee JT Jr, Langsjoen P. Coenzyme Q10 increases T4/T8 ratios of lymphocytes in ordinary subjects and relevance to patients having the AIDS related complex. *Biochem Biophys Res Commun*. 1991;176:786-791.

295. Gazdík F, Gvozdjáková A, Nádvorníková R, et al. Decreased levels of coenzyme Q(10) in patients with bronchial asthma. *Allergy*. 2002;57:811-814.

296. Gvozdjáková A, Kucharská J, Bartkovjaková M, Gazdíková K, Gazdík FE. Coenzyme Q10 supplementation reduces corticosteroids dosage in patients with bronchial asthma. *Biofactors*. 2005;25(1-4):235-240.

297. Birdsall TC. 5-Hydroxytryptophan: a clinically-effective serotonin precursor. *Altern Med Rev*. 1998;3:271-280.

298. Genazzani AR, Sandrini G, Facchinetti F, et al. Effects of L-5HTP with and without carbidopa on plasma beta-endorphin and pain perception. Possible implications in migraine prophylaxis. *Cephalalgia*. 1986;6:241-245.

299. Sarzi Puttini P, Caruso I. Primary fibromyalgia syndrome and 5-hydroxy-L-tryptophan: a 90-day open study. *J Int Med Res*. 1992;20:182-189.

300. Caruso I, Sarzi Puttini P, Cazzola M, Azzolini V. Double-blind study of 5-hydroxytryptophan versus placebo in the treatment of primary fibromyalgia syndrome. *J Int Med Res*. 1990;18:201-209.

301. Titus F, Davalos A, Alom J, Codina A. 5-Hydroxytryptophan versus methysergide in the prophylaxis of migraine. Randomized clinical trial. *Eur Neurol*.1986;25:327-329.

302. Ribeiro CA. L-5-Hydroxytryptophan in the prophylaxis of chronic tension-type headache: a double-blind, randomized, placebo-controlled study. For the Portuguese Head Society. *Headache*. 2000;40:451-456.

303. De Benedittis G, Massei R. Serotonin precursors in chronic primary headache. A double-blind cross-over study with L-5-hydroxytryptophan vs. placebo. *J Neurosurg Sci*. 1985;29:239-248.

304. Russell AL, McCarty MF. DL-phenylalanine markedly potentiates opiate analgesia - an example of nutrient/pharmaceutical up-regulation of the endogenous analgesia system. *Med Hypotheses*. 2000;55:283-288.

305. Battistella PA, Bordin A, Cernetti R, et al. beta-endorphin in plasma and monocytes in juvenile headache. *Headache*. 1996;36:91-94.

306. Ehrenpreis S. D-phenylalanine and other enkephalinase inhibitors as pharmacological agents: implications for some important therapeutic application. *Acupunct Electrother Res*. 1982;7(2-3):157-172.

307. Ehrenpreis S. Pharmacology of enkephalinase inhibitors: animal and human studies. *Acupunct Electrother Res*. 1985;10:203-208.

308. Kitade T, Odahara Y, Shinohara S, et al. Studies on the enhanced effect of acupuncture analgesia and acupuncture anesthesia by D-phenylalanine (2nd report): schedule of administration and clinical effects in low back pain and tooth extraction. *Acupunct Electrother Res*. 1990;15:121-135.

309. Curran JN, Winter DC, Bouchier-Hayes D. Biological fate and clinical implications of arginine metabolism in tissue healing. *Wound Repair Regen*. 2006;14:376-386.

310. Witte MB, Barbul A. Arginine physiology and its implication for wound healing. *Wound Repair Regen*. 2003;11:419-423.

311. Kirk SJ, Hurson M, Regan MC, Holt DR, Wasserkrug HL, Barbul A. Arginine stimulates wound healing and immune function in elderly human beings. *Surgery*. 1993;114:155-159.

312. Barbul A, Lazarou SA, Efron DT, Wasserkrug HL, Efron G. Arginine enhances wound healing and lymphocyte immune responses in humans. *Surgery*. 1990;108:331-336.

313. Desneves KJ, Todorovic BE, Cassar A, Crowe TC. Treatment with supplementary arginine, vitamin C and zinc in patients with pressure ulcers: a randomised controlled trial. *Clin Nutr*. 2005;24:979-987.

314. Mischoulon D, Fava M. Role of S-adenosyl-L-methionine in the treatment of depression: a review of the evidence. *Am J Clin Nutr*. 2002;76:1158S-1161S.

315. Harmand MF, Vilamitjana J, Maloche E, Duphil R, Ducassou D. Effects of S-adenosylmethionine on human articular chondrocyte differentiation. An in vitro study. *Am J Med*. 1987;83(5A):48-54.

316. Barceló HA, Wiemeyer JC, Sagasta CL, Macias M, Barreira JC. Effect of S-adenosylmethionine on experimental osteoarthritis in rabbits. *Am J Med*. 1987;83(5A):55-59.

317. Vetter G. Double-blind comparative clinical trial with S-adenosylmethionine and indomethacin in the treatment of osteoarthritis. *Am J Med*. 1987;83(5A):78-80.

318. Maccagno A, Di Giorgio EE, Caston OL, Sagasta CL. Double-blind controlled clinical trial of oral S-adenosylmethionine versus piroxicam in knee osteoarthritis. *Am J Med*. 1987;83(5A):72-77.

319. König B. A long-term (two years) clinical trial with S-adenosylmethionine for the treatment of osteoarthritis. *Am J Med*. 1987;83(5A):89-94.

320. Volkmann H, Nørregaard J, Jacobsen S, Danneskiold-Samsøe B, Knoke G, Nehrdich D. Double-blind, placebo-controlled cross-over study of intravenous S-adenosyl-L-methionine in patients with fibromyalgia. *Scand J Rheumatol*. 1997;26:206-211.

321. Jacobsen S, Danneskiold-Samsøe B, Andersen RB. Oral S-adenosylmethionine in primary fibromyalgia. Double-blind clinical evaluation. *Scand J Rheumatol*. 1991;20:294-302.

322. Tavoni A, Vitali C, Bombardieri S, Pasero G. Evaluation of S-adenosylmethionine in primary fibromyalgia. A double-blind crossover study. *Am J Med*. 1987;83(5A):107-110.

323. Gatto G, Caleri D, Michelacci S, Sicuteri F. Analgesizing effect of a methyl donor (S-adenosylmethionine) in migraine: an open clinical trial. *Int J Clin Pharmacol Res*. 1986;6:15-17.

324. Mischoulon D, Fava M. Role of S-adenosyl-L-methionine in the treatment of depression: a review of the evidence. *Am J Clin Nutr*. 2002;76:1158S-1161S.

325. Lawrence JR, Peter R, Baxter GJ, Robson J, Graham AB, Paterson JR. Urinary excretion of salicyluric and salicylic acids by non-vegetarians, vegetarians, and patients taking low dose aspirin. *J Clin Pathol.* 2003;56:651-653.
326. Paterson JR, Lawrence JR. Salicylic acid: a link between aspirin, diet and the prevention of colorectal cancer. *QJM.* 2001;94:445-448.
327. Hare LG, Woodside JV, Young IS. Dietary salicylates. *J Clin Pathol.* 2003;56:649-650.
328. Clauson KA, Santamarina ML, Buettner CM, Cauffield JS. Evaluation of presence of aspirin-related warnings with willow bark. *Ann Pharmacother.* 2005;39:1234-1237.
329. Vasquez A, Muanza DN. Comment: Evaluation of presence of aspirin-related warnings with willow bark. *Ann Pharmacotherapy.* 2005;39:1763.
330. Boullata JI, McDonnell PJ, Oliva CD. Anaphylactic reaction to a dietary supplement containing willow bark. *Ann Pharmacother.* 2003;37:832-835.
331. Nahrstedt A, Schmidt M, Jäggi R, Metz J, Khayyal MT. Willow bark extract: the contribution of polyphenols to the overall effect. *Wien Med Wochenschr.* 2007;157:348-351.
332. Chrubasik S, Eisenberg E, Balan E, Weinberger T, Luzzati R, Conradt C. Treatment of low-back pain exacerbations with willow bark extract: a randomized double-blind study. *Am J Med.* 2000;109:9-14.
333. Chrubasik S, Kunzel O, Model A, Conradt C, Black A. Treatment of low-back pain with a herbal or synthetic anti-rheumatic: a randomized controlled study. Willow bark extract for low-back pain. *Rheumatology* (Oxford). 2001;40:1388-1393.
334. Safayhi H, Mack T, Sabieraj J, Anazodo MI, Subramanian LR, Ammon HP. Boswellic acids: novel, specific, nonredox inhibitors of 5-lipoxygenase. *J Pharmacol Exp Ther.* 1992;261:1143-1146.
335. Takada Y, Ichikawa H, Badmaev V, Aggarwal BB. Acetyl-11-keto-beta-boswellic acid potentiates apoptosis, inhibits invasion, and abolishes osteoclastogenesis by suppressing NF-kappa B and NF-kappa B-regulated gene expression. *J Immunol.* 2006;176:3127-3140.
336. Cuaz-Pérolin C, Billiet L, Baugé E, et al. Antiinflammatory and antiatherogenic effects of the NF-{kappa}B inhibitor acetyl-11-keto-{beta}-boswellic acid in LPS-challenged ApoE-/- mice. *Arterioscler Thromb Vasc Biol.* 2008;28:272-277.
337. Kimmatkar N, Thawani V, Hingorani L, Khiyani R. Efficacy and tolerability of Boswellia serrata extract in treatment of osteoarthritis of knee: a randomized double blind placebo controlled trial. *Phytomedicine.* 2003;10:3-7.
338. Gupta I, Parihar A, Malhotra P, et al. Effects of Boswellia serrata gum resin in patients with ulcerative colitis. *Eur J Med Res.* 1997;2:37-43.
339. Gupta I, Parihar A, Malhotra P, et al. Effects of gum resin of Boswellia serrata in patients with chronic colitis. *Planta Med.* 2001;67:391-395.
340. Moussaieff A, Shohami E, Kashman Y, et al. Incensole acetate, a novel anti-inflammatory compound isolated from Boswellia resin, inhibits nuclear factor-kappa B activation. *Mol Pharmacol.* 2007;72:1657-1664.
341. Shin MC, Chang HK, Jan MH, Kim CJ, Kim Y, Kim EH. Modulation of Harpagophytum procumbens on ion channels in acutely dissociated periaquideuctal gray neurons of rats. *Korean Journal of Meridian and Acupoint.* 2003;20;17-29.
342. Huang TH, Tran VH, Duke RK, et al. Harpagoside suppresses lipopolysaccharide-induced iNOS and COX-2 expression through inhibition of ^{NF}-kappa B activation. *J Ethnopharmacol.* 2006;104(1-2):149-155.
343. Moussard C, Alber D, Toubin MM, Thevenon N, Henry JC. A drug used in traditional medicine, harpagophytum procumbens: no evidence for NSAID-like effect on whole blood eicosanoid production in human. *Prostaglandins Leukot Essent Fatty Acids.* 1992;46:283-286.
344. Chrubasik S, Thanner J, Kunzel O, Conradt C, Black A, Pollak S. Comparison of outcome measures during treatment with the proprietary Harpagophytum extract doloteffin in patients with pain in the lower back, knee or hip. *Phytomedicine.* 2002;9:181-194.
345. Chantre P, Cappelaere A, Leblan D, Guedon D, Vandermander J, Fournie B. Efficacy and tolerance of Harpagophytum procumbens versus diacerhein in treatment of osteoarthritis. *Phytomedicine.* 2000;7:177-183.
346. Chrubasik S, Model A, Black A, Pollak S. A randomized double-blind pilot study comparing Doloteffin and Vioxx in the treatment of low back pain. *Rheumatology* (Oxford). 2003;42:141-148.
347. Chrubasik S, Junck H, Breitschwerdt H, Conradt C, Zappe H. Effectiveness of Harpagophytum extract WS 1531 in the treatment of exacerbation of low back pain: a randomized, placebo-controlled, double-blind study. *Eur J Anaesthesiol.* 1999;16:118-129.
348. Brien S, Lewith GT, McGregor G. Devil's Claw (Harpagophytum procumbens) as a treatment for osteoarthritis: a review of efficacy and safety. *J Altern Complement Med.* 2006;12:981-993.
349. Lanhers MC, Fleurentin J, Mortier F, Vinche A, Younos C. Anti-inflammatory and analgesic effects of an aqueous extract of Harpagophytum procumbens. *Planta Med.* 1992;58:117-123.
350. Srivastava KC, Mustafa T. Ginger (Zingiber officinale) in rheumatism and musculoskeletal disorders. *Med Hypotheses.* 1992;39:342-348.
351. Srivastava KC, Mustafa T. Ginger (Zingiber officinale) and rheumatic disorders. *Med Hypotheses.* 1989;29:25-28.
352. Altman RD, Marcussen KC. Effects of a ginger extract on knee pain in patients with osteoarthritis. *Arthritis Rheum.* 2001;44:2531-2538.
353. Bliddal H, Rosetzsky A, Schlichting P, e tal. A randomized, placebo-controlled, cross-over study of ginger extracts and ibuprofen in osteoarthritis. *Osteoarthritis Cartilage.* 2000;8:9-12.
354. Vutyavanich T, Kraisarin T, Ruangsri R. Ginger for nausea and vomiting in pregnancy: randomized, double-masked, placebo-controlled trial. *Obstet Gynecol.* 2001;97:577-582.
355. Sheehan P. Hyperemesis gravidarum: assessment and management. *Aust Fam Physician.* 2007;36:698-701.
356. Hardin SR. Cat's claw: an Amazonian vine decreases inflammation in osteoarthritis. *Complement Ther Clin Pract.* 2007;13:25-28.
357. Piscoya J, Rodriguez Z, Bustamante SA, Okuhama NN, Miller MJ, Sandoval M.Efficacy and safety of freeze-dried cat's claw in osteoarthritis of the knee: mechanisms of action of the species Uncaria guianensis. *Inflamm Res.* 2001;50:442-448.
358. Mur E, Hartig F, Eibl G, Schirmer M. Randomized double blind trial of an extract from the pentacyclic alkaloid-chemotype of uncaria tomentosa for the treatment of rheumatoid arthritis. *J Rheumatol.* 2002;29:678-681.
359. McCleane G. Topical application of doxepin hydrochloride, capsaicin and a combination of both produces analgesia in chronic human neuropathic pain: a randomized, double-blind, placebo-controlled study. *Br J Clin Pharmacol.* 2000;49:574-579.
360. Biesbroeck R, Bril V, Hollander P, et al. A double-blind comparison of topical capsaicin and oral amitriptyline in painful diabetic neuropathy. *Adv Ther.* 1995;12:111-120.
361. Robbins WR, Staats PS, Levine J, et al. Treatment of intractable pain with topical large-dose capsaicin: preliminary report. *Anesth Analg.* 1998;86:579-583.
362. Kim KS, Kim DW, Yu YK. The effect of capsicum plaster in pain after inguinal hernia repair in children. *Paediatr Anaesth.* 2006;16:1036-1041.
363. Kim KS, Nam YM. The analgesic effects of capsicum plaster at the Zusanli point after abdominal hysterectomy. *Anesth Analg.* 2006;103:709-713.
364. Frerick H, Keitel W, Kuhn U, Schmidt S, Bredehorst A, Kuhlmann M. Topical treatment of chronic low back pain with a capsicum plaster. *Pain.* 2003;106(1-2):59-64.

365. Marks DR, Rapoport A, Padla D, et al. A double-blind placebo-controlled trial of intranasal capsaicin for cluster headache. *Cephalalgia*. 1993;13:114-116.

366. Fusco BM, Barzoi G, Agrò F. Repeated intranasal capsaicin applications to treat chronic migraine. *Br J Anaesth*. 2003;90:812.

367. Stiles JC, Sparks W, Ronzio RA. The inhibition of Candida albicans by oregano. *J Applied Nutr*. 1995;47:96-102.

368. Force M, Sparks WS, Ronzio RA. Inhibition of enteric parasites by emulsified oil of oregano in vivo. *Phytother Res*. 2000;14:213-214.

369. Berberine. *Altern Med Rev*. 2000;5:175-177.

370. Kong W, Wei J, Abidi P, et al. Berberine is a novel cholesterol-lowering drug working through a unique mechanism distinct from statins. *Nat Med*. 2004;10:1344-1351.

371. Gulliver WP, Donsky HJ. A report on three recent clinical trials using Mahonia aquifolium 10% topical cream and a review of the worldwide clinical experience with Mahonia aquifolium for the treatment of plaque psoriasis. *Am J Ther*. 2005;12:398-406.

372. Dien TK, de Vries PJ, Khanh NX, et al. Effect of food intake on pharmacokinetics of oral artemisinin in healthy Vietnamese subjects. *Antimicrob Agents Chemother*. 1997;41:1069-1072.

373. Gordi T, Huong DX, Hai TN, Nieu NT, Ashton M. Artemisinin pharmacokinetics and efficacy in uncomplicated-malaria patients treated with two different dosage regimens. *Antimicrob Agents Chemother*. 2002;46:1026-1031.

374. Giao PT, Binh TQ, Kager PA, et al. Artemisinin for treatment of uncomplicated falciparum malaria: is there a place for monotherapy? *Am J Trop Med Hyg*. 2001;65:690-695.

375. Karunajeewa HA, Manning L, Mueller I, Ilett KF, Davis TM. Rectal administration of artemisinin derivatives for the treatment of malaria. *JAMA*. 2007;297:2381-2390.

376. Lynch DM. Cranberry for prevention of urinary tract infections. *Am Fam Physician*. 2004;70:2175-2177.

377. Ebringer A, Rashid T. Rheumatoid arthritis is an autoimmune disease triggered by Proteus urinary tract infection. *Clin Dev Immunol*. 2006;13:41-48.

378. Ebringer A, Rashid T, Wilson C. Rheumatoid arthritis: proposal for the use of anti-microbial therapy in early cases. *Scand J Rheumatol*. 2003;32:2-11.

379. El Baz MA, Morsy TA, El Bandary MM, Motawea SM. Clinical and parasitological studies on the efficacy of Mirazid in treatment of schistosomiasis haematobium in Tatoon, Etsa Center, El Fayoum Governorate. *J Egypt Soc Parasitol*. 2003;33:761-776.

380. Abo-Madyan AA, Morsy TA, Motawea SM. Efficacy of Myrrh in the treatment of schistosomiasis (haematobium and mansoni) in Ezbet El-Bakly, Tamyia Center, El-Fayoum Governorate, Egypt. *J Egypt Soc Parasitol*. 2004;34:423-446.

381. Yarnell E. Botanical medicines for the urinary tract. *World J Urol*. 2002;20:285-293.

382. Wang L, Del Priore LV. Bull's-eye maculopathy secondary to herbal toxicity from uva ursi. *Am J Ophthalmol*. 2004;137:1135-1137.

383. Saxena VN, Dogra J. Long-term use of penicillin for the treatment of chronic plaque psoriasis. *Eur J Dermatol*. 2005;15:359-362.

384. Simanek V, Kren V, Ulrichova J, Gallo J. The efficacy of glucosamine and chondroitin sulfate in the treatment of osteoarthritis: are these saccharaides drugs or nutraceuticals? *Biomed Papers*. 2005;149:51-56.

385. Morrison LM. Treatment of coronary arteriosclerotic heart disease with chondroitin sulfate A: preliminary report. *J Am Geriatr Soc*. 1968;16:779-785.

386. Morrison LM, Branwood AW, Ershoff BH, et al. The prevention of coronary arteriosclerotic heart disease with chondroitin sulfate A: preliminary report. *Exp Med Surg*. 1969;27:278-289.

387. Morrison LM, Bajwa GS. Absence of naturally occurring coronary atherosclerosis in squirrel monkeys (Saimiri sciurea) treated with chondroitin sulfate A. *Experientia*. 1972;28:1410-1411.

388. Morrison LM, Enrick N. Coronary heart disease: reduction of death rate by chondroitin sulfate A. *Angiology*. 1973;24:269-287.

389. Adams ME. Hype about glucosamine. *Lancet*. 1999;354(9176):353-354.

390. Scroggie DA, Albright A, Harris MD. The effect of glucosamine-chondroitin supplementation on glycosylated hemoglobin levels in patients with type 2 diabetes mellitus: a placebo-controlled, double-blinded, randomized clinical trial. *Arch Intern Med*. 2003;163:1587-1590.

391. Reginster JY, Deroisy R, Rovati LC, et al. Long-term effects of glucosamine sulphate on osteoarthritis progression: a randomised, placebo-controlled clinical trial. *Lancet*. 2001;357(9252):251-256.

392. Tallia AF, Cardone DA. Asthma exacerbation associated with glucosamine-chondroitin supplement. *J Am Board Fam Pract*. 2002;15:481-484.

393. Singh G. Recent considerations in nonsteroidal anti-inflammatory drug gastropathy. *Am J Med*. 1998;105(1B):31S-38S.

394. Ray WA, Griffin MR, Stein CM. Cardiovascular toxicity of valdecoxib. *N Engl J Med*. 2004;351:2767.

395. *FDA Statement on the Halting of a Clinical Trial of the COX-2 Inhibitor Celebrex*. U.S. Food and Drug Administration. December 17, 2004. Available online at: http://www.fda.gov/bbs/topics/news/2004/NEW01144.html.

396. Vlad SC, LaValley MP, McAlindon TE, Felson DT. Glucosamine for pain in osteoarthritis: why do trial results differ? *Arthritis Rheum*. 2007;56:2267-2277.

397. McAlindon TE, LaValley MP, Gulin JP, Felson DT. Glucosamine and chondroitin for treatment of osteoarthritis: a systematic quality assessment and meta-analysis. *JAMA*. 2000;283:1469-1475.

398. Richy F, Bruyere O, Ethgen O, Cucherat M, Henrotin Y, Reginster JY. Structural and symptomatic efficacy of glucosamine and chondroitin in knee osteoarthritis: a comprehensive meta-analysis. *Arch Intern Med*. 2003;163:1514-1522.

399. Reginster JY, Deroisy R, Rovati LC, et al. Long-term effects of glucosamine sulphate on osteoarthritis progression: a randomised, placebo-controlled clinical trial. *Lancet*. 2001;357(9252):251-256.

400. Muller-Fassbender H, Bach GL, Haase W, Rovati LC, Setnikar I. Glucosamine sulfate compared to ibuprofen in osteoarthritis of the knee. *Osteoarthritis Cartilage*. 1994;2:61-69.

401. Pavelka K, Gatterova J, Olejarová M, Machacek S, Giacovelli G, Rovati LC. Glucosamine sulfate use and delay of progression of knee osteoarthritis: a 3-year, randomized, placebo-controlled, double-blind study. *Arch Intern Med*. 2002;162:2113-2123.

402. Bruyere O, Pavelka K, Rovati LC, et al. Glucosamine sulfate reduces osteoarthritis progression in postmenopausal women with knee osteoarthritis: evidence from two 3-year studies. *Menopause*. 2004;11:138-143.

403. Herrero-Beaumont G, Ivorra JA, Del Carmen Trabado M, et al. Glucosamine sulfate in the treatment of knee osteoarthritis symptoms: a randomized, double-blind, placebo-controlled study using acetaminophen as a side comparator. *Arthritis Rheum*. 2007;56:555-567.

404. Mazières B, Hucher M, Zaïm M, Garnero P. Effect of chondroitin sulphate in symptomatic knee osteoarthritis: a multicentre, randomised, double-blind, placebo-controlled study. *Ann Rheum Dis*. 2007;66:639-645.

405. Vlad SC, LaValley MP, McAlindon TE, Felson DT. Glucosamine for pain in osteoarthritis: why do trial results differ? *Arthritis Rheum.* 2007;56:2267-2277.

406. Clegg DO, Reda DJ, Harris CL, et al. Glucosamine, chondroitin sulfate, and the two in combination for painful knee osteoarthritis. *N Engl J Med.* 2006;354:795-808.

407. Vasquez A. *Integrative Orthopedics.* 2nd ed. Fort Worth, Tex: Integrative and Biological Medicine Research and Consulting; 2007.

408. Mehta K, Gala J, Bhasale S, et al. Comparison of glucosamine sulfate and a polyherbal supplement for the relief of osteoarthritis of the knee: a randomized controlled trial [ISRCTN25438351]. *BMC Complement Altern Med.* 2007;7:34.

409. Beard J. The action of trypsin upon the living cells of Jensen's mouse-tumour. *Br Med J.* 1906; 4:140-141.

410. Cutfield A. Trypsin treatment in malignant disease. *Br Med J.* 1907;5:525.

411. Wiggin FH. Case of multiple fibrosarcoma of the tongue, with remarks on the use of trypsin and amylopsin in the treatment of malignant disease. *JAMA.* 1906;47:2003-2008.

412. Goeth RA. Pancreatic treatment of cancer, with report of a cure. *JAMA.* 1907;48:1030.

413. Campbell JT. Trypsin treatment of a case of malignant disease. *JAMA.* 1907;48:225-226.

414. Gotze H, Rothman SS. Enteropancreatic circulation of digestive enzymes as a conservative mechanism. *Nature.* 1975;257(5527):607-609.

415. Liebow C, Rothman SS. Enteropancreatic circulation of digestive enzymes. *Science.* 1975; 189(4201):472-474.

416. Taub SJ. The use of bromelains in sinusitis: a double-blind clinical evaluation. *Eye Ear Nose Throat Mon.* 1967;46:361-365.

417. Trickett P. Proteolytic enzymes in treatment of athletic injuries. *Appl Ther.* 1964;30:647-652.

418. Walker AF, Bundy R, Hicks SM, Middleton RW. Bromelain reduces mild acute knee pain and improves well-being in a dose-dependent fashion in an open study of otherwise healthy adults. *Phytomedicine.* 2002;9:681-686.

419. Brien S, Lewith G, Walker AF, Middleton R, Prescott P, Bundy R. Bromelain as an adjunctive treatment for moderate-to-severe osteoarthritis of the knee: a randomized placebo-controlled pilot study. *QJM.* 2006;99:841-850.

420. Klein G, Kullich W, Schnitker J, Schwann H. Efficacy and tolerance of an oral enzyme combination in painful osteoarthritis of the hip. A double-blind, randomised study comparing oral enzymes with non-steroidal anti-inflammatory drugs. *Clin Exp Rheumatol.* 2006;24:25-30.

421. Akhtar NM, Naseer R, Farooqi AZ, Aziz W, Nazir M. Oral enzyme combination versus diclofenac in the treatment of osteoarthritis of the knee--a double-blind prospective randomized study. *Clin Rheumatol.* 2004;23:410-415.

422. Kerkhoffs GM, Struijs PA, de Wit C, Rahlfs VW, Zwipp H, van Dijk CN. A double blind, randomised, parallel group study on the efficacy and safety of treating acute lateral ankle sprain with oral hydrolytic enzymes. *Br J Sports Med.* 2004;38:431-435.

423. Tilwe GH, Beria S, Turakhia NH, Daftary GV, Schiess W. Efficacy and tolerability of oral enzyme therapy as compared to diclofenac in active osteoarthrosis of knee joint: an open randomized controlled clinical trial. *J Assoc Physicians India.* 2001;49:617-621.

424. Leipner J, Iten F, Saller R. Therapy with proteolytic enzymes in rheumatic disorders. *BioDrugs.* 2001;15:779-789.

425. Brien S, Lewith G, Walker A, Hicks SM, Middleton D. Bromelain as a treatment for osteoarthritis: a review of clinical studies. *Evidence-Based Complementary and Alternative Medicine.* 2004;1:251-257.

426. Leach RA, ed. *The Chiropractic Theories: A Textbook of Scientific Research.* 4th ed. Baltimore, Md: Lippincott, Williams & Wilkins; 2004.

427. Hammer WI. *Functional Soft Tissue Examination and Treatment by Manual Methods.* 3rd ed. Sudbury: Jones & Bartlett Publishers; 2007.

428. Peterson DH, Bergman TF. *Chiropractic Technique.* Mosby; 2002.

429. Maigne JY, Vautravers P. Mechanism of action of spinal manipulative therapy. *Joint Bone Spine.* 2003;70:336-341.

430. Boal RW, Gillette RG. Central neuronal plasticity, low back pain and spinal manipulative therapy. *J Manipulative Physiol Ther.* 2004;27:314-326.

431. Dabbs V, Lauretti WJ. A risk assessment of cervical manipulation vs. NSAIDs for the treatment of neck pain. *J Manipulative Physiol Ther.* 1995;18:530-536.

432. Rosner AL. Evidence-based clinical guidelines for the management of acute low-back pain: response to the guidelines prepared for the Australian Medical Health and Research Council. *J Manipulative Physiol Ther.* 2001;24:214-220.

433. Oliphant D. Safety of spinal manipulation in the treatment of lumbar disk herniations: a systematic review and risk assessment. *J Manipulative Physiol Ther.* 2004;27:197-210.

434. Manga P, Angus DE, Papadopoulos C, Swan WR. *The Effectiveness and Cost-Effectiveness of Chiropractic Management of Low-Back Pain.* Richmond Hill, Ontario: Kenilworth Publishing; 1993.

435. Licciardone JC, Brimhall AK, King LN. Osteopathic manipulative treatment for low back pain: a systematic review and meta-analysis of randomized controlled trials. *BMC Musculoskelet Disord.* 2005;6:43.

436. Meade TW, Dyer S, Browne W, Townsend J, Frank AO. Low-back pain of mechanical origin: randomised comparison of chiropractic and hospital outpatient treatment. *BMJ.* 1990;300(6737):1431-1437.

437. Meade TW, Dyer S, Browne W, Frank AO. Randomised comparison of chiropractic and hospital outpatient management for low-back pain: results from extended follow up. *BMJ.* 1995;311(7001):349-351.

438. Leboeuf-Yde C, Axen I, Ahlefeldt G, Lidefelt P, Rosenbaum A, Thurnherr T. The types and frequencies of improved nonmusculoskeletal symptoms reported after chiropractic spinal manipulative therapy. *J Manipulative Physiol Ther.* 1999;22:559-564.

439. Nielson NH, Bronfort G, Bendix T, Madsen F, Wecke B. Chronic asthma and chiropractic spinal manipulation: a randomized clinical trial. *Clin Exp Allergy.* 1995;25:80-88.

440. Mein EA, Greenman PE, McMillin DL, Richards DG, Nelson CD. Manual medicine diversity: research pitfalls and the emerging medical paradigm. *J Am Osteopath Assoc.* 2001;101:441-444.

441. Balon J, Aker PD, Crowther ER, et al. A comparison of active and simulated chiropractic manipulation as adjunctive treatment for childhood asthma. *N Engl J Med.* 1998;339:1013-1020.

442. Bronfort G, Evans RL, Kubic P, Filkin P. Chronic pediatric asthma and chiropractic spinal manipulation: a prospective clinical series and randomized clinical pilot study. *J Manipulative Physiol Ther.* 2001;24:369-377.

443. Guiney PA, Chou R, Vianna A, Lovenheim J. Effects of osteopathic manipulative treatment on pediatric patients with asthma: a randomized controlled trial. *J Am Osteopath Assoc.* 2005;105:7-12.

444. Stephens D, Pollard H, Bilton D, Thomson P, Gorman F. Bilateral simultaneous optic nerve dysfunction after periorbital trauma: recovery of vision in association with chiropractic spinal manipulation therapy. *J Manipulative Physiol Ther.* 1999;22:615-621.

445. Stephens D, Gorman F, Bilton D. The step phenomenon in the recovery of vision with spinal manipulation: a report on two 13-yr-olds treated together. *J Manipulative Physiol Ther.* 1997;20:628-633.

446. Stephens D, Gorman F. The association between visual incompetence and spinal derangement: an instructive case history. *J Manipulative Physiol Ther*. 1997;20:343-350.

447. Stephens D, Gorman RF. Does 'normal' vision improve with spinal manipulation? *J Manipulative Physiol Ther*. 1996;19:415-418.

448. Gorman RF. Monocular scotomata and spinal manipulation: the step phenomenon. *J Manipulative Physiol Ther*. 1996;19:344-349.

449. Gorman RF. Monocular visual loss after closed head trauma: immediate resolution associated with spinal manipulation. *J Manipulative Physiol Ther*. 1995;18:308-314.

450. Gorman RF. The treatment of presumptive optic nerve ischemia by spinal manipulation. *J Manipulative Physiol Ther*. 1995;18:172-177.

451. Gorman RF. Automated static perimetry in chiropractic. *J Manipulative Physiol Ther*. 1993;16:481-487.

452. Elster EL. Treatment of bipolar, seizure, and sleep disorders and migraine headaches utilizing a chiropractic technique. *J Manipulative Physiol* Ther. 2004;27:E5.

453. Alcantara J, Heschong R, Plaugher G, Alcantara J. Chiropractic management of a patient with subluxations, low-back pain and epileptic seizures. *J Manipulative Physiol Ther*. 1998;21:410-418.

454. Giesen JM, Center DB, Leach RA. An evaluation of chiropractic manipulation as a treatment of hyperactivity in children. *J Manipulative Physiol Ther*. 1989;12:353-363.

455. Bastecki AV, Harrison DE, Haas JW. Cervical kyphosis is a possible link to attention-deficit/hyperactivity disorder. *J Manipulative Physiol Ther*. 2004;27:e14.

456. Elster EL. Upper cervical chiropractic management of a patient with Parkinson's disease: a case report. *J Manipulative Physiol Ther*. 2000;23:573-577.

457. Brennan PC, Triano JJ, McGregor M, Kokjohn K, Hondras MA, Brennan DC. Enhanced neutrophil respiratory burst as a biological marker for manipulation forces: duration of the effect and association with substance P and tumor necrosis factor. *J Manipulative Physiol Ther*. 1992;15:83-89.

458. Brennan PC, Kokjohn K, Kaltinger CJ, et al. Enhanced phagocytic cell respiratory burst induced by spinal manipulation: potential role of substance P. *J Manipulative Physiol Ther*. 1991;14:399-408.

459. Bakris G, Dickholtz M Sr, Meyer PM, et al. Atlas vertebra realignment and achievement of arterial pressure goal in hypertensive patients: a pilot study. *J Hum Hypertens*. 2007;21:347-352.

460. Lewit K, Simons DG. Myofascial pain: relief by post-isometric relaxation. *Arch Phys Med Rehabil*. 1984;65:452-456.

461. Ingber RS. Iliopsoas myofascial dysfunction: a treatable cause of "failed" low-back syndrome. *Arch Phys Med Rehabil*. 1989;70:382-386.

462. Diego MA, Field T, Hernandez-Reif M, et al. Aggressive adolescents benefit from massage therapy. *Adolescence*. 2002;37(147):597-607.

463. Mainous RO. Infant massage as a component of developmental care: past, present, and future. *Holist Nurs Pract*. 2002;16(5):1-7.

464. Hernandez-Reif M, Martinez A, Field T, Quintero O, Hart S, Burman I. Premenstrual symptoms are relieved by massage therapy. *J Psychosom Obstet Gynaecol*. 2000;21:9-15.

465. Hernandez-Reif M, Field T, Krasnegor J, Theakston H. Lower back pain is reduced and range of motion increased after massage therapy. *Int J Neurosci*. 2001;106(3-4):131-145.

466. Knebl JA, Shores JH, Gamber RG, Gray WT, Herron KM. Improving functional ability in the elderly via the Spencer technique, an osteopathic manipulative treatment: a randomized, controlled trial. *J Am Osteopath Assoc*. 2002;102:387-396.

467. Bergman GJ, Winters JC, Groenier KH, et al. Manipulative therapy in addition to usual medical care for patients with shoulder dysfunction and pain: a randomized, controlled trial. *Ann Intern Med*. 2004;141:432-439.

468. Guiney PA, Chou R, Vianna A, Lovenheim J. Effects of osteopathic manipulative treatment on pediatric patients with asthma: a randomized controlled trial. *J Am Osteopath Assoc*. 2005;105:7-12.

469. Eisenhart AW, Gaeta TJ, Yens DP. Osteopathic manipulative treatment in the emergency department for patients with acute ankle injuries. *J Am Osteopath Assoc*. 2003;103:417-421

470. Plotkin BJ, Rodos JJ, Kappler R, et al. Adjunctive osteopathic manipulative treatment in women with depression: a pilot study. *J Am Osteopath Assoc*. 2001;101:517-523.

471. Noll DR, Shores JH, Gamber RG, Herron KM, Swift J Jr. Benefits of osteopathic manipulative treatment for hospitalized elderly patients with pneumonia. *J Am Osteopath Assoc*. 2000;100:776-782.

472. Sucher BM, Hinrichs RN, Welcher RL, Quiroz LD, St Laurent BF, Morrison BJ. Manipulative treatment of carpal tunnel syndrome: biomechanical and osteopathic intervention to increase the length of the transverse carpal ligament: part 2. Effect of sex differences and manipulative "priming." *J Am Osteopath Assoc*. 2005;105:135-143.

473. O-Yurvati AH, Carnes MS, Clearfield MB, Stoll ST, McConathy WJ. Hemodynamic effects of osteopathic manipulative treatment immediately after coronary artery bypass graft surgery. *J Am Osteopath Assoc*. 2005;105:475-481.

Chapter 3

Clinical Focus: Migraine

Introduction

Headaches are a common symptom-based diagnosis with a wide variety of underlying causes ranging from commonplace and benign (e.g., muscle tension headache) to catastrophic (e.g., meningitis or stroke). This section deals only with the pathophysiology and amelioration of routine benign headaches (migraine, cluster, allergic, tension, and cervicogenic); emphasis is placed on migraine headaches as the prototype for these disorders.

Clinical Presentation and Assessment

The differential diagnosis of headache by history, examination, and laboratory and imaging assessments should be familiar to clinicians. In particular, the neurological examination should include psycho-emotional assessment, as well as cranial nerve and fundoscopic examination, and any new headache symptoms, even in a patient with a history of headaches, must receive due diligence on the part of the clinician. Once serious pathological causes of headache have been excluded, the headache can be treated with symptom-suppressing drugs or by biological interventions that address the underlying causative mechanisms.

Pathophysiology

The sensation of headache pain results from activation and sensitization of sensory trigeminal pain neurons that service intracranial blood vessels and meninges. The debate continues as to whether *vasculogenic* or *neurogenic* influences predominate, and most if not all headaches appear to involve both of these main components, thus allowing for the consensus that headaches are *neurovascular* in origin. That said, the weight of evidence increasingly supports the neurological origin of headaches in general and migraines in particular. "Brain-initiated events" such as cortical spreading depression culminate in the release of nociceptive substances including hydrogen ions and arachidonate metabolites, which irritate trigeminovascular sensory neurons surrounding pial vessels.[1,2] Neurogenic inflammation (e.g., the release of neuropeptides from trigeminal nerve [cranial nerve V] neurons to local blood vessels and meninges) is also important and contributes to a vicious cycle of pain and inflammation.[3] Elevated intracellular calcium levels that trigger inflammatory pathways can be promoted by arachidonate, secondary hyperparathyroidism due to vitamin D deficiency, a relative insufficiency of magnesium, and mitochondrial impairment.

Mast cell degranulation releases inflammatory mediators such as serotonin, prostaglandin I-2, and histamine, which induce local inflammation and activation of meningeal nociceptors[4,5] and might serve as a pathophysiological link between emotional stress or allergen exposure and headache (i.e., the link between environmental stressors and headache pain). Mast cells can also be activated by neuropeptides that originate from neurons in the brain parenchyma. Further substantiating the role of local inflammation in migraine is the finding of increased activity of nuclear transcription factor-kappa B (NF-κB) in jugular blood of migraine patients during migraine episode[6]; NF-κB is an important mediator of inflammation through its ability to enhance transcription of genes that encode for inflammatory mediators.[7] This model provides for the often observed continuum between external and biopsychosocial factors such as exposure to bright lights, hypoglycemia, stress, anxiety, allergen exposure, and hormonal fluctuations with the triggering of new or recurrent headaches.

An appreciation for the intraneuronal genesis of headaches such as migraines sharpens our focus on events occurring within the neuronal cell, in particular mitochondrial bioenergetics, intraneuronal calcium homeostasis, and the elaboration of inflammatory mediators derived from polyunsaturated fatty acids. With the realization of mitochondrial and eicosanoid contributions to headache, clinicians can intervene with nutritional intervention and fatty acid supplementation to enhance mitochondrial function and modulate eicosanoid production, respectively. Failure to appreciate these underlying pathophysiological mechanisms forces clinicians and patients to rely on pharmacological symptom suppression while the underlying processes remain unaddressed.

Standard Medical Treatment

For benign headaches including migraine, standard medical treatment is targeted at the alleviation of symptoms. To this end, analgesics and anti-inflammatory drugs such as acetaminophen, aspirin, ibuprofen, naproxen, and ketoprofen are the medical mainstays. Antidepressant drugs ranging from amitriptyline to fluoxetine also might be used for both migraine and tension headaches. Other drugs used for migraine include beta-adrenergic blockers such as propanolol, calcium-channel antagonists such as verapamil, anticonvulsants such as gabapentin and topirmate, and serotonin-modulating drugs such as methysergide and sumatriptan, as well as monoamine oxidase inhibitors and angiotensin-2 receptor blockers. Treatments unique to cluster headaches include inhaled oxygen, lithium carbonate, and prednisone. Migraine patients may become dependent on prescription narcotic drugs, which carry inherent risks of dependence and abuse.

Topiramate (Topomax®) is one of the most commonly used pharmaceutical drugs for the treatment of migraine, and a brief description of its efficacy and expense is warranted in order to provide clinical perspective. A recent clinical trial in a leading headache journal concluded that topiramate "resulted in statistically significant improvements" and that the drug is "safe and generally well tolerated"[8]; these statements would appear to support clinical use of the drug. However, more than 10% of patients stopped using the drug due to adverse effects, and the statistically significant benefit largely consisted of a reduction in headache days by 1.5 days per 91 days of treatment compared to placebo. The out-of-pocket cost for 3 months of this drug treatment (not including physician fees, recommended laboratory monitoring, and management of adverse effects) is in the range of $400 to $600. Thus, for a yearly cost of approximately $2000, the total reduction in headache days over placebo would be approximately 6 days per year. This study was funded by the company that makes the drug, and 11 of the 13 authors received funding, employment, or direct payment from Ortho-McNeil Neurologics, Inc.

Functional Medicine Considerations and Interventions

Functional medicine clinicians appreciate the myriad of triggering factors and underlying biochemical and nutritional imbalances that contribute to headache frequency, intensity, and duration. An understanding of the *mitochondrial model for headache and migraine* described herein will help readers of this monograph appreciate how seemingly divergent research generally points toward nutritional intervention for the alleviation of neurogenic inflammation triggered by *genotropic* and *envirotropic* mitochondrial dysfunction; this model applies particularly, though not exclusively, to migraine-type headaches. Functional medicine clinicians are careful to search for underlying causes of headache that are otherwise easy to overlook; for example, hypothyroidism[9] and hemochromatosis[10,11] are common and readily treatable causes of chronic headaches. The mitochondrial model incorporates the research literature showing that migraine patients have defects in mitochondrial function.[12] In general, with regard to migraine headaches, functional medicine treatment plans commonly focus on the combination of: (1) avoidance of headache triggers, (2) nutritional support of mitochondrial function (*mitochondrial resuscitation*), and (3) amelioration of neurogenic inflammation with diet modification and nutritional supplementation. Some overlap exists among the categories and the interventions therein, as will be discussed below.

Food Allergy Avoidance and Management

Food allergy is among the most common triggers of headaches, particularly migraine-type headaches and those that do not respond to drug treatments. While the foods most commonly implicated are the same foods that commonly trigger other allergic problems, the inciting cephalgenic food(s) need to be identified individually *per patient*. In a 1979 study by Grant,[13] the following foods were identified as the most common headache triggers: wheat (78%), orange (65%), eggs (45%), tea and coffee (40% each), chocolate and milk (37% each), beef (35%), corn, cane sugar, and yeast (33% each); when an average of 10 triggering foods were avoided, patients experienced a "dramatic fall in the number of headaches per month, 85% of patients becoming headache-free." Food allergen identification via the elimination and challenge technique is accurate and inexpensive, and problem-causing foods are then eliminated from the daily diet. In addition to food allergen avoidance, immunomodulatory and anti-inflammatory techniques can be used (including hormonal correction, eradication of gastrointestinal dysbiosis, and supplementation with vitamin C, mixed tocopherols, balanced combination fatty acids, probiotics, vitamin B12, bioflavonoids, pancreatic/proteolytic enzymes, honey, calcium and magnesium butyrate, and cromolyn and other prescription agents) as has been reviewed elsewhere.[14]

> **Clinical Pearl:**
>
> Most food-sensitive headache patients are sensitive to more than one food; often as many as 10 foods must be avoided to attain maximal relief.

Avoidance of Food Additives

Red wine, aged cheeses, sardines, sausage, bacon, and monosodium glutamate (MSG) -containing foods are common triggers for headache and migraine in susceptible patients and should therefore be avoided. Most of these foods contain tyramine, nitrites, or other neuroexcitatory or vasoactive substances, in addition to components (allergens) to which migraine patients tend to be immunologically sensitized.

Magnesium Supplementation

Magnesium deficiency is common, affecting approximately 30% of different populations in various industrialized nations.[15,16,17,18] Regardless of headache etiology or classification, magnesium deficiency is more common in headache patients than in headache-free controls. Magnesium deficiency directly contributes to headache by at least 4 mechanisms: (1) facilitating brain cortex hyperexcitability and hypesthesia due to a reduction in the partial blockade of N-methyl-D-aspartate (NMDA) neurotransmitter receptor sites by magnesium[19], (2) impairing cellular energy production, (3) promoting vasoconstriction, and (4) promoting increased muscle tension, with the latter 2 mechanisms caused in part by impaired energy production, as well as altered intracellular calcium-to-magnesium ratios. Conversely, adequate magnesium nutriture and use of magnesium supplementation help prevent headaches by modulation of NMDA receptor sensitivity and support of energy production, vasorelaxation, and myorelaxation.

Given the excellent overall benefits, safety, and low cost, magnesium supplementation should be offered to all headache patients unless contraindicated.[20,21,22,23,24,25] A reasonable clinical approach is to: (1) evaluate each patient with a history, physical examination, and screening laboratory tests to exclude contraindications such as renal insufficiency (assess with BUN, creatinine, and urinalysis), (2) assess for possible drug interactions, and then (3) start with 200 mg elemental magnesium (citrate or malate) and increase the dose by 200 mg every 1 to 2 days until bowel tolerance is reached; reduce the dose if excessively loose stools or diarrhea occur. Findings common in patients with magnesium deficiency are muscle cramps, bruxism, constipation, and cravings for sweets/candies, especially chocolate. Magnesium status can be objectively assessed by measuring intracellular magnesium levels in leukocytes and erythrocytes.

> **Clinical Pearl:**
>
> Efficacy of magnesium supplementation is enhanced with concomitant pyridoxine supplementation (e.g., 50–250 mg/d of vitamin B6 taken with food) and consumption of a Paleolithic-Mediterranean diet,[26] which promotes alkalinization[27] and thereby facilitates renal magnesium retention[28] and increases intracellular magnesium levels.[29]

Vitamin D3 (cholecalciferol)

Several case reports have documented the effectiveness of vitamin D supplementation in the treatment and prevention of migraine.[30,31] Vitamin D is anti-inflammatory and immunomodulatory,[32] and it relaxes vascular tone by reducing intracellular calcium levels.[33] Reasonable replacement doses are 2000 IU/d for children and 4000 IU/d for adults; monitoring serum calcium ensures safety as described by Vasquez, Manso, and Cannell.[34]

Fatty Acid Supplementation

American diets are notoriously deficient in omega-3 fatty acids; modern-day intake of these fatty acids is approximately 1 g/d, in contrast to the 7 g/d consumed by traditional hunter-gatherer societies. The omega-3 fatty acids studied for use in migraine include alpha-linolenic acid (ALA) from flaxseed oil and eicosapentaenoic acid (EPA) and docosahexaenoic acid (DHA) from fish oil. In addition, omega-6 gamma-linolenic acid (GLA) from borage and evening primrose seed oils and omega-9 oleic acid found in olive oil have been studied. Supplementation with GLA and ALA—along with the use of a multivitamin-multimineral supplement and avoidance of dietary arachidonic acid—has been shown to significantly reduce the intensity, frequency, and duration of migraine headaches.[35] Similarly, significant reductions in migraine burden follow supplementation with fish oil or olive oil,[36] and combination fatty acid therapy with ALA, EPA, DHA, GLA, and oleic acid can be used clinically.

Spinal Manipulation

Myofascial, arthrogenic, and dyskinetic contributions to headache are significant, and these cervicogenic problems can be addressed with manual spinal and myofascial manipulation. Spinal manipulation safely alleviates headaches with efficacy comparable to commonly used first-line prophylactic prescription medications for tension-type headache and migraine headache.[37,38] Spinal manipulation should be performed only by professionals with graduate and postgraduate training in relevant spinal biomechanics, patient assessment, and manipulative technique.[39,40,41,42]

Treatment of Cervical Myofascial Trigger Points

Myofascial trigger points (MFTP) are much more common in migraine patients[43] than in non-headache controls, and they are an important cervicogenic contribution to chronic headaches.[44] MFTP are easily addressed with in-office

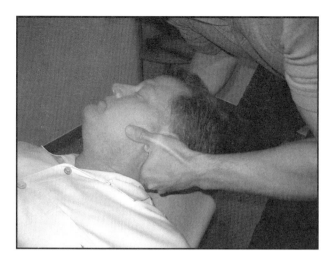 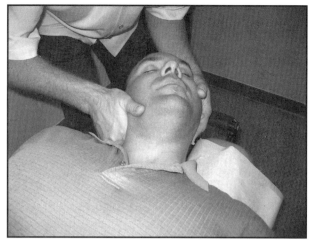

Figure 3.1—Examples of Cervical Spine Manipulation

These photos demonstrate typical premanipulative positioning in treatment of the upper cervical spine. Left, the patient is receiving a rotational manipulation to the atlas. Right, the patient is being treated with a technique that emphasizes lateral bending. Photos reprinted with permission from Vasquez A. *Integrative Orthopedics*. 2nd ed. Fort Worth, Tex: Integrative and Biological Medicine Research and Consulting; 2007.

and at-home treatments; such measures greatly reduce headache frequency, duration, and intensity in affected patients without the risks and expense of pharmaceutical drugs.[45]

Ginger

Components of ginger reduce production of the leukotriene LTB4 (by inhibiting 5-lipoxygenase) and reduce production of the prostaglandin PG-E2 (by inhibiting cyclooxygenase). With its dual reduction of prostaglandins and leukotrienes, NF-κB-blocking actions, and ability to interfere with vanilloid receptor-mediated pain reception, ginger root (either as food or supplement) can safely mitigate musculoskeletal pain[46] and migraine headaches.[47]

Relaxation, Rational Motive Therapy, and Biofeedback

Biofeedback with rational emotive therapy is effective in the prevention of recurrent migraine.[48] Relaxation and stress management are more effective than drug treatment with metoprolol for pediatric migraine.[49]

5-Hydroxytryptophan

5-hydroxytryptophan (5-HTP) is a natural constituent of the human body: it is also found in some plants and is thus available as a nutritional supplement. Altered serotonin metabolism has been observed in headache patients, and this observation serves to support the use of selective serotonin reuptake inhibitors (SSRIs) in headache patients, while supplementation with 5-HTP increases serotonin levels naturally. (For a summary of evidence, see *Protein and Amino Acids* in Chapter 2.)

Among various types of headache, migraine would be expected to show the best response to 5-HTP because the conversion of serotonin to melatonin would extend the benefits of serotonin-mediated analgesia to include the protection of mitochondrial function, an important benefit of melatonin. Conversion of serotonin to melatonin occurs in non-migraine headaches but is of lesser therapeutic importance since these disorders (cluster headaches excepted) are not associated directly with mitochondrial dysfunction.

Hydroxocobalamin (hydroxylated form of vitamin B12)

Hydroxocobalamin (hydroxycobalamin) is a nitric oxide scavenger that appears to benefit the majority of migraine patients when administered intranasally in an aqueous spray solution.[50] If the route of administration is unimportant, as the authors of the trial imply, then high-dose oral supplementation with 2000 mcg/d may prove to be just as effective as nasal/parenteral administration, according to comparable research using orally administered cyanocobalamin.[51]

Feverfew (Tanacetum parthenium)

Results of numerous studies support the use of feverfew for the safe and cost-effective treatment and prevention of migraine headaches. Feverfew has several mechanisms of action including antithrombosis and inhibition of NF-κB. Feverfew products are generally concentrated to 0.2% to 0.7% parthenolide, and a reasonable starting dose is 250 mcg/d of parthenolide; lower doses can be used within a context of multicomponent treatment. Feverfew can be used alone, with other nutrients, or with other botanical medicines. The combination of ginger and feverfew has shown efficacy for halting incipient migraine attacks when started within 2 hours of pain onset.[52] Similarly, the combination of feverfew and willow extract was shown to be remarkably safe and effective in preventing and reducing migraine.[53]

Eradication of Dysbiosis (including gastrointestinal dysbiosis due to Helicobacter Pylori)

Migraine patients have a higher than average prevalence of gastric colonization with *Helicobacter pylori*, and significant symptomatic improvement can be obtained following eradication of *Helicobacter pylori* (according to 3 studies,[54,55,56] but refuted by 2 others[57,58]). For patients with recalcitrant headaches (and for those seeking comprehensive, whole-patient health care), assessment of digestion, absorption, and gastrointestinal microecology is a reasonable component of evaluation that can help guide treatment. Although *Helicobacter pylori* is a common inhabitant of the human gastrointestinal tract (found in more than 50% of Americans over age 50), immunologic responses to the organism can range from nonreactive on one end of the spectrum to diverse diseases like chronic gastritis, chronic urticaria, autoimmune thrombocytopenia, or reactive arthritis on the more severe and systemic end of the spectrum. Thus, the host-microbe relationship is of greater significance than the identity and microbiological characteristics of the microbe.

Surgical Closure of Patent Foramen Ovale

While the prevalence of patent foramen ovale in the general adult population is approximately 20% to 30%, patients with migraine—especially migraine with aura—show a higher prevalence (55–65%) of this physiological cardiopulmonary shunt. Surgical closure of a patent foramen ovale can provide relief from headache in many migraine patients.[59,60] If the cardiopulmonary shunt is severe enough to result in reduced blood oxygenation, it can exacerbate the already reduced energy production caused by the aforementioned mitochondrial dysfunction. More likely, bypassing the lungs results in failure of pulmonary degradation of proinflammatory mediators. The lungs inactivate proinflammatory mediators such as prostaglandins E1, E2, and F2-alpha, all of the leukotrienes, and norepinephrine (30% reduction). Thus, surgical closure of the patent foramen ovale stops inflammatory mediators from bypassing the lungs and may provide a systemic anti-inflammatory benefit that reduces migraine severity. While most practitioners of functional medicine are clinicians rather than surgeons or interventionists, the use of surgical intervention to correct a functional physiological shunt is wholly consistent with the functional medicine model.

Lifestyle Modification

Patients with cluster headaches show a greater percentage of increased work-related stress, self-employment, tobacco smoking, and alcohol use or abuse. These concerns should be addressed per patient as indicated. Lifestyle factors such the standard American diet, overconsumption of caffeine and alcohol, and use of tobacco can result in mitochondrial impairment through various mechanisms, not the least of which are nutrient (especially magnesium) deficiency and accumulation of cyanide, a known mitochondrial poison and constituent of tobacco smoke.

Melatonin

Melatonin levels are low in patients with migraine and cluster headache. According to case reports and studies with small numbers of patients, 10 mg of melatonin taken at night relieves cluster headaches in approximately 50% of patients, with results beginning 3 to 5 days after the start of treatment and continuing for the duration of treatment.[61,62] Melatonin is generally administered at night in doses ranging from 3 to 10 mg, although studies in cancer patients have safely used doses as high as 20 to 40 mg and have shown antitumor and pro-survival benefits. Melatonin has antioxidant and immunomodulatory actions in addition to its ability to preserve mitochondrial function, which is particularly relevant to migraine and cluster headaches (see below).

> **Clinical Pearl:**
>
> Clinical trials using melatonin in migraine patients have shown consistently positive results, with a significant number of patients becoming completely migraine-free.[63]

Hormonal Correction (orthoendocrinology) and the Role of Sex Hormone Deficiency in Cluster Headache

Low testosterone levels have been observed in men with cluster headache, but whether the hypogonadism was caused by or causative to the cluster headache syndrome was not initially clear. However, two reports have now documented the effectiveness of testosterone replacement in hypogonadal patients with cluster headache.[64, 65] The more recent of these studies, conducted by Stillman,[65] showed that testosterone supplementation in men and combined testosterone-estrogen supplementation in women resulted in important clinical improvements even among patients who had previously not responded to drug treatment, melatonin, oxygen, verapamil, antiepileptic agents, and parenteral serotonin agonists.

Intranasal Capsaicin

Intranasal capsaicin (300 mcg/100 mcL) is remarkably well studied in the treatment and prevention of cluster headaches, beginning with the first report published by Sicuteri et al in 1989.[66] Treatment of active cluster headache with intranasal capsaicin (compared with placebo) reduced severity after 7 days of treatment.[67] In a small controlled clinical trial, patients stated that intranasal capsaicin alleviated chronic migraine suffering by 50% to 80%.[68] Burning pain, sneezing, and increased nasal secretions induced by topical capsaicin application are intense for the first few applications but decrease over time, generally within a week or so; clinical benefits generally begin on the eighth day of consecutive treatment. Episodic cluster headache patients appear to benefit more than do chronic cluster headache patients. Cluster headaches are typically unilateral, and capsaicin should be applied to the nostril on the same side as the head pain.

Oxygen

One hundred percent oxygen delivered by facial mask at 8 L/min for 10 minutes can help abort an attack of cluster headache. Oxygen is the required terminal component of the mitochondrial electron transport chain (ETC) for ATP production; thus, supraphysiological oxygen, like supraphysiological doses of mitochondria-specific nutrients, generally improves mitochondrial energy (ATP) production.

Acupuncture

Acupuncture is effective symptomatic treatment for migraine and tension headaches, with cost-effectiveness comparable to standard medical treatment.[69,70,71] Acupuncture is known to affect regional blood flow, and the neurophysiological mechanisms involved include increased release of endogenous analgesics such as endomorphin-1, beta-endorphin, encephalin, and serotonin.[72] In a head-to-head study of acupuncture versus drug treatment with metoprolol, "two of 59 patients randomized to acupuncture withdrew prematurely from the study compared to 18 of 55 randomized to metoprolol.... The proportion of responders was 61% for acupuncture and 49% for metoprolol. Both physicians and patients reported fewer adverse effects in the acupuncture group."[73] While pain relief is an important benefit, it should not be the primary goal in treatment if an underlying physiological or biochemical disturbance (including nutritional deficiencies or imbalances) can be corrected.

Nutritional Support and Enhancement of Mitochondrial Function (mitochondrial resuscitation)

Migraine patients have defects in energy production due to impairments in mitochondrial enzymatic reactions and in several components of the ETC. Specifically, the energy production steps that are affected include reduced activity of NADH dehydrogenase, citrate synthase, and cytochrome-c-oxidase; defects in NADH-cytochrome c reductase appear to be specific to migraine with aura.[74] Genotropic enzyme defects often result in decreased binding affinity between the enzyme and its coenzyme, resulting in a lower rate of reaction, and many such diseases "can be remedied or ameliorated by the administration of high doses of the vitamin component of the corresponding coenzyme, which at least partially restores enzymatic activity."[75] Supplementation with nutrients intimately involved with ATP production has shown impressive efficacy in the treatment and prevention of migraine; all of these nutrients, including magnesium, are extremely safe and are appropriate for use in children and adults.

Niacin — High-dose niacin alleviates migraine headaches and headaches of various etiologies, whether administered orally, intramuscularly, or intravenously; niacin can also be used to halt acute migraine attacks.[76,77] Niacinamide adenine dinucleotide (NADH) is an essential component of the first stage (Complex 1) of the ETC, a step that is commonly defective in migraine patients. High-dose niacin facilitates this step and thus enhances energy production. Another anti-migraine benefit of high-dose niacin is its sparing effect on tryptophan, allowing its conversion to serotonin. Niacin also has a vasodilating action and may thereby address the vasculogenic component of headache.

Efficacious oral doses of niacin can range from 300 to 1500 mg/d; lower doses are used for children. High-dose niacin, particularly in time-released tablets, presents some risk for hepatic damage, and thus, safer forms of niacin such as plain niacin, slow-release niacin (e.g., Niaspan®), and inositol hexaniacinate are preferred; niacinamide and NADH might also be efficacious but neither has vasodilating actions provided by the other forms of niacin. Doses of niacin exceeding 500 to 1000 mg/d are probably unnecessary in headache patients if other treatments such as coenzyme Q10 (CoQ10), vitamin D, and fatty acids are being used; before implementing high-dose niacin, patients should be selected, informed, and monitored appropriately.

Coenzyme Q10 — As an essential component of the mitochondrial ETC, CoQ10 is both endogenously produced and available in very small amounts from fish and meat. CoQ10 shuttles electrons from Complex 1 to Complex 2 and from Complex 2 to Complex 3; thus, CoQ10 supplementation helps to bypass defects in Complexes 1 and 2.

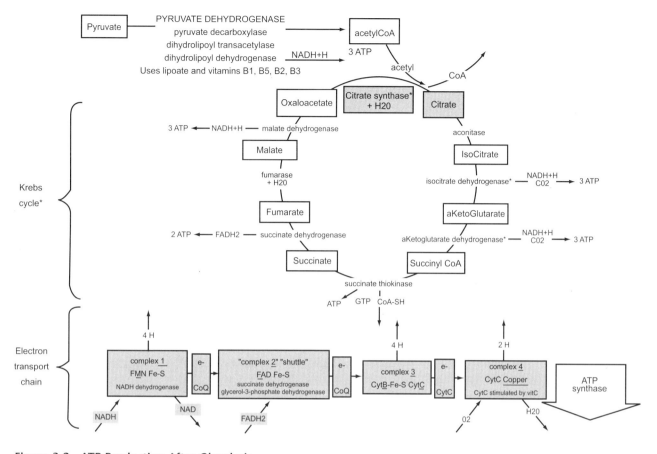

Figure 3.2—ATP Production After Glycolysis

Schematic diagram of ATP production after glycolysis, starting with the pyruvate dehydrogenase complex and proceeding to the ETC. Items shaded or bolded are particularly relevant for migraine pathogenesis and treatment. Diagram adapted with permission from Vasquez A. *Integrative Orthopedics*. 2nd ed. Fort Worth, Tex: Integrative and Biological Medicine Research and Consulting; 2007.

Note: Many of the enzymes in the Krebs cycle require magnesium as a cofactor.

Abbreviations: ATP: adenosine triphosphate; CoQ: coenzyme Q10; CytB, CytC: cytochromes B and C, respectively; FAD, FADH: flavin adenine dinucleotide (derived from vitamin B2); Fe-S: iron and sulfur; FMN: flavin mononucleotide (derived from vitamin B2); GTP: guanine triphosphate; Lipoate: lipoic acid; NADH: niacinamide adenine dinucleotide (derived from vitamin B3); Vit C: vitamin C.

In addition to its antioxidant and ETC roles, CoQ10 is immunomodulatory and may have a role in the treatment of allergic disease, chronic viral infections, and cancer.[78,79,80,81,82] (For more information, see *Vitamin and Mineral Supplements* in Chapter 2.) CoQ10 probably has at least 4 separate yet synergistic anti-headache mechanisms, namely modulation of cell membrane dynamics, inhibition of NF-κB, protection of mitochondrial function, and antiallergy immunomodulation. CoQ10 supplementation has been shown to significantly reduce migraine headache frequency, duration, and intensity.[83] Research published in 2007 showed that a large subset of pediatric and adolescent patients with migraine have primary deficiency of CoQ10 and that CoQ10 supplementation normalizes serum levels and results in significant reductions in headache frequency and headache-related disability.[84] The most commonly used clinical doses are in the range of 100 to 300 mg/d, but some patients will respond to as little as 30 mg/d while others may need 1000 mg/d, depending on condition, antioxidant status, and body weight. To enhance absorption and therefore clinical effectiveness, CoQ-10 should be pre-emulsified or taken with fatty food.

Riboflavin (vitamin B2) — Flavin adenine dinucleotide is required at Complex 2 of the ETC. High-dose vitamin B2 (400 mg/d) shows high efficacy, excellent tolerability, and low cost in the prevention of migraine headaches, as demonstrated by several open and placebo-controlled trials.[85]

Lipoic acid — Lipoic (thiotic) acid is an essential component of the pyruvate dehydrogenase complex. A placebo-controlled clinical trial showed benefit of lipoic acid (600 mg/d) supplementation in migraine patients.[86] Lipoic acid also inhibits NF-κB activation and thus may have at least 2 separate anti-headache mechanisms: promotion of ATP production and inhibition of NF-κB-activated inflammation.

Melatonin — As mentioned previously, melatonin is a potent protector of mitochondrial function, which has been demonstrated in experimental models of mitochondrial inhibition by bacterial endotoxin. As a powerful antioxidant, melatonin scavenges oxygen and nitrogen-based reactants generated in mitochondria and thereby limits the loss of the intramitochondrial glutathione; this prevents mitochondrial protein and DNA damage. Melatonin increases the activity of Complexes 1 and 4 of the ETC, improving mitochondrial respiration and increasing ATP synthesis under various physiological and experimental conditions.[87]

Carnitine — The amino acid carnitine is necessary for fatty acid transport into the mitochondria for oxidative metabolism and energy production. Deficiency of or metabolic inability to use carnitine can precipitate or perpetuate migraine headaches, which can be alleviated by carnitine supplementation.[88] As a natural component of the human diet, carnitine has a wide safety margin, and supplemental doses ranging from 300 to 2000 mg/d are commonly used.

Other mitochondrial nutrients — Copper, vitamin C, iron, and sulfur are also necessary components of the mitochondrial ETC.

Conclusion and Clinical Approach

Standard medical treatment for headaches is expensive and fraught with adverse effects, drug dependence, and suboptimal efficacy. Further, such symptom-suppressive treatment fails to address the causative food intolerances, nutritional deficiencies, and mitochondrial defects that are common in headache patients and migraineurs. Following the exclusion of serious underlying disease, headache patients should be counseled on allergen identification (free and highly efficacious) and should receive nutritional supplementation with combination fatty acids (e.g., ALA, GLA, EPA, DHA) and therapeutic doses of vitamins and minerals, particularly riboflavin, vitamin D3, and magnesium. CoQ10, 5-HTP, melatonin, spinal manipulation, post-isometric stretching, and the other treatments listed above can be used in combination as appropriate per patient to optimize the therapeutic response.

References

1. Moskowitz MA. Pathophysiology of headache: past and present. *Headache*. 2007;47(Suppl 1):S58-63.
2. Moskowitz MA. Genes, proteases, cortical spreading depression and migraine: impact on pathophysiology and treatment. *Funct Neurol*. 2007;22:133-136.
3. Tierney ML, McPhee SJ, Papadakis MA, eds. *Current Medical Diagnosis and Treatment 2006. 45th ed*. New York, NY: Lange Medical Books; 2006: 31-33.
4. Levy D, Burstein R, Kainz V, Jakubowski M, Strassman AM. Mast cell degranulation activates a pain pathway underlying migraine headache. *Pain*. 2007;130(1-2):166-176.
5. Zhang XC, Strassman AM, Burstein R, Levy D. Sensitization and activation of intracranial meningeal nociceptors by mast cell mediators. *J Pharmacol Exp Ther*. 2007;322:806-812.
6. Sarchielli P, Floridi A, Mancini ML, et al. NF-kappaB activity and iNOS expression in monocytes from internal jugular blood of migraine without aura patients during attacks. *Cephalalgia*. 2006;26:1071-1079.
7. Tak PP, Firestein GS. NF-kappaB: a key role in inflammatory diseases. *J Clin Invest*. 2001;107:7-11.
8. Silberstein SD, Lipton RB, Dodick DW, et al. Efficacy and safety of topiramate for the treatment of chronic migraine: a randomized, double-blind, placebo-controlled trial. *Headache*. 2007;47:170-180.
9. Moreau T, Manceau E, Giroud-Baleydier F, Dumas R, Giroud M. Headache in hypothyroidism. Prevalence and outcome under thyroid hormone therapy. *Cephalalgia*. 1998;18:687-689.
10. Hagen K, Stovner LJ, Asberg A, Thorstensen K, Bjerve KS, Hveem K. High headache prevalence among women with hemochromatosis: the Nord-Trondelag health study. *Ann Neurol*. 2002;51:786-789.
11. Stovner LJ, Hagen K, Waage A, Bjerve KS. Hereditary haemochromatosis in two cousins with cluster headache. *Cephalalgia*. 2002;22:317-319.
12. Okada H, Araga S, Takeshima T, Nakashima K. Plasma lactic acid and pyruvic acid levels in migraine and tension-type headache. *Headache*. 1998;38:39-42.

13. Grant EC. Food allergies and migraine. *Lancet*. 1979;1(8123):966-969.
14. Vasquez A. Improving neuromusculoskeletal health by optimizing immune function and reducing allergic reactions: a review of 16 treatments and a 3-step clinical approach. *Nutritional Perspectives*. October 2005: 27-35, 40. Available online at: http://optimalhealthresearch.com/part5.
15. Innerarity S. Hypomagnesemia in acute and chronic illness. *Crit Care Nurs Q*. 2000;23(2):1-19.
16. Frankel H, Haskell R, Lee SY, Miller D, Rotondo M, Schwab CW. Hypomagnesemia in trauma patients. *World J Surg*. 1999;23:966-969.
17. Fox CH, Ramsoomair D, Mahoney MC, Carter C, Young B, Graham R. An investigation of hypomagnesemia among ambulatory urban African Americans. *J Fam Pract*. 1999;48:636-639.
18. Schimatschek HF, Rempis R. Prevalence of hypomagnesemia in an unselected German population of 16,000 individuals. *Magnes Res*. 2001;14:283-290.
19. Boska MD, Welch KM, Barker PB, Nelson JA, Schultz L. Contrasts in cortical magnesium, phospholipid and energy metabolism between migraine syndromes. *Neurology*. 2002;58:1227-1233.
20. Mazzotta G, Sarchielli P, Alberti A, Gallai V. Intracellular Mg++ concentration and electromyographical ischemic test in juvenile headache. *Cephalalgia*. 1999;19:802-809.
21. Mishima K, Takeshima T, Shimomura T, et al. Platelet ionized magnesium, cyclic AMP, and cyclic GMP levels in migraine and tension-type headache. *Headache*. 1997;37:561-564.
22. Peikert A, Wilimzig C, Kohne-Volland R. Prophylaxis of migraine with oral magnesium: results from a prospective, multi-center, placebo-controlled and double-blind randomized study. *Cephalalgia*. 1996;16:257-263.
23. Mauskop A, Altura BT, Cracco RQ, Altura BM. Intravenous magnesium sulfate rapidly alleviates headaches of various types. *Headache*. 1996;36:154-160.
24. Wang F, Van Den Eeden SK, Ackerson LM, Salk SE, Reince RH, Elin RJ. Oral magnesium oxide prophylaxis of frequent migrainous headache in children: a randomized, double-blind, placebo-controlled trial. *Headache*. 2003;43:601-610.
25. Grazzi L, Andrasik F, Usai S, Bussone G. Magnesium as a preventive treatment for paediatric episodic tension-type headache: results at 1-year follow-up. *Neurol Sci*. 2007;28:148-150.
26. Vasquez A. A five-part nutritional protocol that produces consistently positive results. *Nutritional Wellness*. September 2005. Available online at: http://optimalhealthresearch.com/protocol.
27. Sebastian A, Frassetto LA, Sellmeyer DE, Merriam RL, Morris RC Jr. Estimation of the net acid load of the diet of ancestral preagricultural Homo sapiens and their hominid ancestors. *Am J Clin Nutr*. 2002;76:1308-1316.
28. Rylander R, Remer T, Berkemeyer S, Vormann J.Acid-base status affects renal magnesium losses in healthy, elderly persons. *J Nutr*. 2006; 136:2374-2377.
29. Vormann J, Worlitschek M, Goedecke T, Silver B. Supplementation with alkaline minerals reduces symptoms in patients with chronic low back pain. *J Trace Elem Med Biol*. 2001;15(2-3):179-183.
30. Thys-Jacobs S. Alleviation of migraines with therapeutic vitamin D and calcium. *Headache*. 1994;34:590-592.
31. Thys-Jacobs S. Vitamin D and calcium in menstrual migraine. *Headache*. 1994;34:544-546.
32. Timms PM, Mannan N, Hitman GA, et al. Circulating MMP9, vitamin D and variation in the TIMP-1 response with VDR genotype: mechanisms for inflammatory damage in chronic disorders? *QJM*. 2002;95:787-796.
33. Vasquez A. Intracellular hypercalcinosis: A functional nutritional disorder with implications ranging from myofascial trigger points to affective disorders, hypertension and cancer. *Naturopathy Digest*. September 2006. Available online at: http://www.naturopathydigest.com/archives/2006/sep/vasquez.php
34. Vasquez A, Manso G, Cannell J. The clinical importance of vitamin D (cholecalciferol): A paradigm shift with implications for all healthcare providers. *Altern Ther Health Med*. 2004;10:28-37.
35. Wagner W, Nootbaar-Wagner U. Prophylactic treatment of migraine with gamma-linolenic and alpha-linolenic acids. *Cephalalgia*. 1997;17:127-130.
36. Harel Z, Gascon G, Riggs S, Vaz R, Brown W, Exil G. Supplementation with omega-3 polyunsaturated fatty acids in the management of recurrent migraines in adolescents. *J Adolesc Health*. 2002;31:154-161.
37. Bronfort G, Assendelft WJ, Evans R, Haas M, Bouter L. Efficacy of spinal manipulation for chronic headache: a systematic review. *J Manipulative Physiol Ther*. 2001;24:457-466.
38. Tuchin PJ, Pollard H, Bonello R. A randomized controlled trial of chiropractic spinal manipulative therapy for migraine. *J Manipulative Physiol Ther*. 2000;23:91-95.
39. Kirk CR, Lawrence DJ, Valvo NL. *States Manual of Spinal, Pelvic, and Extravertebral Technics*. 2nd ed. Lombard, Ill: National College of Chiropractic; 1985.
40. Kimberly PE. *Outline of Osteopathic Manipulative Procedures. The Kimberly Manual 2006*. Mardeline, Mo: Walsworth Publishing.
41. Bergmann TF, Peterson DH, Lawrence DJ. *Chiropractic Technique*. New York, NY: Churchill Livingstone; 1993.
42. Gatterman MI. *Chiropractic Management of Spine Related Disorders*. Baltimore, Md: Williams and Wilkins; 1990.
43. Calandre EP, Hidalgo J, Garcia-Leiva JM, Rico-Villademoros F. Trigger point evaluation in migraine patients: an indication of peripheral sensitization linked to migraine predisposition? *Eur J Neurol*. 2006;13:244-249.
44. Borg-Stein J. Cervical myofascial pain and headache. *Curr Pain Headache Rep*. 2002;6:324-330.
45. Davidoff RA. Trigger points and myofascial pain: toward understanding how they affect headaches. *Cephalalgia*. 1998;18:436-448.
46. Grzanna R, Lindmark L, Frondoza CG. Ginger: an herbal medicinal product with broad anti-inflammatory actions. *J Med Food*. 2005;8:125-132.
47. Mustafa T, Srivastava KC. Ginger (Zingiber officinale) in migraine headache. *J Ethnopharmacol*. 1990;29:267-273.
48. Lake A, Rainey J, Papsdorf JD. Biofeedback and rational-emotive therapy in the management of migraine headache. *J Appl Behav Anal*. 1979;12:127-140.
49. Sartory G, Muller B, Metsch J, Pothmann R. A comparison of psychological and pharmacological treatment of pediatric migraine. B*ehav Res Ther*. 1998;36:1155-1170.
50. van der Kuy PH, Merkus FW, Lohman JJ, ter Berg JW, Hooymans PM. Hydroxocobalamin, a nitric oxide scavenger, in the prophylaxis of migraine: an open, pilot study. *Cephalalgia*. 2002; 22:513-519.
51. Kuzminski AM, Del Giacco EJ, Allen RH, Stabler SP, Lindenbaum J. Effective treatment of cobalamin deficiency with oral cobalamin. *Blood*. 1998;92:1191-1198.

52. Cady RK, Schreiber CP, Beach ME, Hart CC. Gelstat Migraine (sublingually administered feverfew and ginger compound) for acute treatment of migraine when administered during the mild pain phase. *Med Sci Monit*. 2005;11(9):PI65-69.
53. Shrivastava R, Pechadre JC, John GW. Tanacetum parthenium and Salix alba (Mig-RL) combination in migraine prophylaxis: a prospective, open-label study. *Clin Drug Investig*. 2006;26:287-296.
54. Gasbarrini A, De Luca A, Fiore G, et al. Beneficial effects of Helicobacter pylori eradication on migraine. *Hepatogastroenterology*. 1998;45:765-770.
55. Tunca A, Turkay C, Tekin O, Kargili A, Erbayrak M. Is Helicobacter pylori infection a risk factor for migraine? A case-control study. *Acta Neurol Belg*. 2004;104:161-164.
56. Yiannopoulou KG, Efthymiou A, Karydakis K, Arhimandritis A, Bovaretos N, Tzivras M. Helicobacter pylori infection as an environmental risk factor for migraine without aura. *J Headache Pain*. 2007;8:329-333.
57. Pinessi L, Savi L, Pellicano R, et al. Chronic Helicobacter pylori infection and migraine: a case-control study. *Headache*. 2000;40:836-839.
58. Ciancarelli I, Di Massimo C, Tozzi-Ciancarelli MG, De Matteis G, Marini C, Carolei A. Helicobacter pylori infection and migraine. *Cephalalgia*. 2002;22:222-225.
59. Rigatelli G, Braggion G, Aggio S, Chinaglia M, Cardaioli P. Primary patent foramen ovale closure to relieve severe migraine. *Ann Intern Med*. 2006;144:458-460.
60. Dubiel M, Bruch L, Schmehl I, et al. Migraine headache relief after percutaneous transcatheter closure of interatrial communications. *J Interv Cardiol*. 2008;21:32-37.
61. Leone M, D'Amico D, Moschiano F, Fraschini F, Bussone G. Melatonin versus placebo in the prophylaxis of cluster headache: a double-blind pilot study with parallel groups. *Cephalalgia*. 1996;16:494-496.
62. Peres MF, Rozen TD. Melatonin in the preventive treatment of chronic cluster headache. *Cephalalgia*. 2001;21:993-995.
63. Vogler B, Rapoport AM, Tepper SJ, Sheftell F, Bigal ME. Role of melatonin in the pathophysiology of migraine: implications for treatment. *CNS Drugs*. 2006;20:343-350.
64. Klimek A. Use of testosterone in the treatment of cluster headache. *Eur Neurol*. 1985;24:53-56.
65. Stillman MJ. Testosterone replacement therapy for treatment refractory cluster headache. *Headache*. 2006;46:925-933.
66. Sicuteri F, Fusco BM, Marabini S, et al. Beneficial effect of capsaicin application to the nasal mucosa in cluster headache. *Clin J Pain*. 1989;5:49-53.
67. Marks DR, Rapoport A, Padla D, et al. A double-blind placebo-controlled trial of intranasal capsaicin for cluster headache. *Cephalalgia*. 1993;13:114-116.
68. Fusco BM, Barzoi G, Agrò F. Repeated intranasal capsaicin applications to treat chronic migraine. *Br J Anaesth*. 2003;90:812.
69. Endres HG, Bowing G, Diener HC, et al. Acupuncture for tension-type headache: a multicentre, sham-controlled, patient-and observer-blinded, randomised trial. *J Headache Pain*. 2007;8:306-314.
70. Vickers AJ, Rees RW, Zollman CE, et al. Acupuncture of chronic headache disorders in primary care: randomised controlled trial and economic analysis. *Health Technol Assess*. 2004;8(48):iii, 1-35.
71. Wonderling D, Vickers AJ, Grieve R, McCarney R. Cost effectiveness analysis of a randomised trial of acupuncture for chronic headache in primary care. *BMJ*. 2004;328(7442):747.
72. Cabyoglu MT, Ergene N, Tan U. The mechanism of acupuncture and clinical applications. *Int J Neurosci*. 2006;116:115-125.
73. Streng A, Linde K, Hoppe A, et al. Effectiveness and tolerability of acupuncture compared with metoprolol in migraine prophylaxis. *Headache*. 2006;46:1492-1502.
74. Sangiorgi S, Mochi M, Riva R, et al. Abnormal platelet mitochondrial function in patients affected by migraine with and without aura. *Cephalalgia*. 1994;14:21-23.
75. Ames BN, Elson-Schwab I, Silver EA. High-dose vitamin therapy stimulates variant enzymes with decreased coenzyme binding affinity (increased K(m)): relevance to genetic disease and polymorphisms. *Am J Clin Nutr*. 2002;75:616-658.
76. Velling DA, Dodick DW, Muir JJ. Sustained-release niacin for prevention of migraine headache. *Mayo Clin Proc*. 2003;78(6):770-771.
77. Prousky J, Seely D. The treatment of migraines and tension-type headaches with intravenous and oral niacin (nicotinic acid): systematic review of the literature. *Nutr J*. 2005;4:3.
78. Ye CQ, Folkers K, Tamagawa H, Pfeiffer C. A modified determination of coenzyme Q10 in human blood and CoQ10 blood levels in diverse patients with allergies. *Biofactors*. 1988;1:303-306.
79. Gaby AR. The role of coenzyme Q10 in clinical medicine, part I. *Altern Med Rev*. 1996;1:11-17.
80. Gaby AR. The role of coenzyme Q10 in clinical medicine, part II. Cardiovascular disease, hypertension, diabetes mellitus and infertility. *Altern Med Rev*. 1996;1:168-175.
81. Ebadi M, Sharma SK, Wanpen S, Amornpan A. Coenzyme Q10 inhibits mitochondrial complex-1 down-regulation and nuclear factor-kappa B activation. *J Cell Mol Med*. 2004;8:213-222.
82. Gvozdjáková A, Kucharská J, Bartkovjaková M, Gazdíková K, Gazdík FE. Coenzyme Q10 supplementation reduces corticosteroids dosage in patients with bronchial asthma. *Biofactors*. 2005;25(1-4):235-240.
83. Rozen TD, Oshinsky ML, Gebeline CA, et al. Open label trial of coenzyme Q10 as a migraine preventive. *Cephalalgia*. 2002;22:137-141.
84. Hershey AD, Powers SW, Vockell AL, et al. Coenzyme Q10 deficiency and response to supplementation in pediatric and adolescent migraine. *Headache*. 2007;47:73-80.
85. Boehnke C, Reuter U, Flach U, Schuh-Hofer S, Einhaupl KM, Arnold G. High-dose riboflavin treatment is efficacious in migraine prophylaxis: an open study in a tertiary care centre. *Eur J Neurol*. 2004;11:475-477.
86. Magis D, Ambrosini A, Sandor P, Jacquy J, Laloux P, Schoenen J. A randomized double-blind placebo-controlled trial of thioctic acid in migraine prophylaxis. *Headache*. 2007;47:52-57.
87. León J, Acuña-Castroviejo D, Escames G, Tan DX, Reiter RJ. Melatonin mitigates mitochondrial malfunction. *J Pineal Res*. 2005;38:1-9.
88. Kabbouche MA, Powers SW, Vockell AL, LeCates SL, Hershey AD. Carnitine palmityltransferase II (CPT2) deficiency and migraine headache: two case reports. *Headache*. 2003;43:490-495.

Chapter 4

Clinical Focus: Low Back Pain

Introduction

Chronic low back pain is common in clinical practice, yet aside from ascriptions to disc herniations and muscle spasm, the condition is often viewed as enigmatic and idiopathic. Up to 80% of the adult population is affected by back pain at one time or another, and at any one time, approximately 20% of working adults in the United States suffer from chronic low back pain, defined as pain in the lumbar spine and paraspinal tissues lasting more than 3 months. Annual economic and societal costs in America related to low back pain are estimated at $26 billion in direct healthcare costs and $50 billion in indirect healthcare costs, including doctor's fees, drugs, surgery, nonpharmacological and nonsurgical treatments, lost days from work, and reduced productivity. [1,2,3] Adverse effects and high costs due to pharmaceutical and surgical treatments are also significant. Nonpharmacological and nonsurgical interventions are generally of lower cost and less risk, but despite their often equivalent or higher efficacy and cost-effectiveness compared with standard medical treatments, these interventions are not commonly used in conventional medicine.

A wide range of problems, both serious and benign, can cause or contribute to chronic low back pain, and therefore, keen diagnostic acumen on behalf of the clinician is of paramount importance. This chapter will discuss acute causes of low back pain such as fracture or intervertebral disc herniation and pathological causes such as infection or cancer in order to remind clinicians of these important considerations. In October 2007, new clinical practice guidelines for the management of low back pain (hereafter: "LBP guidelines") were published by the American College of Physicians and the American Pain Society.[1] These new LBP guidelines, as well as other sources of information and the clinician's professional training, should be integrated with this monograph since the purpose of this monograph is not to review the management of low back pain *per se*, but rather to highlight the uniqueness and advantages of the functional medicine approach.

Pathophysiology

Low back pain contributors and causes can be grouped within 4 categories: (1) anatomical, (2) functional (metabolic, nutritional, dyskinetic), (3) neurocompressive, and (4) pathological. This 4-part categorization differs from the 3-part categorization used in the LBP guidelines because it divides *nonspecific low back pain* based on anatomical and functional contributors; such nonspecific pain accounts for more than 85% of low back complaints.[1] The descriptor *nonspecific low back pain* fails to appreciate the very specific nuances and perturbations that are identifiable and remediable. Nonspecific descriptions lead to nonspecific treatments and thereby promote clinical confusion and therapeutic failure.

Anatomical structures of the lumbar spine capable of producing pain include the vertebrae, facet (zygapophysial) joints, and the paraspinal ligaments, tendons, and muscles. Intervertebral discs are generally considered insensitive to pain. However, injury or degeneration of the discs can alter spinal biomechanics and result in increased pain due to, for example, increased weight bearing on the posterior facet joints, which are highly innervated and pain sensitive. Further, the inflammatory and healing response to disc injury or chronic segmental hypermobility may result in nociceptor sensitization and neoinnervation in the vertebral end plate and periphery of the annulus fibrosis. Thus, in contrast to their healthy predecessors and neighbors, degenerative discs may evolve to become a significant source of spinal pain.[4] Spasm, hypertonicity, and myofascial trigger points (MFTP) in paraspinal musculature, particularly including the quadratus lumborum and psoas, are clearly major causes of chronic spinal pain, which are ameliorated only through physical means such as post-isometric stretching and which are unserviceable by anti-inflammatory treatments and vertebral surgery.[5] Pain originating from the periosteum of the lumbar vertebrae is an underappreciated cause of chronic low back pain, a fact that has been made plain by research showing that vitamin D deficiency triggers periosteal pain and leads to chronic skeletal pain.

In addition to vitamin D status, other important nutritional and metabolic considerations include vitamin B12 nurture, fatty acid balance, and acid-base balance, particularly as related to the chronic subclinical *metabolic acidosis* resultant from the American/Western diet pattern. Also related to the American/Western diet pattern is the proinflammatory state resultant from overconsumption of carbohydrates and proinflammatory fatty acids and underconsumption of phytonutrients and the vitamins, minerals, and fatty acids that have additive and synergistic anti-inflammatory activity.

Postural and ergonomic contributors to pain are generally apparent with specific questioning and physical examination. Chronic facet joint irritation secondary to lumbar hyperlordosis can be caused by tight hip flexors (psoas and iliacus), weakened and relaxed rectus abdominis, and/or abdominal obesity. Subtle aberrations in paraspinal muscle coordination that allow recurrent microtrauma are common in patients with low back pain; these proprioceptive and kinesthetic defects are also seen in patients with chronic pain and recurrent injuries involving the knee and ankle. Most of these problems will be discussed in greater detail below under *Clinical Applications*.

Pathological causes of low back pain are common enough to warrant routine consideration during initial and follow-up evaluation and treatment. Viscerosomatic pain referral from cancerous, injured, infected, or inflamed internal organs such as the pancreas (acute or chronic pancreatitis), kidneys (nephrolithiasis or pyelonephritis), or an aneurismal aorta is notorious for causing back pain. Primary and metastatic cancerous involvement of vertebrae is an important consideration, particularly as patients reach later adulthood or if there is a history of cancer. Fungal and bacterial infections of vertebrae are more common among patients who are immunocompromised (e.g., due to pharmacological immunosuppression, human immunodeficiency virus infection, or primary immune deficiency), and vertebral osteomyelitis and infectious discitis may not present with the expected classic manifestations of infection such as fever or elevated leukocyte count. Radicular pain due to nerve root compromise, physical compression, and/or inflammatory chemical irritation typically presents in a dermatomal distribution, is exacerbated by nerve root tension tests, and may be characterized by segmental sensory, motor, and reflex deficits. Cauda equina syndrome secondary to massive disc herniation may present acutely or chronically with altered bowel or bladder function, bilateral or unilateral sciatica, and perineal-genital numbness; cauda equina syndrome is an unequivocal surgical emergency. Central and lateral recess stenosis are also noteworthy considerations in the differential assessment of low back pain, particularly in older patients with bilateral or unilateral sciatica. Rheumatic conditions characteristically afflicting the low back include ankylosing spondylitis, reactive arthritis, psoriatic arthritis, and enteropathic spondyloarthropathy. Trauma opens a Pandora's box of possibilities and complications, including spinal fracture, dislocation, internal hemorrhage, and damage to viscera or spinal and paraspinal tissues.

Clinical Presentation, Evaluation, and Diagnosis

Diagnosis of low back pain is founded on the subjective report of the patient, and the clinician has the responsibility to determine and address the cause(s) of the pain and to exclude pathological conditions (e.g., visceral disease, spinal infection, cancer, rheumatic disease) and urgent situations (e.g., fracture, cauda equina syndrome). The patient's history and nuances of presentation and clinical findings are of paramount importance; all patients require physical examination including blood pressure, pulse rate, temperature, neurological exam (reflexes, strength, sensory), and regional examination of the thoracolumbar spine, abdomen, bony pelvis, and sacroiliac joints (SIJ). Psychosocial factors, particularly depression and pending medicolegal compensation, should be considered; the depression associated with low back pain may have an organic biochemical (nutritional) basis, as will be discussed below. The pelvis and lower extremity can be examined for biomechanical faults and anatomical discrepancy. Imaging and laboratory assessments typically play secondary roles except in recalcitrant and potentially pathological or urgent cases.

Standard Medical Treatment

The LBP guidelines note that "more than 85% of patients who present to primary care have low back pain that cannot reliably be attributed to a specific disease or spinal abnormality (nonspecific low back pain)." This inability on the part of clinicians to identify the cause of the patient's pain is often ascribed to the inherent enigmatic and idiopathic nature of the condition, whereas the problem may more accurately lie with inadequacies in musculoskeletal training in medical schools and residency programs.[6,7,8] Standard medical treatment is mostly pharmacological, with surgical interventions being reserved for more recalcitrant, painful, or neurocompressive cases. Many pharmacological and surgical treatments are characterized by high cost, inefficacy, acute and chronic adverse effects, therapeutic passivity, treatment dependency, and addiction.

Drug treatment centers on nonsteroidal anti-inflammatory drugs (NSAIDs), skeletal muscle relaxants, tricyclic antidepressants, benzodiazepines, oral/injected corticosteroids, and opioid narcotics. Among the more notorious adverse effects of NSAIDs are gastric ulceration and hemorrhage,[9] increased cardiovascular mortality,[10,11] and inhibition of cartilage repair and maintenance leading to perpetuation and exacerbation of joint pain and destruction.[12,13,14,15] Liver and kidney damage are more common among patients who use acetaminophen and NSAIDs; NSAID hepatotoxicity and nephrotoxicity show dose-dependent predictability. More than 17 000 Americans per year die from NSAID use.[16] The cyclooxygenase-2 (COX-2) inhibitors (coxibs) were supposed to deliver pain relief without the typical gastric irritation and antithrombotic effects of classic NSAIDs; however, their clinical applicability is limited due to their disappointing clinical efficacy, cardiovascular toxicity, minimal side benefits, and exorbitant costs for long-term use ($100–200 per month). The COX-2 inhibitor rofecoxib (Vioxx) is estimated to have killed as many as 55,000 patients and injured up to 139,000 Americans who took the drug for benign musculoskeletal pain.[17] All skeletal muscle relaxants cause sedation or other adverse central nervous system effects, and several of these drugs including dantrolene, tizanidine, and chlorzaoxazone are known for their hepatotoxicity; dantrolene carries a black box warning for potentially fatal hepatotoxicity. Opioid narcotics are commonly used in the treatment of chronic low back pain despite their unproven long-term efficacy and proclivity for misuse and addition.[18] Numerous surgical interventions exist for spinal disorders, ranging from microdiscectomy and decompressive laminectomy to relieve pressure caused by large disc herniations, to segmental spinal fusion, to the implantation of artificial discs; these treatments are reserved more for major orthopedic problems, severe intractable pain, and neurocompression and have variable levels of risk and long-term efficacy.

Nonpharmalogical and nonsurgical treatments traditionally utilized within standard medical protocols include the use of heating pads, bed rest, and general advice for exercise. Impressively and consistent with clinical practice and research results, the new LBP guidelines include recommendations for the use of spinal manipulation in the treatment of acute and chronic low back pain, as well as exercise, massage, acupuncture, yoga, cognitive-behavioral therapy, and progressive relaxation in the treatment of chronic low back pain. Not surprisingly, these guidelines fail to mention concepts and interventions such as nutritional supplementation, proprioceptive rehabilitation, evaluation and treatment of sacroiliac dysfunction and MFTP, and sclerosant prolotherapy. The LBP guidelines note that "herbal therapies, such as devil's claw, willow bark, and capsicum, seem to be safe options for acute exacerbations of chronic low back pain, but benefits range from small to moderate"; these 3 botanical treatments will be detailed below under *Biochemical, Phytonutrient, and Psycho-Emotional Interventions.*

Functional Medicine Considerations

When viewed through the lens of standard medicine, chronic low back pain appears to exist largely as an enigma and conundrum. A paradox exists for this condition, which afflicts such a high percentage of the population and yet which is so poorly understood and often treated with only cursory and transient efficacy. This leads one to wonder whether the problem is with the condition itself or with the lens through which clinicians view the condition. Musculoskeletal competency examinations among physicians trained only in standard medicine have consistently shown the need for increased training in the diagnosis and management of musculoskeletal disorders.[19,20] This monograph serves as a concise introductory review of many evidence-based diagnostic and therapeutic considerations; readers desiring information on other clinical disorders are referred to the outpatient orthopedics text by this author.[21]

How can a common and important problem such as low back pain have remained so enigmatic and recalcitrant to standard medical treatment? The answer to this question must reside in the fact that the solutions to this chronic problem lie outside of the standard *pharmaco-surgical* paradigm. The sole reliance on drugs and surgery for the treatment of this (or any other) condition presupposes that the condition results from a need for those interventions. When doctors are trained to think only about the diagnosis and the corresponding drug, and when doctors fail to seek answers to their clinical questions,[22] the range of considerations for effective management of a particular patient's problem becomes too narrow. When the question asked is, "What is the correct drug or surgery for this patient's low back pain?" then the only answers that will be considered are drugs and surgery. But what if the best answer lies outside this narrow pharmaco-surgical paradigm? With a broadened perspective, we find different questions and therefore different solutions. Let us now explore four questions that open the door to new answers and thus new clinical solutions.

1. **Could chronic low back pain result from undiagnosed vitamin deficiency?** Clearly, the answer to this question is "yes" as demonstrated in the numerous clinical studies showing increased prevalence of vitamin D deficiency among patients with chronic musculoskeletal pain. More impressive than the prevalence and concordance data is the research showing that vitamin D supplementation in deficient patients resolves their pain safely and with efficacy rates greater than 95%. As we would expect, skeletal pain caused by vitamin D deficiency is not amenable to treatment with NSAIDs or surgery, nor would drug and surgical treatment be appropriate for a problem caused by nutritional deficiency that can be treated directly, safely, and inexpensively through correction of the deficiency.

2. **Could chronic low back pain result from undiagnosed fatty acid deficiency or imbalance?** The American/Western diet is notoriously imbalanced with regard to fatty acid intake; the high consumption of saturated, *trans*, and omega-6 fatty acids and the low consumption of omega-3 fatty acids lead to a dramatically skewed ratio.[23] Numerous sources of scientific research in many fields indicate that this dietary pattern contributes to manifold overt and subtle clinical disorders, one of which is chronic low back pain. Several studies have already demonstrated the anti-inflammatory and analgesic benefits of increased omega-3 fatty acid consumption, either via food such as cold-water fish or via supplementation with fish oil. Recently, a clinical trial specific to chronic low back pain was conducted, and results showed that fish oil supplementation as a source of omega-3 eicosapentaenoic acid (EPA) and docosahexaenoic acid (DHA) produced marked reductions in pain and drug use. Shapiro[24] reviewed evidence showing that an important mechanism of action of omega-3 fatty acids is their central neurological effects, such as inhibiting eicosanoid production in glial cells, blocking voltage-gated sodium channels, inhibiting neuronal protein kinases, increasing serotonergic activity, and modulating gene expression; these mechanisms contribute to the observed mood-stabilizing, analgesic, and sympatholytic effects. Thus, by the simple provision of a nutrient lacking in our modern diets, chronic pain is alleviated, and the use of potentially harmful and expensive drugs is likewise reduced.[25]

3. **Could chronic low back pain result from undiagnosed mineral deficiency or acid-alkaline imbalance?** The American/Western diet produces a state of chronic metabolic acidosis resultant from the high consumption of acidogenic foods such as wheat, milk, and chloride (from sodium chloride) and the relatively low consumption of alkalinizing fruits and vegetables.[26] Adverse physiological effects of this diet-induced chronic metabolic acidosis[27] are manifold and significant. Conversely, benefits of a more pH-balanced diet include

prevention and treatment of osteoporosis, age-related muscle wasting, calcium kidney stones, hypertension, exercise-induced asthma, and age- and disease-related chronic renal insufficiency.[28] An acidogenic diet can lead to increased urinary loss of minerals such as calcium and magnesium; the relevance of this finding to the treatment of chronic pain lies in the realization that skeletal and central pain phenomena can result from deficiency of these minerals. Proof of this principle is provided in the pain-relieving effect of alkalinizing, plant-based diets in the treatment of conditions characterized by chronic pain, such as rheumatoid arthritis and fibromyalgia; however, attribution of the analgesic effect of plant-based diets to the restoration of acid-base balance is complicated by the manifold benefits of these diets on (anti)inflammatory, (anti)oxidant, and intestinal microflora status. Thus, a clinical trial of alkalinization *without* dietary change would be necessary to prove that alkalinization alone effected an analgesic benefit. Such a study was conducted by Vormann et al[29] in 2001, in which use of a low-potency, alkalinizing mineral supplement resulted in a 49% reduction in the Arhus low back pain rating scale in 76 of 82 patients with chronic low back pain. Objectively, blood pH-buffering capacity and blood pH both increased slightly but significantly, while intracellular magnesium increased by 11% despite the lack of high-dose magnesium supplementation. As discussed in Chapter 2, magnesium has an analgesic and anti-hyperalgesic function through its ability to partially block N-methyl-D-aspartate-type glutamate receptors, which are important in pain mediation.[30] The researchers were therefore justified in concluding, "The results show that a disturbed acid-base balance may contribute to the symptoms of low back pain. The simple and safe addition of an alkaline multimineral [preparation] was able to reduce the pain symptoms in these patients with chronic low back pain." Outpatient therapeutic alkalinization can be achieved and sustained by use of diet modification and nutritional supplementation via methods detailed by Vasquez[31] and by Minich and Bland.[32]

4. **Could subtle aberrations in proprioceptive function, neuromuscular coordination, and joint motion contribute to chronic low back pain even in patients who are apparently normal, have no history of neurological or musculoskeletal trauma, and whose findings on standard physical examination are normal?** Classic research by Janda and colleagues[33] showed that patients with chronic low back pain have proprioceptive and coordinative deficits in gluteal muscles and that these deficits were readily amenable to in-office training on labile surfaces. These proprioceptive and coordinative deficits in the gluteal muscles are representative of similar deficits in paraspinal muscles, and the reduced pelvic and paraspinal stabilization leads to accumulative microtrauma to the lumbar spine, while also reducing the input from mechanoreceptor neurons which block nociception. The cause of this dynamic *discoordination* is not only the chronic under-training induced by sedentary lifestyles, but also the aforementioned vitamin D deficiency that is common in patients with low back pain. Vitamin D deficiency results in a subtle discoordination effect on the neuromusculoskeletal system, and vitamin D replenishment improves balance and coordination. Indeed, part of the anti-fracture benefit of vitamin D in older patients stems from its dual ability to improve both dynamic and static/postural neuromuscular coordination.[34] Subtle aberrations in proprioception are seen in patients with persistent back pain,[35] and the benefits of manual therapeusis such as chiropractic manipulative therapy may reside at least in part in the ability of these interventions to favorably alter neurocortical processing and proprioceptive-kinesthetic coordination.[36,37,38]

This small sampling of only 4 questions takes us far beyond the restrictions of the pharmaco-surgical paradigm of low back pain treatment. Furthermore, this evidence highlights the error of sole reliance on drugs and surgery for the treatment of low back pain, a condition that more commonly originates from subtle aberrations in function and nutritional status than it does from a disease state requiring external pharmaceutical control or surgical intervention.

Clinical Applications

The above mentioned considerations, along with other interventions, will now be discussed in a clinically oriented format. Taken together, they outline an expanded paradigm for understanding the etiopathogenesis of chronic low back pain, thus illuminating paths for its prevention and amelioration. The 2 broadest categories of treatment are physical and biochemical; in any particular patient, some of these considerations will be more or less relevant or appropriate than others. Generally, several carefully chosen and skillfully implemented interventions should be used simultaneously for maximum improvement.

Biochemical, Phytonutrient, and Psycho-Emotional Interventions

The first large category to be surveyed focuses on biochemical and psycho-emotional considerations, with an emphasis on nutritional status.

Diet, lifestyle, and psycho-emotional considerations — Poor dietary habits can contribute to low back pain via physical (quantitative) and biochemical (qualitative) mechanisms. Quantitative excess of calories increases overall body weight and adiposity (percentage of body weight as adipose tissue). Overweight patients, particularly those with body mass index above 25 kg/m^2 and those who are overweight from a young age, show an increased risk for lumbar intervertebral disc herniation.[39] Obesity changes spinal biomechanics by promoting lumbar hyperlordosis and subsequent increased weight bearing on the facet joints, which are not designed for weight bearing and which become increasingly pain sensitive when stressed. Overweight patients are also more likely than their lean counterparts to lead unhealthy lifestyles characterized by physical inactivity (results in muscle weakness and lack of proprioceptive/sensorimotor coordination),[40] increased use of alcohol (increases risk of nutritional deficiencies), increased use of tobacco (contributes to antioxidant depletion and increased atherosclerosis, which delays healing and reduces tissue maintenance),[41] and mental depression and social isolation[42,43]—each of these factors has shown positive correlation with low back pain.[44,45] The dyslipidemia associated with caloric excess and obesity has been shown to predict and contribute to low back pain via the resultant atherosclerosis; this condition leads to a relative tissue hypoxia and reduced nutrient delivery, thus impairing tissue repair and maintenance and promoting lumbar disc herniation.[46] Adipose tissue elaborates proinflammatory cytokines (*adipokines*) such as tumor necrosis factor-alpha and interleukin-6 and is thus correlated with induction of a low-level chronic inflammatory state.

Thus, obesity, physical inactivity, caloric excess, and unhealthy lifestyle habits synergize to promote pain, inflammation, and physical degeneration—a phenomenon documented for more than 60 years.[47] While each of these factors must be corrected and addressed directly, the overall lifestyle and psycho-emotional outlook must often be "upgraded" in favor of one that promotes and preserves optimal health. Patients frequently face many logistical, financial, and occupational obstacles to their pursuit of health; however, with professional guidance, each patient can also learn to make better choices and to use time and resources in ways that are consistent with the pursuit of health rather than disease. Addressing the psycho-emotional determinants of self-care behavior and general outlook is of paramount importance in the initiation and long-term continuation of health-promoting lifestyle habits.[48] Pain, inflammation, and depression can be promoted by nutritional and lifestyle deficiencies, such as lack of vitamin D, omega-3 fatty acids, magnesium, and exercise; conversely, the incorporation of these factors into the therapeutic regimen can help alleviate physical pain and mental depression without the need for combined antidepressant, anti-inflammatory, and analgesic drugs.

Avoidance of proinflammatory foods — Foods can induce transcription of proinflammatory genes, induce endogenous oxidative stress, and/or provide precursors (especially arachidonate) for the production of proinflammatory mediators. Inducers of genotropic inflammation and oxidative stress include saturated fat such as from cream,[49,50] polyunsaturated fatty acids from corn oil,[51] high-glycemic-index foods such as sugary drinks,[53,52,53] and high-fat, high-carbohydrate fast food meals.[54] Cow's milk, beef, liver, pork, and lamb are rich sources of arachidonic acid, which is the precursor to the inflammatory and hyperalgesic prostaglandins, leukotrienes, and isoprostanes. The easiest means by which to reduce intake of saturated fatty acids and arachidonate is consumption of a vegetarian, pesco-vegetarian, or Paleo-Mediterranean diet; such dietary patterns are consistently associated with reduced overall mortality and morbidity due to inflammation-related disorders.

Consumption of an anti-inflammatory diet — Plant-based diets provide ample quantity and diversity of phytonutrients, which generally have antioxidant and anti-inflammatory benefits; these effects are additive and synergistic, and thus, diversity and quantity are both important determinants of overall effect.[55] Generous consumption of fruits, vegetables, nuts, berries, and seeds should be seen as the foundation of any health-promoting diet, with preference, allergenicity, and caloric considerations modified per patient. Consumption of high-quality protein should be emphasized, with a daily target range between 0.5 and 0.9 g of protein per pound of body weight; the upper range is most appropriate for athletes and those recovering from injury.[56] Low-arachidonate and low-saturated-fat sources of protein include fish, soy, and soy protein and whey protein isolates. Olive oil can be used generously and is a source of natural anti-inflammatory phytochemicals including the fatty acids oleic acid and squalene, in addition to powerful phenolic antioxidants and the compound oleocanthal, which has anti-inflammatory, ibuprofen-like cyclooxygenase-inhibiting activity.[57] The end result is a whole-foods, plant-based, protein-abundant diet with characteristics of the Mediterranean diet and the Paleolithic diet. Atop this foundational diet can be added selected supplements such as vitamin D, fatty acids, and probiotics for the completion of the *supplemented Paleolithic-Mediterranean diet*.[58] For most patients, this dietary pattern corrects the subclinical, pathogenic, chronic, diet-induced metabolic acidosis that results from the typical American/Western diet pattern characterized by acidifying food components such as milk, grains, and chloride.[31] Benefits of alkalinization include enhanced urinary xenobiotic excretion,[59] reduced serum cortisol levels, reduced bone resorption,[30] and alleviation of chronic low back pain.[32]

Fatty acid balance — As mentioned previously, the American/Western diet is notoriously imbalanced when it comes to the types of fatty acids consumed. The most prominent and consistent problems include overconsumption of *trans* and saturated fatty acids in general and linolenic and arachidonic acids in particular. Insufficient consumption of alpha-linolenic acid (ALA), gamma-linolenic acid (GLA), EPA, DHA, and oleic acids exacerbates this imbalance and contributes to a diet-induced proinflammatory state.[60] Correction of this imbalance via the combination of proper diet and supplementation leads to a marked, sustainable, and clinically significant reduction in systemic inflammation and improved clinical outcomes, as demonstrated in patients with inflammation-related conditions ranging from rheumatoid arthritis to cardiovascular disease.

Dietary interventions should emphasize reduced intake of linolenic acid from grain oils and arachidonic acid from animal products (meat and milk), which activate inflammatory pathways and serve as the precursor to prostaglandins and leukotrienes, respectively. Supplementation with GLA provides an anti-inflammatory benefit via inhibition of inflammatory gene transcription, as well as reduced proinflammatory leukotriene formation. Effective doses of GLA used to treat rheumatoid arthritis range from 500 to 3000 mg/d. Consumption of ALA from flaxseed oil and EPA and DHA from fish oil provides important anti-inflammatory effects, with the latter (EPA and DHA) being more potent than the former (ALA). The dose of combined EPA and DHA for adults is generally 1000 mg/d for prevention and 3000 mg/d for intervention. In a recent open trial with data from 125 patients with discogenic low back pain in a neurosurgical practice, 1200 to 2400 mg/d of EPA and DHA was shown to alleviate low back pain. Further, 59% of patients were able to discontinue NSAID use thanks to pain relief from fish oil supplementation; 80% of patients were satisfied with their improvement, and 88% chose to continue treatment.[61] Thus, increased consumption of or supplementation with EPA and DHA safely provides numerous health benefits and helps alleviate inflammatory musculoskeletal pain including low back pain. Ideally, GLA should be coadministered with fish oil to prevent the reduction in GLA and its anti-inflammatory benefits that occurs when only EPA and DHA are administered.[62]

> **Clinical Pearl:**
>
> Many studies using fish oil supplementation have shown that correction of fatty acid deficiency alleviates mental depression and enhances well-being; thus, EPA and DHA deficiency may partly explain the often reported link between mental depression and chronic low back pain.

Vitamin D3 (cholecalciferol) — Patients with chronic low back pain often have balance and proprioceptive deficits, and such deficits may be contributed to by vitamin D deficiency. In these cases, pain may be caused by a combination of peripheral and central mechanisms, but the peripheral mechanisms have been more clearly articulated, namely that vitamin D deficiency causes a failure of mineralization of periosteum and endosteum, both of which are then subject to hydration, swelling, and subsequent compression of highly sensitive nerve fibers.[63] Acting centrally, vitamin D deficiency causes a discoordination effect on the neuromuscular system, resulting in deficits in balance and sensorimotor/proprioceptive coordination that can contribute to microtrauma and falls. Further, the effectiveness of vitamin D in treating pain and depression likely also stems from its benefits on serotonergic and other neurotransmitter pathways.

Vitamin D3 supplementation has been shown to improve sensorimotor coordination, functional performance, reaction time, and balance and thereby prevent falls and recurrent microtrauma.[64] (Vitamin D3 is the human nutrient while vitamin D2 [ergocalciferol] is produced from the irradiation of fungi and should not be used due to its comparatively poor efficacy.[65]) At least 3 studies using vitamin D3 supplementation have shown that correction of deficiency alleviates mental depression and enhances well-being; thus, vitamin D deficiency may partly explain the often reported link between mental depression and chronic low back pain. The retail cost for 3 months of this safe and highly effective intervention (excluding physician fees and any laboratory tests) ranges between $7 and $20; additional benefits of such supplementation include alleviation of hypertension and migraine headaches, as well as an overall reduction in risk for cancer and autoimmune diseases. The physiological requirement for vitamin D3 is approximately 4000 IU/d in adult men.[66] Because dietary sources of vitamin D are insufficient for the provision of physiological amounts of vitamin D3, vitamin D sufficiency can be ensured only by supplementation (approximately 4000 IU to 10 000 IU/d for adults) or full-body sun exposure (20-60 min/d, depending on latitude, cloud cover, and skin pigmentation). (For a review of evidence, as well as the range of optimal serum 25-hydroxy vitamin D3 (25[OH]D) levels, see *Vitamin and Mineral Supplements* in Chapter 2.)

Vitamin C — Generally speaking, people consuming an American/Western diet do not consume sufficient quantities and varieties of fruits and vegetables, which are the primary dietary sources of vitamin C, as well as phytonutrients that have additive and synergistic antioxidant and anti-inflammatory benefits. Vitamin C (ascorbic acid) is required for collagen formation and the healing of injuries, and supplemental vitamin C has proven beneficial in the promotion of wound healing when used alone[67,68] or with other nutrients such as zinc and arginine.[69] James Greenwood, MD, FACS, former clinical professor of neurosurgery at Baylor College of Medicine, reported his experience with over 500 patients with low back pain.[70] Patients were administered up to 1000 mg of vitamin C, either with or without surgical treatment for low back pain. Greenwood wrote, "It can be stated with reasonable assurance that a significant percentage of patients with early disc lesions were able to avoid surgery by the use of large doses of vitamin C … The number of reoperations on the same patients for recurrent at the same level or a new disc lesion at a different level has been greatly reduced." Clinically, we can use more than 1000 mg/d of vitamin C, and we can combine supplemental vitamin C (dose range from 3000 mg to bowel tolerance) with other nutrients such as arginine, copper, and zinc and bioflavonoids and other phytonutrients for an improved tissue-healing, anti-inflammatory, and antioxidant benefit.[71] A large, long-term, 4-arm study comparing ascorbate, ascorbate+phytonutrients, ascorbate+phytonutrients+minerals, and placebo is needed in order to determine effect size and comparable efficacy.

Vitamin B12 — High-dose nutritional supplementation has benefits that extend beyond the mere correction of deficiency; potent metabolic, neurological, and analgesic benefits can often be realized.[72,73] In a double-blind, randomized, placebo-controlled trial involving 60 patients, Mauro et al[74] showed that intramuscular vitamin B12 was safe and effective in the treatment of low back pain among patients with no signs of nutritional deficiency. Compared with placebo, vitamin B12 produced sustained reductions in pain, disability, and paracetamol/acetaminophen use. Vitamin B12 has a wide margin of safety when administered orally or parenterally; allergy and anaphylaxis have rarely been reported.

Botanical medicines and supplements — High doses of botanical preparations have shown efficacy in the nonpharmacological and nonsurgical management of low back pain.

- *Salix* **species (willow bark)** — Numerous studies have validated the analgesic and anti-inflammatory benefits of willow bark extract. Willow bark contains salicylates (also commonly found in fruits, vegetables, teas, and spices) and other phytonutrients with potent anti-inflammatory activity. A double-blind, placebo-controlled study of 210 patients experiencing an exacerbation of chronic low back pain at 5 or more (out of

10) on a visual analog scale found a dose-response relationship with *Salix* treatment (containing 120 mg or 240 mg of salicin); patients in the high-dose group benefited in the first week, and 39% were pain-free by the fourth week, compared to 21% in the low-dose group and only 6% in the placebo group.[75] Another study found 240 mg of salicin to be comparable in effectiveness to 12.5 mg rofecoxib, with the former being 40% less expensive[76] and the latter being withdrawn from the market due to unacceptable cardiovascular risk.[13] Many of the proposed warnings against the use of willow bark[77] have been overinflated and are not based on scientific fact.[78] Aspirin/salicylate allergy is the main and perhaps sole contraindication to willow bark supplementation.

- *Harpagophytum procumbens* (**devil's claw**) — *Harpagophytum* has a long history of use for various ailments including musculoskeletal pain, particularly osteoarthritis and chronic low back pain. Mechanisms of action appear to include a central analgesic action localized at the periaqueductal gray[79] and a peripheral anti-inflammatory effect mediated by inhibition of inflammatory gene transcription via suppression of nuclear factor-kappa B.[80] Harpagoside is generally considered the potent component, yet other cofactors probably also contribute to the botanical's efficacy. (For a review of evidence, see *Botanical Medicines* in Chapter 2.)

- **Topical application of capsaicin** — Capsaicin is the pungent component of *Capsicum annuum* and *Capsicum frutescens,* more commonly known as cayenne pepper or chili pepper. Controlled clinical trials have demonstrated capsaicin's ability to deplete sensory fibers of substance P, thus reducing pain in diabetic neuropathy, chronic low back pain, chronic neck pain, osteoarthritis, rheumatoid arthritis, notalgia paresthetica, reflex sympathetic dystrophy, and cluster headache. In a double-blind, randomized, placebo-controlled, multicenter parallel group study, 320 patients with low back pain were randomly assigned to treatment or placebo groups (160 subjects each); active treatment with capsicum showed superiority that was clinically relevant and highly statistically significant.[81]

- **Intravenous colchicine (extract from *Colchicum autumnale*, autumn crocus, meadow saffron)** — Colchicine is FDA approved for the treatment of gout, familial Mediterranean fever, secondary amyloidosis(AA), and scleroderma. Michael Rask, MD, has been the strongest advocate of the use of intravenous colchicine for the treatment of herniated spinal discs, and his monograph "Colchicine use in 6000 patients with disk disease and other related resistantly-painful spinal disorders"[82] is required reading for any physician interested in implementing this technique clinically. Notably, as part of the intravenous colchicine protocol for patients with disc herniation, Rask advocates (1) treatment of MFTP, (2) weight loss, (3) cessation of alcohol, tobacco, and caffeine, (4) avoidance of *Solanaceae* plants such as eggplant, potato, tomato, and green and red peppers, (5) avoidance of sugars and junk foods, and (6) a strict vegan diet, especially for patients who are overweight. Although Rask notes that colchicine is extremely effective and safe, other authors[83] have been less optimistic, noting that the benefit was often of short duration. Given that intravenous colchicine has been associated with complications such as pancytopenia, organ failure, and death,[84] it is not a treatment to be taken lightly, nor should inexperienced physicians administer it. Intravenous colchicine deserves further study in the treatment of low back pain, particularly as an alternative to surgery in patients with disc herniations. Colchicine preparations for intravenous administration must be manufactured properly in order to avoid complications that can arise from inadvertent overdose.[85]

Physical Interventions

Interventions such as postural correction, muscle stretching, massage, manipulation, proprioceptive/sensorimotor rehabilitation, prolotherapy, and acupuncture may be used in the treatment of chronic low back pain. As with the nutritional and botanical interventions, several of these can be used simultaneously to optimize clinical outcomes.

Maintenance of good posture — Patients with low back pain should be reminded to maintain a relaxed yet erect posture throughout the day while sitting, standing, and doing other activities. Poor posture leads to poor proprioception and impaired sensorimotor coordination. Both Wilson and Granata[86] and Dolan and Green[87] found that after normal subjects sat in a slouched posture for several minutes, their spinal repositioning ability was significantly impaired. This suggests that habituation to a poor posture may contribute directly to impaired sensorimotor coordination, which results in recurrent microtrauma and increased cortical sensitivity to painful stimuli; these adverse effects of impaired sensorimotor coordination will be discussed further below.

Correction of leg-length discrepancy (LLD) — This condition can promote chronic low back pain in some patients by adversely changing spinal biomechanics and inducing a lateral curvature, asymmetric twisting, and compressive forces into all motions undertaken while standing, walking, running, and lifting. LLD is generally categorized as either anatomical or functional, and each must be treated differently. Anatomical discrepancies may occur in the femur, tibia, or talus-calcaneus; mild discrepancies are easily corrected with the use of a heel lift or foot lift applied to the short limb only. A clinical trial found that correction of LLD by use of a heel-lift shoe insert significantly reduced both pain intensity and disability in patients with chronic low back pain, leading the authors to conclude, "Shoe inserts appear to reduce chronic low back pain and functional disability in patients with LLDs of 10 mm or less. Shoe inserts are simple, noninvasive, and inexpensive therapeutic means that can be added to the treatment of chronic low back pain."[88] Functional discrepancies may arise from pelvic torsion, since posterior-inferior rotation of one ilia (referenced to the posterior superior iliac spine) or anterior-superior rotation of the opposite ilia can result in elevation or depression, respectively, of the acetabulum and thus functional shortening or lengthening of the corresponding lower extremity; these cases are treated with manipulation or mobilization of the pelvis to restore symmetry. Although pelvic torque (pelvic obliquity) can be assessed radiographically,[89] clinicians trained in palpatory diagnosis and manipulative medicine can assess pelvic asymmetry with manual and clinical methods that generally obviate the need for and cost and risks of radiographic imaging. As will be discussed below, dysfunction of SIJ is a significant contributor to chronic low back pain via functional LLD induced by pelvic torque.

Therapeutic muscle stretching and treatment of MFTP — Although these trigger points are a well-established clinical entity, their consideration, detection, and treatment are commonly overlooked, perhaps due to the time and effort involved or physicians' lack of training in musculoskeletal diagnosis and treatment.[90] The most simple and effective approach relies on palpatory diagnosis followed by post-isometric stretching. Diagnostic palpatory characteristics of MFTP include the triad of: (1) a tender nodule within a taut band of muscle, (2) exacerbation of pain and referred pain with palpatory provocation, and (3) twitch response following palpatory provocation, which is consistent with the finding of spontaneous electromyographic activity.[91] From a practical clinical standpoint, 2 of these criteria (generally #1 and #2) are sufficient for intervention; a proposed fourth characteristic of positive response to treatment could also substitute. The most common muscles involved by MFTP in patients with chronic low back pain are the gluteus maximus, gluteus medius, psoas, quadratus lumborum, and erector spinae and intrinsic spinal muscles. Tightness of and pain referral from the piriformis can resemble sciatica and is termed *piriformis syndrome*, which can also result from compression or irritation of the nearby sciatic nerve.

Post-isometric stretching was described by Lewit and Simons[92] as follows: "The post-isometric relaxation technique begins by placing the muscle in a stretched position. Then an isometric contraction is exerted against minimal resistance. Relaxation and then gentle stretch follow as the muscle releases." The patient contracts the targeted muscle against resistance for 30 to 60 seconds; the patient then fully relaxes as the muscle is effectively stretched to the maximum safe and tolerable length allowed. This process is repeated 3 to 6 times per session, with deeper and progressive stretching of the muscle serving to relieve the self-perpetuating cycle of muscle contraction and secondary autonomic involvement. MFTP may be adjunctively treated with dietary intervention and nutritional supplementation,[24] dry needling and acupuncture, and injection of saline or anesthetic such as lidocaine or procaine.[93]

Clinical Pearl:

Post-isometric stretching taught by the clinician and then performed autonomously by the patient is an effective and cost-effective treatment that minimizes the cost, psychological and technical dependency, patient passivity, and risk associated with physician-performed and invasive interventions.

Massage — Massage is a popular manual therapy consisting of techniques such as effleurage, petrissage, friction, passive stretching, tapotement, vibration, and compression. In a study comparing the effectiveness of relaxation (n = 12) versus massage (n = 12) for the treatment of chronic low back pain, patients in the massage group achieved less pain, depression, and anxiety; simultaneously, improvements in sleep and range of motion, as well as increased serotonin and dopamine levels (measured in urine), were documented.[94] A randomized controlled trial compared comprehensive massage therapy (n = 25), soft-tissue manipulation only (n = 25), remedial exercise with posture education only (n = 22), or a placebo of sham laser therapy (n = 26); the comprehensive massage therapy (soft-tissue manipulation, remedial exercise, and posture education) group showed improved function and less pain compared with the other 3 groups.[95] Thus, massage therapy is subjectively and objectively effective in reducing pain, stress hormone (neurotransmitter) patterns, functional limitations, and symptoms associated with chronic low back pain. Given the high safety of massage, adverse effects are virtually nonexistent.

Spinal manipulation — Spinal manipulation is a component of the core curriculum in all osteopathic, chiropractic, and naturopathic colleges; students and licensure candidates must demonstrate cognitive and clinical proficiency in manual medicine for graduation and licensure. Osteopathic and naturopathic manipulation places a greater emphasis on low-velocity and soft-tissue techniques, whereas chiropractic manipulation emphasizes high-velocity, low-amplitude procedures directed primarily at restricted articulations. Numerous sources of evidence demonstrate that chiropractic management of low back pain is safer and less expensive than allopathic medical treatment.

- In their extensive review of the literature, Manga et al[96] reported in 1993 that chiropractic management of low back pain is superior to allopathic medical management; they concluded, "There is an overwhelming body of evidence indicating that chiropractic management of low back pain is more cost-effective than medical management" and "there would be highly significant cost savings if more management of low back pain was transferred from medical physicians to chiropractors."
- In a randomized trial involving 741 patients, Meade et al[97] showed that "chiropractic treatment was more effective than hospital outpatient management, mainly for patients with chronic or severe back pain.... The benefit of chiropractic treatment became more evident throughout the follow-up period. Secondary outcome measures also showed that chiropractic was more beneficial." A 3-year follow-up study published by these same authors in 1995,[98] they reported, "at 3 years the results confirm the findings of an earlier report that when chiropractic or hospital therapists treat patients with low back pain as they would in day to day practice, those treated by chiropractic derive more benefit and long term satisfaction than those treated by hospitals."
- In 2004, Legorreta et al[99] reported that the availability of chiropractic care was associated with significant cost savings among 700 000 patients with chiropractic coverage compared to 1 million patients whose insurance coverage was limited to standard medical treatments.
- Dabbs and Lauretti[100] showed that spinal manipulation is safer than NSAIDs in the treatment of neck pain.
- Contrasting the rates of manipulation-associated complications to the risks of pharmacological and surgical treatments for spinal disorders, Rosner[101] noted, "These rates are 400 times lower than the death rates observed from gastrointestinal bleeding due to the use of nonsteroidal anti-inflammatory drugs and 700 times lower than the overall mortality rate for spinal surgery."
- In his review of the literature comparing the safety of chiropractic manipulation in patients with low back pain associated with lumbar disc herniation, Oliphant[102] showed that "the apparent safety of spinal manipulation, especially when compared with other [medically] accepted treatments for [lumbar disk herniation], should stimulate its use in the conservative treatment plan of [lumbar disk herniation]." Of course, manipulative treatment of back pain due to recent disc herniation carries higher risk than manipulative treatment of nondiscogenic back pain; however, the risk-benefit ratio is still favorable for manipulation when performed with proper technique by appropriately trained clinicians.[103,104]

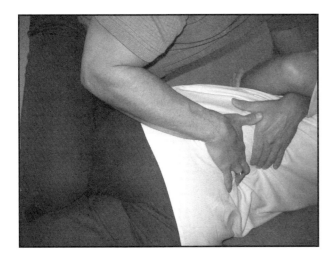 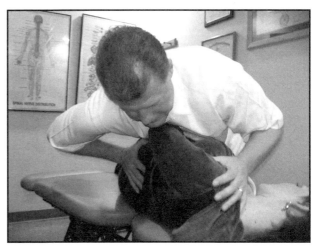

Figure 4.1—Examples of Lumbar Spine Manipulation

These photos demonstrate typical premanipulative positioning in treatment of the lumbar spine. Left, the patient is receiving a level-specific rotational manipulation. Right, the patient is being treated with a technique that delivers a more generalized, nonspecific mobilization of the lumbar spine and paravertebral tissues. Photos reprinted with permission from Vasquez A. *Integrative Orthopedics.*[24]

Spinal manipulation refers to a large, heterogenous group of manual techniques, the implementation of which follows patient history, routine physical examination, neuro-orthopedic examination, and palpatory examination using static and motion palpation for assessment of joint motion, end feel, malpositions, and myofascial lesions such as myospasm, trigger points, tender points, hypertonicity, hypertrophy, atrophy, imbalance, and the detection of somatovisceral or viscerosomatic autonomic phenomena. Segments chosen for manipulative treatment generally show a combination of subjective tenderness and objective aberrancy in motion as determined by the clinician's palpatory skill and experienced judgment. Spinal segmental mobility disturbances (*somatic dysfunction* in the osteopathic literature; *segmental dysfunction* and less commonly *subluxation* in the chiropractic literature[105]) can include segmental rigidity (fixation or motion restriction), segmental hypermobility, and segmental instability; these restrictions or excesses in motion can occur in rotation, flexion, extension, side bending, rotation, or translation at each intervertebral level. Hypermobility and hypomobility can occur in the same segment in different directions. Also, primary segmental dysfunction at one level can be expected to result in a compensatory or secondary dysfunction in a nearby segment; for example, a flexion restriction at L4-L5 might result in a flexion hypermobility/instability at L5-S1 in order to maintain normal range of motion.

Clinicians with training and clinical experience in manual medicine can use specific palpatory manual techniques to detect radiographically documented segmental dysfunction[106,107] and to differentiate the subtlety of treated versus nontreated segments.[108] Palpatory diagnosis provides sufficiently accurate assessment of segmental motion so that patient-specific and dysfunction-specific manipulation or stabilization can be implemented to alleviate pain and improve overall patient outcome.[109] Clinicians can take advantage of the triplanar motion coupling throughout the spine by using manipulative techniques that improve motion in several planes even when delivered primarily through a single plane.[110,111]

High-velocity, low-amplitude spinal manipulation appears to have numerous physical and physiological effects, including but not limited to those listed in Table 4.1. While this list of mechanisms is certainly not exhaustive, for purposes of this discussion, it is sufficient to have established that, indeed, joint manipulation in general and spinal manipulation in particular have objective mechanistic effects that correlate with their clinical benefits. Additional details are provided in numerous published reviews and primary research[112,113,114,115,116,117,118,119] and by Leach,[120] whose extensive documentation of the clinical application of spinal manipulative therapy is unsurpassed. The audible popping or clicking sound common to high-velocity, low-amplitude joint manipulation is due to cavitation (formation of a gas bubble due to the manipulation-induced transient reduction in pressure inside the joint); the sound indicates that rapid mobilization of the joint has occurred, but the sound itself is neither necessary nor sufficient for manipulative success.[121,122]

Table 4.1—Spinal Manipulation: Mechanistic Considerations

- Releasing entrapped intraarticular menisci and synovial folds
- Acutely reducing intradiscal pressure, thus promoting replacement of decentralized disc material
- Stretching of deep periarticular muscles to break the cycle of chronic autonomous muscle contraction by lengthening the muscles and thereby releasing excessive actin-myosin binding
- Promoting restoration of proper kinesthesia and proprioception
- Promoting relaxation of paraspinal muscles by stretching facet joint capsules
- Promoting relaxation of paraspinal muscles via post-activation depression, which is the temporary depletion of contractile neurotransmitters
- Temporarily elevating plasma beta-endorphin
- Temporarily enhancing the phagocytic ability of neutrophils and monocytes
- Activating the diffuse descending pain inhibitory system located at the periaqueductal gray
- Improving neurotransmitter balance and reducing pain (soft-tissue manipulation)

Correction of sacroiliac dysfunction, pelvic torque, and sacral base unleveling — SIJ are important contributors to chronic low back pain, and pelvic torque and sacral base unleveling can induce lateral curvature in the lumbar spine (functional scoliosis) that alters spinal biomechanics and increases the propensity for pain and recurrent injury.[123] A detailed history and palpatory examination are sufficient for diagnosis, and treatment is accomplished with manipulation, mobilization, external stabilization, prolotherapy, cryotherapy, or temporary relief by anesthetic injection.[124] Failure by clinicians to diagnose and treat sacroiliac contributions to chronic low back pain is an important cause of the purported recalcitrance of this condition. Exemplification of this point was made by Weksler et al,[125] who assessed the contribution of SIJ dysfunction to chronic low back pain among 50 patients who had both chronic pain along with diagnostic evidence of lumbar disc herniation (viewed by computed tomography or magnetic resonance imaging); average initial pain rated at 7.8 on a 0-10 scale dropped to 1.3 immediately after fluoroscopic-guided, anesthetic, anti-inflammatory injection (bupivacaine and betamethasone) of one or both SIJ, and 46 patients (92%) had pain levels of 0-3 at 12-week follow-up. This study by is important for at least 3 reasons:

- It shows that low back pain with associated disc herniation does not imply that the low back pain is due to the disc herniation.
- It shows that as many as 92% of patients with what appears to be discogenic lumbalgia actually have low back pain caused by SIJ irritation.
- It shows good correlation of SIJ dysfunction with common orthopedic tests: compression test (94%), thigh thrust/posterior shear test (90%), Yeoman's test (prone hip extension, 88%), and FABER/Patrick's test (80%).

Because of different selection criteria and treatment methods (e.g., use of lidocaine and bupivacaine), the study by Maigne et al[126] showed a lower prevalence of SIJ-induced low back pain; in this study of 54 patients, SIJ was incriminated in 19% of patients as a cause or the major contributor to their chronic low back pain. Overall, most studies show that the prevalence of pain originating from SIJ as the cause of chronic low back is approximately 20%, and thus, SIJ dysfunction is a real and important contributor to the burden of chronic low back pain.[127] Clinicians therefore have an obligation to ensure that the SIJ and pelvis are properly assessed and treated among their patients with low back pain. Treatments for SIJ dysfunction include anesthetic and anti-inflammatory injections, regional soft tissue therapy, manipulation, mobilization, stabilization via muscle strengthening and proprioceptive rehabilitation, and use of a compressive SIJ belt to restrict motion in patients with hypermobility. Specific interventions are based on static and motion findings of SIJ in each individual patient.

Exercise — Exercise programs for the alleviation and prevention of low back pain must contain strengthening, stretching, and coordinating activities. Further, patients with physically demanding occupational or recreational requirements should engage in activity-specific exercises to develop strength, coordination, confidence, and proper technique for their specific activities. Strengthening exercises are characterized by progressive increases in resistance and repetitions, with targeted muscles including rectus abdominis, abdominal obliques and transversus, quadratus lumborum, the erector spinae group, and the lateral and posterior glutei which provide pelvic stability. Ideally, patients should be instructed and supervised for the first few sessions in which they are taught how to exercise the targeted muscles with minimal reliance on gym equipment; equipment dependency is an obstacle to compliance whereas training patients to exercise without equipment facilitates lifestyle integration and minimizes cost and time investment. Clinician follow-up is important for encouraging and maintaining compliance. Asking, "Show me how you do your home exercises" (open-ended, performance-based demonstration) is more informative and revealing than asking the close-ended question, "Have you been doing your home exercises?" Clinicians can access sample exercises described and illustrated online.[128,129,130]

Proprioceptive and sensorimotor rehabilitation — Proprioceptive deficits are common in patients with chronic low back pain, neck pain, knee pain and arthritis, and ankle instability. Poor proprioception leaves joints vulnerable to recurrent microtrauma, and lack of proprioceptive inhibition of nociceptors negates the proposed *gate-control mechanism* of pain inhibition and thus heightens the conscious reception of painful stimuli, which would have otherwise been dampened in the spinal cord. Impaired proprioception must of course lead to impaired sensorimotor coordination; these deficits, along with the resultant abnormalities in muscle firing patterns, are well-documented and contributory problems among patients with chronic low back pain. When analyzed during sensorimotor challenges in a research clinical setting, patients with low back pain showed an absence of normal muscle contractions (rectus abdominis) and asymmetry of contractions (erector spinae and rectus abdominis) compared to normal control patients; these perturbations represent altered proprioception and are consistent with "an abnormality of the neuromuscular loop."[131] Patients with recurrent or chronic low back pain appear to show an increased prevalence of lumbar segmental mobility disorders.[132] The combination of lumbar segmental mobility disorders with deficits in proprioception and neuromuscular coordination would be expected to produce a synergistic effect, increasing the likelihood of recurrent microtrauma to spinal tissues and culminating in arthrosis and accelerated intervertebral disc degeneration, perhaps leading ultimately to overt disc herniation.

A complete protocol for the correction of these biomechanical and neuro-coordinative problems includes:

- Spinal manipulation to restore motion in segmental directions that were previously restricted[133]
- Strengthening exercises to enhance overall dynamic stabilization[134]
- Proprioceptive challenge exercises to strengthen and quicken sensorimotor reflex loops[36]
- Spinal manipulation to improve proprioception and sensorimotor coordination[135]
- Functional exercises to prepare for and protect against occupational and recreational activities[136]
- Nutritional repletion—specifically with vitamin D3—to restore balance and neuromuscular coordination[67]

Dextrose prolotherapy — Dextrose prolotherapy involves the injection of dextrose into lax ligaments for the purpose of stimulating fibrosis; the resultant local collagen deposition strengthens weakened and overstretched ligaments and increases joint stability, compensating for previous injury and local hypermobility or instability. Various names including *sclerosant therapy* and *proliferant treatment* have been used to describe prolotherapy, which has been used in various forms since the time of Hippocrates.[137] Dextrose prolotherapy has shown benefit in the treatment of back pain, knee pain,[138] and thumb-finger osteoarthritis.[139] Beyond its ability to stimulate therapeutic fibrosis, hypertonic dextrose may also alleviate pain through chemoneuromodulatory mechanisms; in a clinical trial using biweekly disc space injection of a solution consisting of 50% dextrose and 0.25% bupivacaine, 43.4% of patients achieved sustained improvement, with an average reduction in pain scores of 71%.[140] A pilot study used a combination intradiscal injection of glucosamine, chondroitin sulfate, hypertonic dextrose, and dimethylsulfoxide; 30 patients with chronic, intractable, discography-reproduced discogenic low back pain of 8.5 years' average duration achieved significant reductions in pain and disability at 12-month follow-up with no serious adverse effects from treatment.[141] Overall, the literature suggests that prolotherapy is safe and effective for the treatment of low back pain, and future research will help delineate the specifics of intervention and patient selection to optimize outcomes.[142]

Acupuncture — Acupuncture is a popular, safe, and effective treatment for chronic low back pain. Mechanisms of acupuncture benefit include endorphin and neurophysiological effects; studies in patients with fibromyalgia have demonstrated increased regional blood flow following acupuncture.[143,144] A meta-analysis published in 2005 concluded, "Acupuncture effectively relieves chronic low back pain."[145] A systematic review also published in 2005 concluded, "For chronic low back pain, acupuncture is more effective for pain relief and functional improvement than no treatment or sham treatment immediately after treatment and in the short-term only … The data suggest that acupuncture and dry-needling may be useful adjuncts to other therapies for chronic low back pain."[146]

Yoga — Related to the previous discussion of therapeutic and self-directed stretching is a recent clinical trial that showed yoga to be superior to aerobic and strengthening exercises, which were superior to an educational self-care booklet for the treatment of low back pain.[147] Clinicians should appreciate that authentic yoga practice involves several components that can contribute to the alleviation of chronic back pain, including stretching, strengthening, balancing, stress reduction, stress modulation, and enhanced affect and confidence, especially when practiced in a positive social environment.

Conclusion and Clinical Approach

Many safe and effective treatments for low back pain lie outside the limitations of the conventional pharmaco-surgical paradigm. Evidence reviewed here on individual treatment components almost certainly underestimates the additive and synergistic benefits realized when these components are used in tailored and orchestrated treatment plans, which more truly reflect functional medicine practice. Such treatment plans generally combine numerous interventions such as fatty acid supplementation, correction of vitamin D deficiency, spinal manipulation, treatment of MFTP, and the use of phytonutritional supplements such as willow bark for the safe and effective treatment of low back pain. In the future, now that individual therapies have been validated, clinical trials should include multiple safe and cost-effective interventions so that the research literature more accurately reflects integrative clinical practice. Such research should be designed or supervised by clinicians with appropriate training in these modalities so that the research provides an authentic representation of clinical reality. In the meantime, based on existing research and with consideration of each patient's unique presentation and possible contraindications, clinicians may reasonably address low back pain with a multifaceted functional medicine approach that seeks to alleviate pain first by correcting the numerous underlying contributors and secondarily through safe and effective symptomatic relief.

References

1. Chou R, Qaseem A, Snow V, et al. Diagnosis and treatment of low back pain: a joint clinical practice guideline from the American College of Physicians and the American Pain Society. Ann Intern Med. 2007;147:478-491.
2. Luo X, Pietrobon R, Sun SX, Liu GG, Hey L.Estimates and patterns of direct health care expenditures among individuals with back pain in the United States. *Spine.* 2004;29:79-86.
3. McBeth J, Jones K. Epidemiology of chronic musculoskeletal pain. *Best Pract Res Clin Rheumatol.* 2007;21:403-425.
4. Lotz JC, Ulrich JA. Innervation, inflammation, and hypermobility may characterize pathologic disc degeneration: review of animal model data. *J Bone Joint Surg Am.* 2006;88(Suppl 2):76-82.
5. Lewit K, Simons DG. Myofascial pain: relief by post-isometric relaxation. *Arch Phys Med Rehabil.* 1984;65:452-456.
6. Lynch JR, Schmale GA, Schaad DC, Leopold SS. Important demographic variables impact the musculoskeletal knowledge and confidence of academic primary care physicians. *J Bone Joint Surg Am.* 2006;88:1589-1595.
7. Freedman KB, Bernstein J. The adequacy of medical school education in musculoskeletal medicine. *J Bone Joint Surg Am.* 1998;80:1421-1427.
8. Schmale GA. More evidence of educational inadequacies in musculoskeletal medicine. *Clin Orthop Relat Res.* 2005;(437):251-259.
9. Singh G. Recent considerations in nonsteroidal anti-inflammatory drug gastropathy. *Am J Med.* 1998;105(1B):31S-38S.
10. Topol EJ. Failing the public health: rofecoxib, Merck, and the FDA. *N Engl J Med.* 2004;351:1707-1709.
11. Sooriakumaran P. COX-2 inhibitors and the heart: are all coxibs the same? *Postgrad Med J.* 2006;82(966):242-245.
12. Brandt KD. Effects of nonsteroidal anti-inflammatory drugs on chondrocyte metabolism in vitro and in vivo. *Am J Med.* 1987;83(5A):29-34.
13. Prathapkumar KR, Smith I, Attara GA. Indomethacin induced avascular necrosis of head of femur. *Postgrad Med J.* 2000;76(899):574-575.
14. Newman NM, Ling RS. Acetabular bone destruction related to non-steroidal anti-inflammatory drugs. *Lancet.* 1985;2(8445):11-14.

15. Vidal y Plana RR, Bizzarri D, Rovati AL. Articular cartilage pharmacology: I. In vitro studies on glucosamine and non steroidal antiinflammatory drugs. *Pharmacol Res Commun*. 1978;10:557-569.

16. Singh G. Recent considerations in nonsteroidal anti-inflammatory drug gastropathy. *Am J Med*. 1998;105(1B):31S-38S.

17. Memorandum from David J. Graham, MD, MPH, Associate Director for Science, Office of Drug Safety to Paul Seligman, MD, MPH, Acting Director, Office of Drug Safety entitled, "Risk of Acute Myocardial Infarction and Sudden Cardiac Death in Patients Treated with COX-2 Selective and Non-Selective NSAIDs." September 30, 2004. Available online at: http://www.fda.gov/cder/drug/infopage/vioxx/vioxxgraham.pdf. Accessed December 13, 2007.

18. Martell BA, O'Connor PG, Kerns RD, et al. Systematic review: opioid treatment for chronic back pain: prevalence, efficacy, and association with addiction. *Ann Intern Med*. 2007;146:116-127.

19. Freedman KB, Bernstein J. Educational deficiencies in musculoskeletal medicine. *J Bone Joint Surg Am*. 2002;84-A(4):604-608.

20. Matzkin E, Smith ME, Freccero CD, Richardson AB. Adequacy of education in musculoskeletal medicine. *J Bone Joint Surg Am*. 2005;87-A(2):310-314.

21. Vasquez A. *Integrative Orthopedics*. 2nd ed. Fort Worth, Tex: Integrative and Biological Medicine Research and Consulting; 2007.

22. Ely JW, Osheroff JA, Ebell MH, et al. Analysis of questions asked by family doctors regarding patient care. *BMJ*. 1999;319(7206):358-361.

23. Simopoulos AP. Essential fatty acids in health and chronic disease. *Am J Clin Nutr*. 1999;70(Suppl 3):560S-569S.

24. Shapiro H. Could n-3 polyunsaturated fatty acids reduce pathological pain by direct actions on the nervous system? *Prostaglandins Leukot Essent Fatty Acids*. 2003;68:219-224.

25. Ausman JI. Why omega-3 fatty acids are important to neurosurgeons. *Surg Neurol*. 2006;65:325.

26. Jehle S, Zanetti A, Muser J, Hulter HN, Krapf R. Partial neutralization of the acidogenic Western diet with potassium citrate increases bone mass in postmenopausal women with osteopenia. *J Am Soc Nephrol*. 2006;17:3213-3222.

27. Maurer M, Riesen W, Muser J, Hulter HN, Krapf R. Neutralization of Western diet inhibits bone resorption independently of K intake and reduces cortisol secretion in humans. *Am J Physiol Renal Physiol*. 2003;284(1):F32-40.

28. Cordain L, Eaton SB, Sebastian A, et al. Origins and evolution of the Western diet: health implications for the 21st century. *Am J Clin Nutr*. 2005;81:341-354.

29. Vormann J, Worlitschek M, Goedecke T, Silver B. Supplementation with alkaline minerals reduces symptoms in patients with chronic low back pain. *J Trace Elem Med Biol*. 2001;15(2-3):179-183.

30. Park JH, Niermann KJ, Olsen N. Evidence for metabolic abnormalities in the muscles of patients with fibromyalgia. *Curr Rheumatol Rep*. 2000;2:131-140.

31. Vasquez A. *Integrative Rheumatology*. 2nd ed. Fort Worth, Tex: Integrative and Biological Medicine Research and Consulting; 2007.

32. Minich DM, Bland JS. Acid-alkaline balance: role in chronic disease and detoxification. *Altern Ther Health Med*. 2007;13:62-65.

33. Bullock-Saxton JE, Janda V, Bullock MI. Reflex activation of gluteal muscles in walking. An approach to restoration of muscle function for patients with low back pain. *Spine*. 1993;18:704-708.

34. Bischoff-Ferrari HA, Conzelmann M, Stähelin HB, et al. Is fall prevention by vitamin D mediated by a change in postural or dynamic balance? *Osteoporos Int*. 2006;17:656-663.

35. Gill KP, Callaghan MJ. The measurement of lumbar proprioception in individuals with and without low back pain. *Spine*. 1998;23:371-377.

36. Haavik-Taylor H, Murphy B. Cervical spine manipulation alters sensorimotor integration: a somatosensory evoked potential study. *Clin Neurophysiol*. 2007;118:391-402.

37. Rogers RG. The effects of spinal manipulation on cervical kinesthesia in patients with chronic neck pain: a pilot study. *J Manipulative Physiol Ther*. 1997;20:80-85.

38. Palmgren PJ, Sandström PJ, Lundqvist FJ, Heikkilä H. Improvement after chiropractic care in cervicocephalic kinesthetic sensibility and subjective pain intensity in patients with nontraumatic chronic neck pain. *J Manipulative Physiol Ther*. 2006;29:100-106.

39. Liuke M, Solovieva S, Lamminen A, et al. Disc degeneration of the lumbar spine in relation to overweight. *Int J Obes (Lond)*. 2005;29:903-908.

40. Verbunt JA, Seelen HA, Vlaeyen JW, et al. Disuse and deconditioning in chronic low back pain: concepts and hypotheses on contributing mechanisms. *Eur J Pain*. 2003;7:9-21.

41. John U, Meyer C, Rumpf HJ, Hapke U. Relationships of psychiatric disorders with overweight and obesity in an adult general population. *Obes Res*. 2005;13:101-109.

42. Strauss RS, Pollack HA. Social marginalization of overweight children. *Arch Pediatr Adolesc Med*. 2003;157:746-752.

43. Sjöberg RL, Nilsson KW, Leppert J. Obesity, shame, and depression in school-aged children: a population-based study. *Pediatrics*. 2005;116(3):e389-392.

44. Dunn KM, Croft PR. Epidemiology and natural history of low back pain. *Eura Medicophys*. 2004;40:9-13.

45. Rubin DI. Epidemiology and risk factors for spine pain. *Neurol Clin*. 2007;25:353-371.

46. Leino-Arjas P, Kaila-Kangas L, Solovieva S, Riihimäki H, Kirjonen J, Reunanen A. Serum lipids and low back pain: an association? A follow-up study of a working population sample. *Spine*. 2006;31:1032-1037.

47. Price WA. *Nutrition and Physical Degeneration: A Comparison of Primitive and Modern Diets and Their Effects*. Santa Monica, Calif: Price-Pottinger Nutrition Foundation; 1945.

48. Prochaska JO, Norcross JC, DiClemente CC. *Changing for Good: A Revolutionary Six-Stage Program for Overcoming Bad Habits and Moving Your Life*. New York, NY: William Morrow and Company; 1994.

49. Lee JY, Sohn KH, Rhee SH, Hwang D. Saturated fatty acids, but not unsaturated fatty acids, induce the expression of cyclooxygenase-2 mediated through toll-like receptor 4. *J Biol Chem*. 2001;276(20):16683-16689.

50. Mohanty P, Ghanim H, Hamouda W, Aljada A, Garg R, Dandona P. Both lipid and protein intakes stimulate increased generation of reactive oxygen species by polymorphonuclear leukocytes and mononuclear cells. *Am J Clin Nutr*. 2002;75:767-772.

51. Rusyn I, Bradham CA, Cohn L, et al. Corn oil rapidly activates nuclear factor-kappaB in hepatic Kupffer cells by oxidant-dependent mechanisms. *Carcinogenesis*. 1999;20(11):2095-2100.

52. Mohanty P, Hamouda W, Garg R, Aljada A, Ghanim H, Dandona P. Glucose challenge stimulates reactive oxygen species (ROS) generation by leucocytes. *J Clin Endocrinol Metab*. 2000 Aug;85(8):2970-3.

53. Koska J, Blazicek P, Marko M, Grna JD, Kvetnansky R, Vigas M. Insulin, catecholamines, glucose and antioxidant enzymes in oxidative damage during different loads in healthy humans. *Physiol Res*. 2000;49(Suppl 1):S95-100.

54. Aljada A, Mohanty P, Ghanim H, et al. Increase in intranuclear nuclear factor kappaB and decrease in inhibitor kappaB in mononuclear cells after a mixed meal: evidence for a proinflammatory effect. *Am J Clin Nutr.* 2004;79:682-690.

55. Liu RH. Health benefits of fruit and vegetables are from additive and synergistic combinations of phytochemicals. *Am J Clin Nutr.* 2003;78(Suppl 3):517S-520S.

56. Clark N. The power of protein. *The Physician and Sportsmedicine.* 1996;24. Available online at: http://www.physsportsmed.com/issues/1996/04_96/protein.htm.

57. Beauchamp GK, Keast RS, Morel D, et al. Phytochemistry: ibuprofen-like activity in extra-virgin olive oil. *Nature.* 2005;437(7055):45-46.

58. Vasquez A. A Five-part nutritional protocol that produces consistently positive results. *Nutritional Wellness.* September 2005. Available online: http://optimalhealthresearch.com/protocol.

59. Proudfoot AT, Krenzelok EP, Vale JA. Position Paper on urine alkalinization. *J Toxicol Clin Toxicol.* 2004;42:1-26.

60. Seaman DR. The diet-induced proinflammatory state: a cause of chronic pain and other degenerative diseases? *J Manipulative Physiol Ther.* 2002;25:168-179.

61. Maroon JC, Bost JW. Omega-3 fatty acids (fish oil) as an anti-inflammatory: an alternative to nonsteroidal anti-inflammatory drugs for discogenic pain. *Surg Neurol.* 2006;65:326-331.

62. Cleland LG, Gibson RA, Neumann M, French JK. The effect of dietary fish oil supplement upon the content of dihomo-gammalinolenic acid in human plasma phospholipids. *Prostaglandins Leukot Essent Fatty Acids.* 1990;40:9-12.

63. Holick MF. Vitamin D deficiency: what a pain it is. *Mayo Clin Proc.* 2003;78:1457-1459.

64. Dhesi JK, Jackson SH, Bearne LM, et al. Vitamin D supplementation improves neuromuscular function in older people who fall. *Age Ageing.* 2004;33:589-595.

65. Armas LA, Hollis BW, Heaney RP. Vitamin D2 is much less effective than vitamin D3 in humans. *J Clin Endocrinol Metab.* 2004;89:5387-5391.

66. Heaney RP, Davies KM, Chen TC, Holick MF, Barger-Lux MJ. Human serum 25-hydroxycholecalciferol response to extended oral dosing with cholecalciferol. *Am J Clin Nutr.* 2003;77:204-210.

67. Collins N. Adding vitamin C to the wound management mix. *Adv Skin Wound Care.* 2004;17:109-112.

68. Taylor TV, Rimmer S, Day B, Butcher J, Dymock IW. Ascorbic acid supplementation in the treatment of pressure-sores. *Lancet.* 1974;2(7880):544-546.

69. Desneves KJ, Todorovic BE, Cassar A, Crowe TC. Treatment with supplementary arginine, vitamin C and zinc in patients with pressure ulcers: a randomised controlled trial. *Clin Nutr.* 2005;24:979-987.

70. Greenwood J. Optimum vitamin C intake as a factor in the preservation of disc integrity. *Med Ann Dist Columbia.* 1964;33:274-276.

71. MacKay D, Miller AL. Nutritional support for wound healing. *Altern Med Rev.* 2003;8:359-377.

72. Ames BN, Elson-Schwab I, Silver EA. High-dose vitamin therapy stimulates variant enzymes with decreased coenzyme binding affinity (increased K(m)): relevance to genetic disease and polymorphisms. *Am J Clin Nutr.* 2002;75:616-658.

73. Newbold HL. Vitamin B-12: placebo or neglected therapeutic tool? *Med Hypotheses.* 1989;28:155-164.

74. Mauro GL, Martorana U, Cataldo P, Brancato G, Letizia G. Vitamin B12 in low back pain: a randomised, double-blind, placebo-controlled study. *Eur Rev Med Pharmacol Sci.* 2000;4:53-58.

75. Chrubasik S, Eisenberg E, Balan E, Weinberger T, Luzzati R, Conradt C. Treatment of low back pain exacerbations with willow bark extract: a randomized double-blind study. *Am J Med.* 2000;109:9-14.

76. Chrubasik S, Kunzel O, Model A, Conradt C, Black A. Treatment of low back pain with a herbal or synthetic anti-rheumatic: a randomized controlled study. Willow bark extract for low back pain. *Rheumatology* (Oxford). 2001;40:1388-1393.

77. Vasquez A, Muanza DN. Comment: Evaluation of presence of aspirin-related warnings with willow bark. *Ann Pharmacotherapy.* 2005;39:1763.

78. Clauson KA, Santamarina ML, Buettner CM, Cauffield JS. Evaluation of presence of aspirin-related warnings with willow bark. *Ann Pharmacother.* 2005;39(7-8):1234-1237.

79. Shin MC, Chang HK, Jan MH, Kim CJ, Kim Y, Kim EH. Modulation of Harpagophytum procumbens on ion channels in acutely dissociated periaquideuctal gray neurons of rats. *Korean Journal of Meridian and Acupoint.* 2003;20;17-29.

80. Huang TH, Tran VH, Duke RK, et al. Harpagoside suppresses lipopolysaccharide-induced iNOS and COX-2 expression through inhibition of NF-kappa B activation. *J Ethnopharmacol.* 2006;104(1-2):149-155.

81. Keitel W, Frerick H, Kuhn U, Schmidt U, Kuhlmann M, Bredehorst A. Capsicum pain plaster in chronic non-specific low back pain. *Arzneimittelforschung.* 2001;51:896-903.

82. Rask MR. Colchicine use in 6,000 patients with disk disease and other related resistantly-painful spinal disorders. *Journal of Neurological and Orthopaedic Medicine and Surgery.* 1989;10:291-298.

83. Simmons JW, Harris WP, Koulisis CW, Kimmich SJ. Intravenous colchicine for low back pain: a double-blind study. *Spine.* 1990;15:716-717.

84. Levy M, Spino M, Read SE. Colchicine: a state-of-the-art review. *Pharmacotherapy.* 1991;11:196-211.

85. Centers for Disease Control and Prevention (CDC). Deaths from intravenous colchicine resulting from a compounding pharmacy error: Oregon and Washington, 2007. MMWR Morb Mortal Wkly Rep. 2007;56(40):1050-1052.

86. Wilson SE, Granata KP. Reposition sense of lumbar curvature with flexed and asymmetric lifting postures. *Spine.* 2003;28:513-518.

87. Dolan KJ, Green A. Lumbar spine reposition sense: the effect of a 'slouched' posture. *Man Ther.* 2006;11:202-207.

88. Defrin R, Ben Benyamin S, Aldubi RD, Pick CG. Conservative correction of leg-length discrepancies of 10mm or less for the relief of chronic low back pain. *Arch Phys Med Rehabil.* 2005;86:2075-2080.

89. Fann AV. Validation of postural radiographs as a way to measure change in pelvic obliquity. *Arch Phys Med Rehabil.* 2003;84:75-78.

90. Joy EA, Hala SV. Musculoskeletal curricula in medical education: Filling in the missing pieces. *The Physician and Sportsmedicine.* 2004;32:42-45.

91. Hubbard DR, Berkoff GM. Myofascial trigger points show spontaneous needle EMG activity. *Spine.* 1993;18:1803-1807.

92. Lewit K, Simons DG. Myofascial pain: relief by post-isometric relaxation. *Arch Phys Med Rehabil.* 1984;65:452-456.

93. Alvarez DJ, Rockwell PG. Trigger points: diagnosis and management. *Am Fam Physician.* 2002;65:653-660.

94. Hernandez-Reif M, Field T, Krasnegor J, Theakston H. Lower back pain is reduced and range of motion increased after massage therapy. *Int J Neurosci.* 2001;106(3-4):131-145.

95. Preyde M. Effectiveness of massage therapy for subacute low-back pain: a randomized controlled trial. *CMAJ.* 2000;162:1815-1820.

96. Manga P, Angus DE, Papadopoulos C, Swan WR. *The Effectiveness and Cost-Effectiveness of Chiropractic Management of Low-Back Pain.* Richmond Hill, Ontario: Kenilworth Publishing; 1993.

97. Meade TW, Dyer S, Browne W, Townsend J, Frank AO. Low-back pain of mechanical origin: randomised comparison of chiropractic and hospital outpatient treatment. *BMJ*. 1990;300(6737):1431-1437.

98. Meade TW, Dyer S, Browne W, Frank AO. Randomised comparison of chiropractic and hospital outpatient management for low-back pain: results from extended follow up. *BMJ*. 1995;311(7001):349-345.

99. Legorreta AP, Metz RD, Nelson CF, Ray S, Chernicoff HO, Dinubile NA. Comparative analysis of individuals with and without chiropractic coverage: patient characteristics, utilization, and costs. *Arch Intern Med*. 2004;164:1985-1992.

100. Dabbs V, Lauretti .WJ. A risk assessment of cervical manipulation vs. NSAIDs for the treatment of neck pain. *J Manipulative Physiol Ther*. 1995;18:530-536.

101. Rosner AL. Evidence-based clinical guidelines for the management of acute low-back pain: response to the guidelines prepared for the Australian Medical Health and Research Council. *J Manipulative Physiol Ther*. 2001;24:214-220.

102. Oliphant D. Safety of spinal manipulation in the treatment of lumbar disk herniations: a systematic review and risk assessment. *J Manipulative Physiol Ther*. 2004;27:197-210.

103. Quon JA, Cassidy JD, O'Connor SM, Kirkaldy-Willis WH. Lumbar intervertebral disc herniation: treatment by rotational manipulation. *J Manipulative Physiol Ther*. 1989;12:220-227.

104. Souza TA. *Differential Diagnosis for the Chiropractor: Protocols and Algorithms*. Gaithersburg: Aspen Publications; 1997: 108, 130.

105. Keating JC Jr, Charlton KH, Grod JP, Perle SM, Sikorski D, Winterstein JF. Subluxation: dogma or science? *Chiropr Osteopat*. 2005;13:17.

106. Abbott JH, McCane B, Herbison P, Moginie G, Chapple C, Hogarty T. Lumbar segmental instability: a criterion-related validity study of manual therapy assessment. *BMC Musculoskelet Disord*. 2005;6:56.

107. Humphreys BK, Delahaye M, Peterson CK. An investigation into the validity of cervical spine motion palpation using subjects with congenital block vertebrae as a 'gold standard.' *BMC Musculoskelet Disord*. 2004;5:19.

108. Hansen BE, Simonsen T, Leboeuf-Yde C. Motion palpation of the lumbar spine: a problem with the test or the tester? *J Manipulative Physiol Ther*. 2006;29:208-212.

109. Fritz JM, Whitman JM, Childs JD. Lumbar spine segmental mobility assessment: an examination of validity for determining intervention strategies in patients with low back pain. *Arch Phys Med Rehabil*. 2005;86:1745-1752.

110. Tsung BY, Evans J, Tong P, Lee RY. Measurement of lumbar spine loads and motions during rotational mobilization. *J Manipulative Physiol Ther*. 2005;28:238-244.

111. Lee RY. Kinematics of rotational mobilisation of the lumbar spine. *Clin Biomech (Bristol, Avon)*. 2001;16:481-488.

112. Maigne JY, Vautravers P. Mechanism of action of spinal manipulative therapy. *Joint Bone Spine*. 2003;70:336-341.

113. Brennan PC, Triano JJ, McGregor M, Kokjohn K, Hondras MA, Brennan DC. Enhanced neutrophil respiratory burst as a biological marker for manipulation forces: duration of the effect and association with substance P and tumor necrosis factor. *J Manipulative Physiol Ther*. 1992;15:83-89.

114. Brennan PC, Kokjohn K, Kaltinger CJ, et al. Enhanced phagocytic cell respiratory burst induced by spinal manipulation: potential role of substance P. *J Manipulative Physiol Ther*. 1991;14:399-408.

115. Heikkila H, Johansson M, Wenngren BI. Effects of acupuncture, cervical manipulation and NSAID therapy on dizziness and impaired head repositioning of suspected cervical origin: a pilot study. *Man Ther*. 2000;5:151-157.

116. Rogers RG. The effects of spinal manipulation on cervical kinesthesia in patients with chronic neck pain: a pilot study. *J Manipulative Physiol Ther*. 1997;20:80-85.

117. Bergmann TF, Peterson DH, Lawrence DJ. *Chiropractic Technique*. New York, NY: Churchill Livingstone; 1993.

118. Herzog WH. Mechanical and physiological responses to spinal manipulative treatments. *JNMS*. 1995;3:1-9.

119. Sung PS, Kang YM, Pickar JG. Effect of spinal manipulation duration on low threshold mechanoreceptors in lumbar paraspinal muscles: a preliminary report. *Spine*. 2005;30:115-122.

120. Leach RA, ed. *The Chiropractic Theories: A Textbook of Scientific Research*. 4th ed. Baltimore, Md: Lippincott, Williams & Wilkins; 2004.

121. Flynn TW, Fritz JM, Wainner RS, Whitman JM. The audible pop is not necessary for successful spinal high-velocity thrust manipulation in individuals with low back pain. *Arch Phys Med Rehabil*. 2003;84:1057-1060.

122. Flynn TW, Childs JD, Fritz JM. The audible pop from high-velocity thrust manipulation and outcome in individuals with low back pain. *J Manipulative Physiol Ther*. 2006;29:40-45.

123. Juhl JH, Ippolito Cremin TM, Russell G. Prevalence of frontal plane pelvic postural asymmetry, part 1. *J Am Osteopath Assoc*. 2004;104:411-421.

124. Forst SL, Wheeler MT, Fortin JD, Vilensky JA. The sacroiliac joint: anatomy, physiology and clinical significance. *Pain Physician*. 2006;9:61-67.

125. Weksler N, Velan GJ, Semionov M, et al. The role of sacroiliac joint dysfunction in the genesis of low back pain: the obvious is not always right. *Arch Orthop Trauma Surg*. 2007;127:885-888.

126. Maigne JY, Aivaliklis A, Pfefer F. Results of sacroiliac joint double block and value of sacroiliac pain provocation tests in 54 patients with low back pain. *Spine*. 1996;21:1889-1892.

127. Cohen SP. Sacroiliac joint pain: a comprehensive review of anatomy, diagnosis, and treatment. *Anesth Analg*. 2005;101:1440-1453.

128. Drezner JA, Herring SA. Exercises in the treatment of low-back pain. *Physician and Sportsmedicine Online*. 2001;29. Available online at: http://www.physssportsmed.com/issues/2001/08_01/pa_drezner.htm.

129. Kuritzky L, White J. Extend yourself for low-back pain relief. *Physician and Sportsmedicine Online*. 1997;25. Available online at: http://www.physssportsmed.com/issues/1997/01jan/back_pa.htm.

130. Shiple B. Relieving low-back pain with exercise. *Physician and Sportsmedicine Online*. 1997;25. Available online at: http://www.physssportsmed.com/issues/1997/08aug/shiplepa.htm.

131. Newcomer KL, Jacobson TD, Gabriel DA, Larson DR, Brey RH, An KN. Muscle activation patterns in subjects with and without low back pain. *Arch Phys Med Rehabil*. 2002;83:816-821.

132. Abbott JH, Fritz JM, McCane B, et al. Lumbar segmental mobility disorders: comparison of two methods of defining abnormal displacement kinematics in a cohort of patients with non-specific mechanical low back pain. *BMC Musculoskelet Disord*. 2006;7:45.

133. Haas M, Panzer D, Peterson D, Raphael R. Short-term responsiveness of manual thoracic end-play assessment to spinal manipulation: a randomized controlled trial of construct validity. *J Manipulative Physiol Ther*. 1995;18:582-589.

134. McGill SM. Low back stability: from formal description to issues for performance and rehabilitation. *Exerc Sport Sci Rev*. 2001;29:26-31.

135. Ferreira ML, Ferreira PH, Hodges PW. Changes in postural activity of the trunk muscles following spinal manipulative therapy. *Man Ther*. 2007;12:240-248.

136. Demoulin C, Distrée V, Tomasella M, Crielaard JM, Vanderthommen M. Lumbar functional instability: a critical appraisal of the literature. *Ann Readapt Med Phys*. 2007;50:677-684.

137. Mooney V. Prolotherapy at the fringe of medical care, or is it the frontier? *Spine J*. 2003;3:253-254.

138. Reeves KD, Hassanein K. Randomized prospective double-blind placebo-controlled study of dextrose prolotherapy for knee osteoarthritis with or without ACL laxity. *Altern Ther Health Med*. 2000;6:68-74, 77-80.

139. Reeves KD, Hassanein K. Randomized, prospective, placebo-controlled double-blind study of dextrose prolotherapy for osteoarthritic thumb and finger (DIP, PIP, and trapeziometacarpal) joints: evidence of clinical efficacy. *J Altern Complement Med*. 2000;6:311-320.

140. Miller MR, Mathews RS, Reeves KD. Treatment of painful advanced internal lumbar disc derangement with intradiscal injection of hypertonic dextrose. *Pain Physician*. 2006;9:115-121.

141. Klein RG, Eek BC, O'Neill CW, Elin C, Mooney V, Derby RR. Biochemical injection treatment for discogenic low back pain: a pilot study. *Spine J*. 2003;3:220-226.

142. Dagenais S, Haldeman S, Wooley JR. Intraligamentous injection of sclerosing solutions (prolotherapy) for spinal pain: a critical review of the literature. *Spine J*. 2005;5:310-328.

143. Sandberg M, Larsson B, Lindberg LG, Gerdle B. Different patterns of blood flow response in the trapezius muscle following needle stimulation (acupuncture) between healthy subjects and patients with fibromyalgia and work-related trapezius myalgia. *Eur J Pain*. 2005;9:497-510.

144. Sandberg M, Lindberg LG, Gerdle B. Peripheral effects of needle stimulation (acupuncture) on skin and muscle blood flow in fibromyalgia. *Eur J Pain*. 2004;8:163-171.

145. Manheimer E, White A, Berman B, Forys K, Ernst E. Meta-analysis: acupuncture for low back pain. *Ann Intern Med*. 2005;142:651-663.

146. Furlan AD, van Tulder M, Cherkin D, et al. Acupuncture and dry-needling for low back pain: an updated systematic review within the framework of the cochrane collaboration. *Spine*. 2005;30:944-963.

147. Sherman KJ, Cherkin DC, Erro J, Miglioretti DL, Deyo RA. Comparing yoga, exercise, and a self-care book for chronic low back pain: a randomized, controlled trial. *Ann Intern Med*. 2005;143:849-856.

Chapter 5

Clinical Focus: Fibromyalgia

Introduction

Fibromyalgia is commonly described as an idiopathic syndrome principally characterized by widespread body pain and numerous tender points at specific locations. The condition is most common in women 20 to 50 years old and often presents with associated complaints of fatigue, headaches, subjective numbness, altered sleep patterns, and gastrointestinal disturbances. Fibromyalgia in children and adolescents presents similarly to fibromyalgia in adults except for the comparatively higher prevalence of sleep disturbance and the finding of fewer tender points.[1] Until recently, fibromyalgia was considered a diagnosis of exclusion after inflammation, autoimmunity, or other primary causes were ruled out by clinical and laboratory assessment. However, current criteria base the diagnosis on positive findings of chronic, widespread musculoskeletal pain in characteristic locations; these criteria will be described below. Fibromyalgia shares several clinical and demographic features with chronic fatigue syndrome (CFS) and irritable bowel syndrome (IBS); the reason for these overlaps is not generally understood by most clinicians and researchers but will be made plain here.

The prevailing medical view, expressed by clinicians and the authors of widely cited articles, is that fibromyalgia is idiopathic with strong neuropsychogenic influences and that, since the underlying causes of the condition have not been identified, the best therapeutic approach is symptom suppression via perpetual pharmacotherapy with adjunctive use of psychotherapy and limited exercise.[2,3] The term *syndrome* connotes that a cluster of symptoms is of a nonorganic, psychogenic, or idiopathic nature, whereas *disease* validates the organic and pathophysiological nature of an illness. This author advocates the use of disease rather than syndrome when describing fibromyalgia in appreciation of the real, organic, biochemical, and histopathological findings which clearly indicate that fibromyalgia is a specific disease entity and not simply a psychogenic or enigmatic cluster of symptoms. If fibromyalgia is a real, organic clinical entity (as will be documented here), then the appropriate designation is fibromyalgia disease (FMD) rather than fibromyalgia syndrome (FMS), as previously and commonly used in the biomedical literature. For consistency and clarity within this monograph, the general term *fibromyalgia* will be used.

Pathophysiology

Muscle biopsies from patients with fibromyalgia show numerous histological, ultrastructural, and biochemical abnormalities, including defects in mitochondrial structure and function, reduced numbers of capillaries in skeletal muscle, thickened capillary endothelium, and ragged red fibers consistent with the development of mitochondrial myopathy. The histological finding of rubber-band morphology, with reticular threads connecting neighboring cells in muscle biopsies of fibromyalgia patients, is associated with prolonged contractions in adjacent muscle fibers, resulting in a low-energy state within myocytes.[4] Other studies have shown disorganization of actin filaments, accumulation of lipofuscin bodies consistent with premature muscle aging, accumulation of glycogen and lipids consistent with mitochondrial impairment, significant reductions in the number of mitochondria, increased DNA fragmentation, and focal areas of chronic muscle contraction.[5]

Despite the importance of these histological abnormalities, and consistent with the view that fibromyalgia is a disease of metabolic dysfunction rather than tissue destruction, ultrastructural and biochemical abnormalities appear to be more relevant and consistent than obvious histological changes in skeletal muscle biopsy samples.

- Numerous mitochondrial enzyme defects are seen, including reduced activity of 3-hydroxy-CoA dehydrogenase, citrate synthase, and cytochrome oxidase. Levels of free magnesium have been shown to be reduced by 31%, and levels of complexed ATP-magnesium reduced by 12% in muscle from fibromyalgia patients compared with healthy controls[6]; these defects contribute to rapid-onset fatigue and muscle pain. From a neurological perspective, magnesium deficiency promotes hypersensitivity to pain due to a reduction in the partial blockade of N-methyl-D-aspartate (NMDA) neurotransmitter receptor sites.[6] Reduced perfusion of muscle tissue during exercise results in relative tissue hypoxia, reduced muscle healing, and promotion of muscle soreness due to accumulation of lactate.[7]
- Increased oxidative stress is also seen in fibromyalgia patients,[8] providing additional evidence of the systemic and non-psychogenic nature of the illness.
- Evidence of hypothalamic-pituitary-adrenal disturbance and increased cytokine production (particularly interleukin-8, which promotes sympathetic pain, and interleukin-6, which induces hyperalgesia, fatigue, and depression[9]) further characterizes the systemic and organic nature of this condition and are well documented in the research literature.
- The majority of fibromyalgia patients demonstrate laboratory evidence of occult bacterial overgrowth in the small bowel, and the details and implications of this will be discussed below (see *Conditions that May Mimic or Contribute to Fibromyalgia*).
- Vitamin D deficiency, a recognized cause of chronic widespread pain, is also common in fibromyalgia patients. [10]

These objective and reproducible abnormalities of biochemical, histological, nutritional, and microbiological/ gastrointestinal status force clinicians to appreciate the valid and organic nature of fibromyalgia; likewise, this evidence refutes promulgations espoused within standard medicine that fibromyalgia is an idiopathic condition warranting lifelong pharmaceuticalization with expensive and potentially hazardous analgesic and antidepressant drugs.

Clinical Presentation

Fibromyalgia is common, affecting approximately 2% of the U.S. population, and 10% of affected patients have severe symptoms resulting in partial or total disability.[11] Affected patients report chronic aches, pains, and stiffness, with a proclivity for localization near the neck, shoulders, low back, and hips. Pain and fatigue are typically exacerbated following physical exertion or psychological stress. Associated manifestations include fatigue, sleep disorders (including insomnia, unrestful sleep, and objective abnormalities such as an increase in stage 1 sleep, a reduction in delta sleep, and alpha-delta sleep anomaly), subjective numbness, headaches, and IBS-like gastrointestinal disturbances. Clinical findings shared between fibromyalgia and IBS include abdominal pain and discomfort, changed frequency of stool including diarrhea and/or constipation, abdominal bloating and distension, dyspepsia, heartburn, headaches (including migraine), fatigue, myalgias, restless leg syndrome, anxiety, and depression.[12] The high prevalence (>50%) of migraine-type headaches in fibromyalgia patients suggests an underlying pathogenesis shared between cephalgia and widespread myalgia, namely impaired mitochondrial function.[13] Cognitive symptoms such as brain fog and difficulty with memory and word retrieval, as well as environmental intolerance and multiple chemical sensitivity, are seen in both fibromyalgia and CFS[14]; again, this overlap of shared symptoms suggests a common etiopathogenesis. Routine physical examination and laboratory findings are generally normal, with the exception of fibromyalgia tender points (described below).

Diagnosis

According to the American College of Rheumatology, a diagnosis of fibromyalgia can be made in a patient with inexplicable, widespread myofascial pain of at least 3 months' duration; *inexplicable* denotes normalcy of routine laboratory and physical examination findings and failure to find an alternate explanation or diagnosis, while *widespread* denotes bilateral pain above and below the waist not attributable to trauma or rheumatic disease and with pain at 11 of 18 classic tender points (see Figure 5.1). Fibromyalgia tender points are assessed bilaterally at 9 paired sites: subocciput, low cervical spine, trapezius, supraspinatus, second rib (anterior near costosternal junction), lateral epicondyle, gluteal region, greater trochanter, and medial fat pad of the knees. Tender points are provoked by the clinician's application of approximately 9 pounds of fingertip pressure, which is sufficient to cause blanching of the clinician's nail bed. The tender points of fibromyalgia are distinguished from myofascial trigger points (MFTP, described by Travell[15]) and strain-counterstrain tender points (described in the osteopathic literature by Jones[16]). In contrast to MFTP, which are located toward the center of the muscle fiber and which refer pain and show spontaneous electrocontractile activity,[17] tender points of fibromyalgia are located near the tendinous insertions of muscle to bone and cause local pain only, without pain referral or contractile activity.

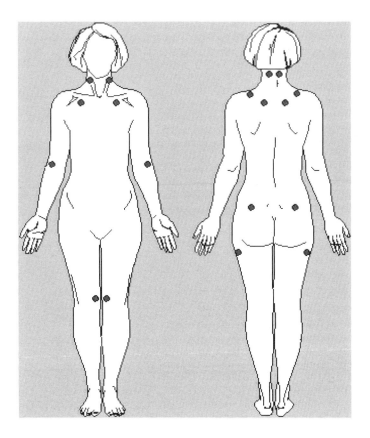

Figure 5.1—Fibromyalgia Tender Points

Illustration shows the 9 paired locations of fibromyalgia tender points. The diagnosis of fibromyalgia is supported when at least 11 out of 18 of these locations are painful following digital compression by the clinician.

C-reactive protein and erythrocyte sedimentation rate should be essentially normal in fibromyalgia patients; abnormalities with these or other common laboratory assessments suggest inflammatory disease, infection, or other concomitant illness. Hypothyroidism is common and can produce widespread myofascial pain similar in initial presentation to fibromyalgia; thus, a complete thyroid evaluation is essential during the initial evaluation of any fibromyalgia-like condition. New-onset fibromyalgia is unlikely over age 50, and the condition never causes fever, significant weight loss, or other objective signs of acute or subacute illness. Common rheumatic conditions such as rheumatoid arthritis and systemic lupus erythematosus (SLE) are excluded by other clinical manifestations and laboratory findings such as anti-cyclic citrullinated protein (CCP) antibodies and antinuclear antibodies (ANA), respectively. Hypophosphatemia must be excluded via demonstration of normal serum phosphate level.

Standard Medical Treatment

Mild exercise and the use of antidepressants, especially those of the tricyclic class, are mainstays of standard medical treatment; these interventions are only partially effective and offer little to no hope of actually curing the disease. Low-intensity aerobic exercise may initially exacerbate symptoms but can result in very modest mental and physical improvement. Cognitive-behavioral therapy can help patients deal with and adapt to the impact of the illness.

In July 2007, the FDA approved pregabalin (Lyrica®) for symptomatic treatment of fibromyalgia[18]; however, because the drug does not address the primary cause(s) of the disease, patients must continue treatment indefinitely. Adverse effects of pregabalin include dizziness, sleepiness, blurred vision, weight gain, dry mouth, swelling of hands and feet, impairment of motor function, and problems with concentration and attention. The most widely used drug for symptomatic treatment of fibromyalgia is amitriptyline (tricyclic antidepressant), which is used "off label" for fibromyalgia and has low efficacy and high potential for adverse effects; up to 20% of patients suffer from weight gain, constipation, orthostatic hypotension, and agitation as a result of the drug. Only 25% to 30% of fibromyalgia patients experience clinically significant improvement with amitriptyline.[19] Other drug treatments, including cyclobenzaprine (muscle relaxant with a tricyclic structure), tramadol (atypical opioid and centrally acting narcotic analgesic), and acetaminophen (centrally acting analgesic), have several important adverse effects and little research supporting their use; none of these treatments favorably alters the course of the disease over the long term.[20]

Functional Medicine Considerations and Interventions

Two fundamental premises of functional medicine are: (1) chronic diseases are a manifestation of chronic dysfunction, and (2) dysfunction can result from a wide range of interconnected genotropic, metabolic, nutritional, microbial, inflammatory, toxic, environmental, and psychological influences. Many of these dysfunctions lie outside the narrow pathology-based and *pharmacocentric* view of standard medicine. The functional medicine approach to each individual fibromyalgia patient is based on the presumption that the condition has an underlying primary cause and that this cause can be identified and addressed. The cause(s) may be manifold and multifaceted and may differ among patients with the same diagnostic label. The functional medicine approach includes the diagnostic and therapeutic considerations of standard medicine but extends far beyond these in assessment, treatment, and understanding.

Functional medicine clinicians appreciate that as a diagnostic label, fibromyalgia is commonly applied to any patient with chronic, widespread pain and that the current trend to limit diagnostic evaluation in such patients will clearly result in failure to identify and address readily diagnosable and treatable problems that can result in widespread pain. In addition to chronic infections such as with hepatitis C and *Borrelia burgdorferi* (Lyme disease), malignant conditions such as multiple myeloma and metastatic disease, and rheumatic diseases such as polymyositis and polymyalgia rheumatica, clinicians should consider other conditions that can precipitate musculoskeletal pain and that are readily diagnosed and treated. A few of the more exemplary conditions to consider in patients with widespread pain are vitamin D deficiency, hypothyroidism, iron overload, and chronic exposure to and accumulation of xenobiotics, perhaps most importantly mercury and lead.

Conditions That May Mimic or Contribute to Fibromyalgia

Vitamin D deficiency — A chronic, widespread pain syndrome[21] associated with mental depression, headaches, systemic inflammation, and numerous other physiological and functional abnormalities can result from vitamin D deficiency. Fibromyalgia patients are commonly deficient in vitamin D, and indeed, Vitamin D deficiency is often misdiagnosed as fibromyalgia, as reported by Holick.[22] Increased severity of the deficiency correlates with worsening depression and anxiety in these patients.[23] Correction of vitamin D deficiency by administration of vitamin D3 (cholecalciferol) in doses of 5000 IU to 10 000 IU/d for several months has resulted in a dramatic alleviation of pain; such intervention among patients with low back pain has resulted in cure rates greater than 95%.[24] Other studies with vitamin D3 doses ranging from 400 to 4000 IU/d have shown that supplementation alleviates depression and enhances well-being.

Vitamin D3 supplementation and adequate endogenous production to meet physiological requirements of approximately 4000 IU/d are remarkably safe and result in numerous major health benefits.[22,25,26] Because use of thiazide diuretics or presence of granulomatous disease (e.g., lymphoma and sarcoidosis) predispose to hypercalcemia, caution and more frequent laboratory monitoring must be employed when using physiological doses of vitamin D3 in these situations. Diagnosis of vitamin D3 deficiency is simple and is based upon measurement of serum 25-hydroxy vitamin D3 (25[OH]D) levels. Supplementation efficacy and safety are monitored by measuring 25(OH)D levels and serum calcium, respectively. (For a review of evidence, as well as the range of optimal serum 25(OH)D levels, see *Vitamin and Mineral Supplements* in Chapter 2.)

Functional hypothyroidism — Both subclinical and overt hypothyroidism are well known in the rheumatology literature as causes of diffuse body pain. Hypothyroidism can mimic fibromyalgia and IBS, and it can contribute to the development of these conditions by causing impaired digestion and delayed intestinal transit, which promote small intestinal bacterial overgrowth (SIBO),[27] a likely cause of both fibromyalgia and IBS (See *Small Intestinal Bacterial Overgrowth* below). Detailed thyroid assessment should include measurements of TSH, free T4, free T3, total T3, reverse T3 (rT3), and antithyroid peroxidase and antithyroglobulin antibodies. (For a more complete discussion of thyroid assessment, see *Laboratory Assessment* in Chapter 2.)

Hemochromatosis and iron overload — Genetic hemochromatosis is a common inherited disease among Caucasians, with a homozygous frequency of approximately 1 in 200 to 250 and a heterozygous frequency of approximately 1 in 7. Various other hereditary iron overload disorders affect all races, with the highest prevalence in persons of African descent (as high as 1 in 80 according to some small studies among hospitalized African-American patients).[28,29] Eighty percent of hemochromatosis patients have chronic musculoskeletal pain, which is commonly the earliest or only presenting complaint.[30] In contrast to the clinical presentation of fibromyalgia, the musculoskeletal manifestations of iron overload are classically arthritic rather than muscular, with the joints of the hands, wrists, hips, and knees most commonly affected. However, due to the widespread distribution of pain and the normalcy of routine laboratory results, iron overload can mimic fibromyalgia. Given the high population prevalence of iron overload and the high frequency with which it presents with musculoskeletal manifestations, all patients with chronic, nontraumatic musculoskeletal pain must be tested for iron overload. Serum ferritin, which can be used alone or with transferrin saturation, is the best single laboratory test; confirmed results greater than 200 mcg/L in women and 300 mcg/L in men necessitate treatment with diagnostic and therapeutic phlebotomy.[31] Additional details about the etiologies, diagnosis, and comprehensive treatment of iron overload are available online.[32]

Accumulation of xenobiotics (including mercury and lead) — Xenobiotic accumulation may occasionally cause widespread pain resembling fibromyalgia, and xenobiotic detoxification (depuration) can alleviate pain in affected patients. Eight percent of American women of childbearing age have sufficiently high levels of mercury in their blood to increase the risk of neurological damage in their children.[33] Americans in general show alarmingly high concentrations and combinations of neurotoxic, carcinogenic, diabetogenic, and immunotoxic xenobiotics.[34] Adverse effects of toxic chemicals (e.g., pesticides, herbicides, solvents, plastics, formaldehyde, petroleum by-products) and heavy metals (especially lead and mercury) are well described throughout the biomedical literature and have been clinically reviewed by Crinnion.[35,36,37,38]

Among toxins with the ability to produce chronic muscle pain, mercury may deserve special recognition given its ubiquitous distribution in the human population and the scientific evidence detailing its numerous adverse effects. [39,40] Whether by metabolic, neurological, or endocrinologic means, occult mercury toxicity may manifest as a syndrome of widespread muscle pain that resembles fibromyalgia. [41] Acrodynia is a subacute peripheral pain syndrome due to mercury toxicity classically seen in children. [42] Acute mercury intoxication can result in severe skeletal muscle damage (rhabdomyolysis). [43] Mercury in organic and inorganic forms interferes with acetylcholine reception and several crucial aspects of the sarcoplasmic reticulum, including calcium-magnesium-ATPase and calcium transport, thus establishing the scientific and molecular basis for a *mercurial myopathy*. [44,45] The toxicity of mercury is greatly increased by simultaneous overaccumulation of lead, elevated levels of which are also common in the U.S. population.

Demonstration of high mercury and lead levels in urine following administration of a chelating agent such as dimercaptosuccinic acid (DMSA) can be used to diagnose chronic mercury or lead overload, and orally administered DMSA is also used for treatment. [46,47,48,49] Failure to preadminister a chelating agent prior to measurement of urine mercury renders the test insensitive for chronic accumulation and can thus give the false impression that mercury is not contributory to fibromyalgia, as concluded by Kotter et al. [50] Orally administered selenium, phytochelatins, a high-fiber diet, and potassium citrate can be used to augment mercury excretion. (Chapter 7, *Case Reports*, will present the case of a woman with chronic progressive muscle pain who was diagnosed with fibromyalgia and who ultimately had complete and permanent remission of all pain following treatment for her elevated lead and mercury.)

Small intestinal bacterial overgrowth — SIBO provides a model for explaining the clinical and pathophysiological manifestations of fibromyalgia. Although commonly underappreciated by many clinicians, SIBO is common in clinical practice, affecting approximately 40% of patients with rheumatoid arthritis, 84% of patients with IBS, and 90% to 100% of patients with fibromyalgia. In a study of 42 fibromyalgia patients, all 42 of them showed evidence of SIBO, and the severity of the bacterial overgrowth correlated positively with the severity of the fibromyalgia, thus indicating the plausibility of a causal relationship. [51]

The links between fibromyalgia and IBS are also strong; most IBS patients meet strict diagnostic criteria for fibromyalgia, and most fibromyalgia patients meet strict criteria for IBS. Lubrano et al [52] showed that fibromyalgia severity correlated with IBS severity among patients who met strict diagnostic criteria for both conditions. The high degree of overlap between these 2 diagnostic labels suggests that these conditions are 2 variations of a common pathophysiological process—SIBO. [53]

SIBO causes altered bowel function, immune activation, and visceral hypersensitivity, and it is one causative explanation for the clinical and pathophysiological manifestations of IBS; see the detailed review by Lin. [54] IBS is characterized by visceral hyperalgesia, just as fibromyalgia is characterized by skeletal muscle hyperalgesia. Given the strong evidence suggesting that IBS is caused by SIBO and that IBS and fibromyalgia are variations of the same pathophysiological process, it follows that fibromyalgia may therefore be caused by SIBO. However, these links and interconnections require substantiation, as provided below.

What is the evidence linking fibromyalgia with SIBO? What are the molecular mechanisms by which absorbed toxins and metabolites from SIBO can contribute to muscle pain and the bioenergetic-mitochondrial defects seen in fibromyalgia patients?

- First, 90% to 100% of fibromyalgia patients show evidence of SIBO, according to the studies cited previously; such a strong correlation and the dose-response relationship imply causality and must be integrated into any science-based model of fibromyalgia.
- Second, fibromyalgia and IBS are strongly convergent, and the evidence indicates that IBS may be caused by SIBO. [54]
- Third, SIBO is associated with overproduction and absorption of bacterial cellular debris (e.g., lipopolysaccharide [LPS], bacterial DNA, peptidoglycans, teichoic acid, exotoxins) and antimetabolites (e.g., D-lactic acid, tyramine, tartaric acid) that are known to impair cellular energy production in ways that accord with

the myopathic metabolic defects seen in skeletal muscle biopsies of fibromyalgia patients. Intestinal gram-negative bacteria produce endotoxin (LPS), which impairs skeletal muscle energy production by stimulating skeletal muscle sodium-potassium-ATPase; endotoxin also raises blood lactate under aerobic conditions in humans.[55] Thus, via direct and indirect effects on mitochondria, chronic low-dose LPS exposure can result in impaired muscle metabolism and reduced ATP synthesis. Intestinal bacteria also produce D-lactate, a well-known metabolic toxin in humans; SIBO often results in variable levels of D-lactate acidosis, severe cases of which can progress from fatigue and malaise to encephalopathy (e.g., confusion, ataxia, slurred speech, altered mental status) and death.[56] Energy/ATP underproduction and lactate overproduction cause muscle fatigue and muscle pain. An additional cellular toxin produced by intestinal bacteria is hydrogen sulfide, which causes DNA damage[57] (noted previously to be increased in fibromyalgia patients) and which impairs cellular energy production, a finding relevant to but not necessarily limited to the pathogenesis of ulcerative colitis.[58,59]

- Fourth, LPS and other antigens absorbed from the intestine during SIBO contribute to a subclinical inflammatory state that results in pain hypersensitivity and increased cytokine release, both of which are characteristics of fibromyalgia. Related to this, Lin wrote, "The immune response to bacterial antigen in SIBO provides a framework for understanding the hypersensitivity in both fibromyalgia and IBS."[54]

- Fifth, somewhat independent from the immune-mediated hyperalgesia induced by LPS is the hyperalgesia mediated by central nervous system responses. The central sensitization seen with fibromyalgia[60] might be explained as being caused by intestinally derived endotoxinemia. Bacterial LPS promotes central sensitization via direct activation of NMDA receptors and by inducing hyperalgesia and anti-analgesia.[61] Accumulated evidence suggests that fibromyalgia may be a disorder of somatic hypersensitivity induced by bacterial toxins derived from quantitative excess or qualitative abnormalities in gut bacteria.[62]

- Sixth, *antimicrobial therapy alleviates fibromyalgia symptoms in direct proportion to the success of bacterial overgrowth eradication, thus adding strong evidence in support of SIBO as a main cause of fibromyalgia.*[63,64] Similarly, recent clinical trials have shown that treatment of the fibromyalgia-related conditions IBS and SIBO by use of the nonabsorbed oral antibiotic rifaximin results in significant diminution of IBS-SIBO symptomatology, with benefits lasting after the discontinuation of therapy.[65,66]

- Seventh, SIBO causes nutrient malabsorption[67] and can thereby contribute to the vitamin D and magnesium deficiencies that promote pain and impair mitochondrial dysfunction and that are common in fibromyalgia.

- Eighth, SIBO can be triggered in humans by reduced mucosal immunity following stressful life events, and this helps explain the link between IBS, fibromyalgia, and psycho-emotional stress.

- Ninth, as will be reviewed below under *Therapeutic Interventions*, essentially all of the most successful therapies for fibromyalgia have effects on intestinal flora, muscle perfusion/contractility, or mitochondrial bioenergetics. This is true for vegetarian diets (which favorably alter gut flora), supplementation with tryptophan/melatonin (which preserve mitochondrial function during LPS exposure), physical treatments such as acupuncture (which restore tissue perfusion), and the use of nutrients such as magnesium, acetyl-L-carnitine (ALC), D-ribose, creatine, and coenzyme Q-10 (which optimize mitochondrial function).

- Tenth and finally, restless leg syndrome occurs in approximately 30% of fibromyalgia patients and can be effectively treated by addressing SIBO with a combination of antibiotics and probiotics.[68]

Thus, the research literature provides compelling evidence linking SIBO with the genesis and perpetuation of fibromyalgia. Chronic low-dose exposure to immunogens and metabolic toxins from SIBO is a plausible cause of impaired cellular energy production that results in chronic, widespread muscle fatigue and soreness and which may precipitate the clinical presentation of fibromyalgia. The individual components of this model have been substantiated by mechanistic studies in animals and/or clinical trials in humans.

CFS also shares many epidemiological and clinical similarities with fibromyalgia, and a similar pathophysiology is highly probable. A consistent report from many CFS and fibromyalgia patients is that of environmental intolerance and multiple chemical sensitivity. This can be explained by SIBO because bacterial LPS and other bacterial products impair hepatic cytochrome P450 detoxification enzymes, resulting in reduced drug metabolism and clearance of xenobiotics.[69] Accumulation of xenobiotics in CFS patients[70] might therefore be explained in part by LPS-induced inhibition of xenobiotic clearance secondary to SIBO. Further, the metabolic and immunologic effects of LPS can also account for the immune activation, neurological dysfunction, and musculoskeletal complaints typical of CFS.

Clinical interventions for the treatment of SIBO include carbohydrate restriction, normalization of gastrointestinal transit time, selective use of probiotic supplements to normalize intestinal flora, support of mucosal immunity, and eradication of bacterial overgrowth with drugs such as ciprofloxacin or metronidazole or natural products such as berberine, artemisia, and oil of oregano, reviewed in greater detail elsewhere[32,71] (also see *Botanical Medicines* in Chapter 2). Failure of any monotherapeutic approach to immediately resolve all manifestations of fibromyalgia is explained by the secondary metabolic, immune, and neurophysiological effects that have generally persisted over periods ranging from years to decades for most patients. The program must be complete in order to facilitate correction of systemic oxidative damage, resultant nutritional deficiencies, immune sensitization and induction of proinflammatory cycles, alterations in neurotransmission and membrane receptor function, and the inflammation-induced disturbances in pain reception and hypothalamic-pituitary-endocrine function.

> **Clinical Pearl:**
> Patients treated for SIBO who do not positively change their diets and lifestyles (which probably promoted the genesis and perpetuation of the disease in the first place) are subject to continual recurrence until such changes are implemented and faithfully maintained.

Following the exclusion of diagnosable and treatable conditions that can contribute to or mimic fibromyalgia, functional medicine clinicians can design treatment plans based on the previously reviewed pathogenesis, standard medical treatments, and the following pathogenic and therapeutic considerations.

Therapeutic Interventions

Vegetarian diet — Diets high in fruits, vegetables, nuts, berries, and seeds provide ample fiber to promote laxation and can be useful as an adjunctive treatment for gastrointestinal dysbiosis in general and SIBO in particular (i.e., *quantitative* reduction in gastrointestinal dysbiosis). Perhaps more importantly, plant-based diets result in *qualitative* benefits by changing microbial behavior and reducing production of irritants, toxins, and bacterial metabolites, including the bioenergetic-mitochondrial poisons D-lactate and hydrogen sulfide. Fibromyalgia patients who consume a mostly vegetarian diet have experienced significant improvements in function and reductions in fibromyalgia symptomatology.[72] Poorly designed dietary interventions that allow abundant intake of whole-grain bread, pasta, rice, and fruit juice[73] would be expected to fail because such high-carbohydrate diets feed intestinal bacteria with an abundance of substrate and would therefore be expected to sustain or exacerbate SIBO.

Tryptophan and 5-hydroxytryptophan (5-HTP) — Tryptophan is the amino acid precursor to the neurotransmitter serotonin, which has antidepressant, antianxiety, and analgesic properties. Patients with fibromyalgia are known to have low blood levels (i.e., functional nutritional insufficiency) of tryptophan, and the severity of the deficiency correlates with the severity of pain.[74,75,76] Blood levels of serotonin are often below normal in fibromyalgia patients.[77] The accepted medical use of selective serotonin reuptake inhibitors (SSRIs) to treat the pain, depression, and anxiety associated with fibromyalgia supports the use of 5-HTP to raise serotonin levels naturally by correcting the underlying nutritional insufficiency. As an over-the-counter nutritional supplement, the 5-hydroxylated form of tryptophan (5-HTP) has been used clinically and in numerous research studies, and supplementation has been shown to significantly alleviate symptoms of fibromyalgia. An open 90-day study in 50 fibromyalgia patients showed significant improvement in all measured parameters (number of tender points, anxiety, pain intensity, quality of sleep, fatigue) after treatment with 5-HTP; global clinical improvement assessed by the patient and the investigator indicated a "good" or "fair" response in nearly 50% of the patients during the treatment period.[78] A double-blind, placebo-controlled study using 5-HTP in 50 fibromyalgia patients showed significant improvement in all measured parameters, with only mild and transient side effects.[79]

Commonly used doses of 5-HTP range from 50 to 300 mg/d, with larger doses divided throughout the day. If tryptophan rather than 5-HTP is used, results are improved when taken on an empty stomach with carbohydrate to induce insulin secretion, which preferentially promotes uptake of tryptophan into the brain. Magnesium deficiency impairs conversion of 5-HTP into serotonin, and the interventional program must ensure nutritional supra-sufficiency.

Melatonin — Patients with fibromyalgia show decreased nocturnal secretion of melatonin.[80] Melatonin benefits fibromyalgia patients through a wide range of mechanisms, including promotion of restful sleep and reduction in LPS-induced mitochondrial impairment. As a powerful antioxidant, melatonin scavenges oxygen and nitrogen-based reactants generated in mitochondria and thereby limits the loss of intramitochondrial glutathione; this prevents damage to mitochondrial protein and DNA. Melatonin increases the activity of Complexes 1 and 4 of the electron transport chain, improving mitochondrial respiration and increasing ATP synthesis under various physiological and experimental conditions.[81] Melatonin (3–6 mg per night, administered orally 1 hour before bedtime) has been reported to normalize sleep, alleviate pain and fatigue, and alleviate many clinical manifestations of fibromyalgia.[82] Successful treatment with melatonin or its precursor tryptophan/5-HTP should not deter the clinician from addressing other contributing or causative problems such as vitamin D deficiency, gastrointestinal dysbiosis including SIBO, magnesium deficiency, and chronic psycho-emotional stress. In adults, melatonin has a wide therapeutic index and has been used safely and effectively in doses up to 20 to 40 mg nightly.

Magnesium — Magnesium deficiency is epidemic in industrialized societies due to insufficient dietary intake (e.g., from mineral water and leafy green vegetables) and concomitant urinary acidosis, which increases urinary magnesium loss.[83,84] Additional causes of magnesium deficiency in fibromyalgia patients include vitamin D deficiency, malabsorption due to SIBO, and the stress of chronic illness. Magnesium deficiency exacerbates the symptoms of fibromyalgia by contributing to impairment of energy (ATP) production in skeletal muscle, increased muscle tone and spasms (hypomagnesemic tetany), and anxiety and hyperalgesia via NMDA receptor overstimulation and neurocortical hyperexcitability. Magnesium deficiency also promotes constipation, which exacerbates SIBO. Magnesium supplementation (600 mg/d or to bowel tolerance) should be used routinely in fibromyalgia patients. Modest benefits demonstrated in clinical trials with magnesium and malic acid[85] can easily be exceeded with concomitant interventions to address vitamin D deficiency, SIBO, and mitochondrial dysfunction.

Acetyl-L-carnitine (ALC) — A large study with 102 patients showed that ALC (administered by oral and parenteral routes, 1500 mg/d) was beneficial in patients with fibromyalgia.[86] Given the role of ALC in supporting and improving mitochondrial function, this supplement probably benefits fibromyalgia patients by compensating for LPS-induced skeletal muscle dysfunction.

D-ribose — D-ribose is a naturally occurring pentose carbohydrate available as a dietary supplement. When administered orally (5 g three times daily), it provides safe and effective benefit to fibromyalgia patients, according to a recent pilot study with 41 patients.[87] Improvements are seen in energy, sleep, mental clarity, pain intensity, and well-being, as well as global assessment. Among its beneficial mechanisms of action is enhancement of mitochondrial ATP production. Thus, the benefits of D-ribose supplementation may be mediated by restoration or preservation of mitochondrial impairment caused by LPS in fibromyalgia patients.

Creatine monohydrate — Skeletal muscle levels of phosphocreatine and ATP are reduced in patients with fibromyalgia compared with normal controls; thus, oral supplementation with creatine would appear to be an obvious intervention to restore these depressed levels to normal. Although no formal trials have been conducted, Artimal et al[88] reported that a patient with severe refractory fibromyalgia attained sustained alleviation of depression and pain, as well as improvements in sleep and quality of life, following oral administration of creatine monohydrate for 4 weeks (3 g daily in the first week, then 5 g daily). Creatine supplementation has been shown to improve ATP production and oxygen utilization in brain and skeletal muscle in humans.[89]

Ginkgo biloba — This extract is an extensively researched botanical medicine with a long history of safe and effective clinical use for various conditions, especially those associated with reduced blood flow and impaired mitochondrial function. *Ginkgo biloba* provides antioxidant, anti-inflammatory, vasodilatory, and mitochondrial-protective benefits. Given these therapeutic benefits, *Ginkgo* would appear to be a reasonable therapeutic agent to address the secondary pathophysiology in fibromyalgia. As cited below, a recent clinical trial using a 2-component treatment that included *Ginkgo* showed benefit in fibromyalgia patients.

Coenzyme Q10 (CoQ10) — An endogenous antioxidant and essential component of the mitochondrial electron transport chain, oral supplementation with CoQ10 has been used therapeutically in numerous studies for the successful treatment of migraine, heart failure, hypertension, and renal failure. Additional data have shown immunomodulatory roles for CoQ10, and many clinicians employ it as an adjunctive treatment for viral infections, cancer, and allergies.[90,91] In an open trial of 23 fibromyalgia patients, the combination of 200 mg CoQ10 and 200 mg *Ginkgo biloba* (for a total dose of 48 mg flavone glycosides and 12 mg terpene lactones) daily for 84 days was shown to provide clinical benefit in 64% of patients.[92]

Physical modalities (chiropractic, acupuncture, osteopathic manipulation, qigong, balneotherapy) — Chiropractic treatment (including spinal manipulation, stretching, soft tissue treatments, and therapeutic ultrasound) has shown benefit in several fibromyalgia case series and clinical trials.[93,94] Acupuncture (including traditional, nontraditional, and electrical stimulation) also has been found beneficial for fibromyalgia patients.[95,96,97] Acupuncture may relieve fibromyalgia pain by improving regional blood flow, in addition to other mechanisms.[98,99] Because specific needle placement does not appear to be important,[100] the conclusion that true acupuncture is ineffective because it may not differ markedly from the results obtained by sham acupuncture[101] may not be logical. A similar conundrum is seen in other clinical trials involving physical interventions such as osseous manipulation, wherein authentic treatments and sham treatments may both be effective by virtue of common physiological responses.[102] A short-term trial showed that osteopathic manipulative therapy with standard medical care was superior to medical care alone for fibromyalgia patients.[103] Qigong was found helpful for 10 fibromyalgia patients, and benefits were still apparent at 3 months' follow-up.[104] In a randomized controlled clinical trial among 24 female fibromyalgia patients, the intervention of balneotherapy, daily 20-minute sessions 5 days per week for 3 weeks (total of 15 sessions; water temperature: 96.8°F = 36°C), resulted in statistically significant reductions in measured inflammatory mediators (PGE2, interleukin-1, LTB4) and amelioration of clinical symptoms among treated patients.[105] The symptomatic benefits of balneotherapy for fibromyalgia patients have been corroborated in other trials.[106,107,108]

S-adenosylmethionine (SAMe). Studies using oral or intravenous administration of the nutritional supplement SAMe have reported conflicting results; however, the overall trend seems to indicate that SAMe (800 mg/d orally) is safe and beneficial in the treatment of fibromyalgia.[109] SAMe helps maintain mitochondrial function by preserving glutathione, and its contribution of methyl groups is important for the regulation of gene expression and neurotransmitter synthesis.

Chlorella — *Chlorella pyrenoidosa* is a unicellular green alga that grows in fresh water. It is a dense source of nutrients, particularly vitamin D (500 IU vitamin D per 1.35 g *Chlorella*). *Chlorella* may have value in treating some fibromyalgia patients, but overall the efficacy is low.[110] Thus, *Chlorella* should not be used as monotherapy for fibromyalgia, although it may be a useful adjunct either as a source of vitamin D, as a means to help modify gut flora, or as an aid in the detoxification of xenobiotics due to its ability to bind ingested and bile-excreted toxins and prevent their absorption and reabsorption in a manner similar to that of cholestyramine.[111,112,113] This detoxifying effect of *Chlorella* in humans is supported by 2 clinical trials showing that nursing mothers who supplement with *Chlorella* during lactation transfer less dioxin in their breast milk compared to nursing mothers who do not consume *Chlorella*.[114,115]

Probiotics — These are beneficial bacteria that can be consumed in foods or as nutritional supplements to populate the gut, particularly following antibiotic use or long-term dietary neglect. In addition to their availability in capsules and powders, probiotics are widely consumed in the form of yogurt, kefir, and other cultured foods, and they have an excellent record of safety. Probiotic supplements are available in different strengths (quantity), potencies (viability), and combinations of bacteria (single or multiple). Some probiotics also contain fermentable carbohydrates (prebiotics) such as fructooligosaccharides and inulin, which are substrates to nourish the beneficial bacteria. From a practical clinical perspective, the clinician can choose probiotic foods and supplements and instruct the patient to use these on an ongoing, periodic, or rotational basis.

The benefits of probiotic supplementation have been demonstrated in patients with IBS,[116,117] rotavirus infection,[118] eczema and increased intestinal permeability,[119] and SIBO associated with renal failure.[120] To date, no studies using probiotics in the treatment of fibromyalgia have been published.

> **Clinical Pearl:**
>
> Probiotics (i.e., bacteria only) may have a therapeutic advantage over prebiotics or synbiotics (probiotics+prebiotics) when treating SIBO because fermentable carbohydrate may exacerbate the preexisting bacterial overgrowth by providing already overpopulated bacteria with additional substrate.

Conclusion and Clinical Approach

In sum, current research indicates that fibromyalgia may result from impairment of cellular bioenergetics due to absorbed metabolic toxins from bacterial overgrowth of the gastrointestinal tract. Available studies have shown that SIBO is ubiquitous among fibromyalgia patients and that antimicrobial interventions—whether pharmaceutical or nutritional—are efficacious. Secondary physiological effects such as mitochondrial impairment, pain sensitization, nutritional deficiencies, oxidative stress, and reduced tissue perfusion are addressed by combined use of select therapeutics as reviewed previously. Patients presenting with widespread pain should be screened for causative underlying disease; if no other explanation can be found, then the diagnosis of fibromyalgia should be made, and the condition should be treated with the therapeutics discussed above. The first visit can include history, physical examination, and laboratory tests; preliminary interventions include dietary modification, multivitamin-multimineral supplementation (including vitamin D3 and magnesium), tryptophan/5-HTP, and CoQ10. SIBO can be treated empirically, or it can be objectively assessed with stool analysis, culture, microscopy, and parasitology. At follow-up visits, additional assessments and interventions can be used to fine-tune the diagnosis and its contributors and to maximize patient response to treatment.

References

1. Siegel DM, Janeway D, Baum J. Fibromyalgia syndrome in children and adolescents: clinical features at presentation and status at follow-up. *Pediatrics*. 1998;101(3 Pt 1):377-382.
2. Chakrabarty S, Zoorob R. Fibromyalgia. *Am Fam Physician*. 2007;76:247-254.
3. Tierney ML, McPhee SJ, Papadakis MA, eds. *Current Medical Diagnosis and Treatment 2006*. 45th ed. New York, NY: Lange Medical Books; 2006: 820-821.
4. Olsen NJ, Park JH. Skeletal muscle abnormalities in patients with fibromyalgia. *Am J Med Sci*. 1998;315:351-358.
5. Sprott H, Salemi S, Gay RE, et al. Increased DNA fragmentation and ultrastructural changes in fibromyalgic muscle fibres. *Ann Rheum Dis*. 2004;63:245-251.
6. Park JH, Niermann KJ, Olsen N. Evidence for metabolic abnormalities in the muscles of patients with fibromyalgia. *Curr Rheumatol Rep*. 2000;2:131-140.
7. Elvin A, Siosteen AK, Nilsson A, Kosek E. Decreased muscle blood flow in fibromyalgia patients during standardised muscle exercise: a contrast media enhanced colour Doppler study. *Eur J Pain*. 2006;10:137-144.
8. Altindag O, Celik H. Total antioxidant capacity and the severity of the pain in patients with fibromyalgia. *Redox Rep*. 2006;11:131-135.
9. Wallace DJ, Linker-Israeli M, Hallegua D, Silverman S, Silver D, Weisman MH. Cytokines play an aetiopathogenetic role in fibromyalgia: a hypothesis and pilot study. *Rheumatology (Oxford)*. 2001;40:743-749.
10. Huisman AM, White KP, Algra A, et al. Vitamin D levels in women with systemic lupus erythematosus and fibromyalgia. *J Rheumatol*. 2001;28:2535-2539.
11. Simms RW. Nonarticular soft tissue disorders. In Andreoli TE, Carpenter CCJ, Griggs RC, Benjamin IJ, eds. *Cecil Essentials of Medicine*. 7th ed. Philadelphia, Pa; Saunders Elsevier; 2007: 851-852.
12. Triadafilopoulos G, Simms RW, Goldenberg DL. Bowel dysfunction in fibromyalgia syndrome. *Dig Dis Sci*. 1991;36:59-64.
13. Pieczenik SR, Neustadt J. Mitochondrial dysfunction and molecular pathways of disease. *Exp Mol Pathol*. 2007;83:84-92.
14. Brown MM, Jason LA. Functioning in individuals with chronic fatigue syndrome: increased impairment with co-occurring multiple chemical sensitivity and fibromyalgia. *Dyn Med*. 2007;6:6.
15. Simons DG, Travell JG, Simons LS. *Travell & Simons' Myofascial Pain and Dysfunction. The Trigger Point Manual*. Baltimore, Md: Lippincott Williams & Wilkins; 1999.

16. Jones LH, Kusunose R, Goering E. *Jones Strain-Counterstrain*. Carlsbad: Jones Strain Counterstrain Incorporated; 1995.

17. Hubbard DR, Berkoff GM. Myofascial trigger points show spontaneous needle EMG activity. *Spine*. 1993;18:1803-1807.

18. *FDA Approves First Drug for Treating Fibromyalgia*. U.S. Food and Drug Administration. June 21, 2007. Available online at: http://www.fda.gov/bbs/topics/NEWS/2007/NEW01656.html.

19. Leventhal LJ. Management of fibromyalgia. *Ann Intern Med*. 1999;131:850-858.

20. Goldenberg DL, Burckhardt C, Crofford L. Management of fibromyalgia syndrome. *JAMA*. 2004;292:2388-2395.

21. Plotnikoff GA, Quigley JM. Prevalence of severe hypovitaminosis D in patients with persistent, nonspecific musculoskeletal pain. *Mayo Clin Proc*. 2003;78:1463-1470.

22. Holick MF. Vitamin D: importance in the prevention of cancers, type 1 diabetes, heart disease, and osteoporosis. *Am J Clin Nutr*. 2004;79:362-371.

23. Armstrong DJ, Meenagh GK, Bickle I, Lee AS, Curran ES, Finch MB. Vitamin D deficiency is associated with anxiety and depression in fibromyalgia. *Clin Rheumatol*. 2007;26:551-554.

24. Al Faraj S, Al Mutairi K. Vitamin D deficiency and chronic low back pain in Saudi Arabia. *Spine*. 2003;28:177-179.

25. Vieth R. Vitamin D supplementation, 25-hydroxyvitamin D concentrations, and safety. *Am J Clin Nutr*. 1999;69:842-856.

26. Zittermann A. Vitamin D in preventive medicine: are we ignoring the evidence? *Br J Nutr*. 2003;89:552-572.

27. Lauritano EC, Bilotta AL, Gabrielli M, et al. Association between hypothyroidism and small intestinal bacterial overgrowth. *J Clin Endocrinol Metab*. 2007;92:4180-4184.

28. Wurapa RK, Gordeuk VR, Brittenham GM, Khiyami A, Schechter GP, Edwards CQ. Primary iron overload in African Americans. *Am J Med*. 1996;101:9-18.

29. Barton JC, Edwards CQ, Bertoli LF, Shroyer TW, Hudson SL. Iron overload in African Americans. *Am J Med*. 1995;99:616-623.

30. Vasquez A. Musculoskeletal disorders and iron overload disease: comment on the American College of Rheumatology guidelines for the initial evaluation of the adult patient with acute musculoskeletal symptoms. *Arthritis Rheum*. 1996;39:1767-1768.

31. Barton JC, McDonnell SM, Adams PC, et al. Management of hemochromatosis. Hemochromatosis Management Working Group. *Ann Intern Med*. 1998;129:932-939.

32. Vasquez A. *Integrative Rheumatology*. 2nd ed. Fort Worth, Tex: Integrative and Biological Medicine Research and Consulting; 2007: 409-414.

33. Schober SE, Sinks TH, Jones RL, et al. Blood mercury levels in US children and women of childbearing age, 1999-2000. *JAMA*. 2003;289:1667-1674.

34. Schafer KS, Reeves M, Spitzer S, Kegley SE. *Chemical Trespass: Pesticides in Our Bodies and Corporate Accountability*. Pesticide Action Network North America. May 2004. Available online at: http://www.panna.org/campaigns/docsTrespass/chemicalTrespass2004.dv.html.

35. Crinnion WJ. Environmental medicine, part 1: The human burden of environmental toxins and their common health effects. *Altern Med Rev*. 2000;5:52-63.

36. Crinnion WJ. Environmental medicine, part 2: Health effects of and protection from ubiquitous airborne solvent exposure. *Altern Med Rev*. 2000;5:133-143.

37. Crinnion WJ. Environmental medicine, part 3: Long-term effects of chronic low-dose mercury exposure. *Altern Med Rev*. 2000;5:209-223.

38. Crinnion WJ. Environmental medicine, part 4: Pesticides-biologically persistent and ubiquitous toxins. *Altern Med Rev*. 2000;5:432-447.

39. Elemental mercury vapor poisoning: North Carolina, 1988. MMWR Morb Mortal Wkly Rep. 1989;38:770-772, 777.

40. Shih H, Gartner JC Jr. Weight loss, hypertension, weakness, and limb pain in an 11-year-old boy. *J Pediatr*. 2001;138:566-569.

41. Sterzl I, Prochazkova J, Hrda P, Bartova J, Matucha P, Stejskal VD. Mercury and nickel allergy: risk factors in fatigue and autoimmunity. *Neuro Endocrinol Lett*. 1999;20(3-4):221-228.

42. Padlewska KK, Scwartz RA. Acrodynia. Last updated February 15, 2007. Available online at: http://www.emedicine.com/derm/topic592.htm.

43. Chugh KS, Singhal PC, Uberoi HS. Rhabdomyolysis and renal failure in acute mercuric chloride poisoning. *Med J Aust*. 1978;2:125-126.

44. Chiu VC, Mouring D, Haynes DH. Action of mercurials on the active and passive transport properties of sarcoplasmic reticulum. *J Bioenerg Biomembr*. 1983;15:13-25.

45. Shamoo AE, Maclennan DH, Elderfrawi ME. Differential effects of mercurial compounds on excitable tissues. *Chem Biol Interact*. 1976;12:41-52.

46. Kalra V, Dua T, Kumar V, Kaul B. Succimer in symptomatic lead poisoning. *Indian Pediatr*. 2002;39:580-585.

47. Bradstreet J, Geier DA, Kartzinel JJ, Adams JB, Geier MR. A case-control study of mercury burden in children with autistic spectrum disorders. *Journal of American Physicians and Surgeons*. 2003;8:76-79. Available online at: http://www.jpands.org/vol8no3/geier.pdf.

48. Forman J, Moline J, Cernichiari E, et al. A cluster of pediatric metallic mercury exposure cases treated with meso-2,3-dimercaptosuccinic acid (DMSA). *Environ Health Perspect*. 2000;108:575-577.

49. Miller AL. Dimercaptosuccinic acid (DMSA), a non-toxic, water-soluble treatment for heavy metal toxicity. *Altern Med Rev*. 1998;3:199-207.

50. Kotter I, Durk H, Saal JG, Kroiher A, Schweinsberg F. Mercury exposure from dental amalgam fillings in the etiology of primary fibromyalgia: a pilot study. *J Rheumatol*. 1995;22:2194-2195.

51. Pimentel M, Wallace D, Hallegua D, et al. A link between irritable bowel syndrome and fibromyalgia may be related to findings on lactulose breath testing. *Ann Rheum Dis*. 2004;63:450-452.

52. Lubrano E, Iovino P, Tremolaterra F, Parsons WJ, Ciacci C, Mazzacca G. Fibromyalgia in patients with irritable bowel syndrome. An association with the severity of the intestinal disorder. *Int J Colorectal Dis*. 2001;16:211-215.

53. Veale D, Kavanagh G, Fielding JF, Fitzgerald O. Primary fibromyalgia and the irritable bowel syndrome: different expressions of a common pathogenetic process. *Br J Rheumatol*. 1991;30:220-222.

54. Lin HC. Small intestinal bacterial overgrowth: a framework for understanding irritable bowel syndrome. *JAMA*. 2004;292:852-858.

55. Bundgaard H, Kjeldsen K, Suarez Krabbe K, et al. Endotoxemia stimulates skeletal muscle Na+-K+-ATPase and raises blood lactate under aerobic conditions in humans. *Am J Physiol Heart Circ Physiol*. 2003;284(3):H1028-H1034.

56. Vella A, Farrugia G. D-lactic acidosis: pathologic consequence of saprophytism. *Mayo Clin Proc*. 1998;73:451-456.

57. Attene-Ramos MS, Wagner ED, Gaskins HR, Plewa MJ. Hydrogen sulfide induces direct radical-associated DNA damage. *Mol Cancer Res*. 2007;5:455-459.

58. Magee EA, Richardson CJ, Hughes R, Cummings JH. Contribution of dietary protein to sulfide production in the large intestine: an in vitro and a controlled feeding study in humans. *Am J Clin Nutr*. 2000;72:1488-1494.

59. Babidge W, Millard S, Roediger W. Sulfides impair short chain fatty acid beta-oxidation at acyl-CoA dehydrogenase level in colonocytes: implications for ulcerative colitis. *Mol Cell Biochem*. 1998;181(1-2):117-124.

60. Meeus M, Nijs J. Central sensitization: a biopsychosocial explanation for chronic widespread pain in patients with fibromyalgia and chronic fatigue syndrome. *Clin Rheumatol*. 2007;26:465-473.

61. Johnston IN, Westbrook RF. Inhibition of morphine analgesia by LPS: role of opioid and NMDA receptors and spinal glia. *Behav Brain Res*. 2005;156:75-83.

62. Othman M, Agüero R, Lin HC. Alterations in intestinal microbial flora and human disease. *Curr Opin Gastroenterol*. 2008;24:11-16.

63. Wallace DJ, Hallegua DS. Fibromyalgia: the gastrointestinal link. *Curr Pain Headache Rep*. 2004;8:364-368.

64. Pimentel M, Hallegua DS, Wallace DJ, et al. Improvement of symptoms by eradication of small intestinal overgrowth in FMS: a double-blind study [abstract]. *Arthritis Rheum*. 1999;42:S343.

65. Pimentel M, Park S, Mirocha J, Kane SV, Kong Y. The effect of a nonabsorbed oral antibiotic (rifaximin) on the symptoms of the irritable bowel syndrome: a randomized trial. *Ann Intern Med*. 2006;145:557-563.

66. Sharara AI, Aoun E, Abdul-Baki H, Mounzer R, Sidani S, Elhajj I. A randomized double-blind placebo-controlled trial of rifaximin in patients with abdominal bloating and flatulence. *Am J Gastroenterol*. 2006;101:326-333.

67. Elphick HL, Elphick DA, Sanders DS. Small bowel bacterial overgrowth. An underrecognized cause of malnutrition in older adults. *Geriatrics*. 2006;61:21-26.

68. Weinstock LB, Fern SE, Duntley SP. Restless legs syndrome in patients with irritable bowel syndrome: response to small intestinal bacterial overgrowth therapy. *Dig Dis Sci*. 2007 Oct 13 [Epub ahead of print].

69. Shedlofsky SI, Israel BC, McClain CJ, Hill DB, Blouin RA. Endotoxin administration to humans inhibits hepatic cytochrome P450-mediated drug metabolism. *J Clin Invest*. 1994;94:2209-2214.

70. Dunstan RH, Donohoe M, Taylor W, et al. A preliminary investigation of chlorinated hydrocarbons and chronic fatigue syndrome. *Med J Aust*. 1995;163:294-297.

71. Vasquez A. Reducing pain and inflammation naturally, part 6: Nutritional and botanical treatments against "silent infections" and gastrointestinal dysbiosis, commonly overlooked causes of neuromusculoskeletal inflammation and chronic health problems. *Nutritional Perspectives*. January 2006: 5-21.

72. Donaldson MS, Speight N, Loomis S. Fibromyalgia syndrome improved using a mostly raw vegetarian diet: an observational study. *BMC Complement Altern Med*. 2001;1:7.

73. Michalsen A, Riegert M, Lüdtke R, et al. Mediterranean diet or extended fasting's influence on changing the intestinal microflora, immunoglobulin A secretion and clinical outcome in patients with rheumatoid arthritis and fibromyalgia: an observational study. *BMC Complement Altern Med*. 2005;5:22.

74. Moldofsky H, Warsh JJ. Plasma tryptophan and musculoskeletal pain in non-articular rheumatism ("fibrositis syndrome"). *Pain*. 1978;5:65-71.

75. Yunus MB, Dailey JW, Aldag JC, Masi AT, Jobe PC. Plasma tryptophan and other amino acids in primary fibromyalgia: a controlled study. *J Rheumatol*. 1992;19:90-94.

76. Russell IJ, Michalek JE, Vipraio GA, Fletcher EM, Wall K. Serum amino acids in fibrositis/fibromyalgia syndrome. *J Rheumatol Suppl*. 1989;19:158-163.

77. Wolfe F, Russell IJ, Vipraio G, Ross K, Anderson J. Serotonin levels, pain threshold, and fibromyalgia symptoms in the general population. *J Rheumatol*. 1997;24:555-559.

78. Sarzi Puttini P, Caruso I. Primary fibromyalgia syndrome and 5-hydroxy-L-tryptophan: a 90-day open study. *J Int Med Res*. 1992;20:182-189.

79. Caruso I, Sarzi Puttini P, Cazzola M, Azzolini V. Double-blind study of 5-hydroxytryptophan versus placebo in the treatment of primary fibromyalgia syndrome. *J Int Med Res*. 1990;18:201-209.

80. Wikner J, Hirsch U, Wetterberg L, Röjdmark S. Fibromyalgia: a syndrome associated with decreased nocturnal melatonin secretion. *Clin Endocrinol (Oxf)*. 1998;49:179-183.

81. León J, Acuña-Castroviejo D, Escames G, Tan DX, Reiter RJ. Melatonin mitigates mitochondrial malfunction. *J Pineal Res*. 2005;38:1-9.

82. Acuna-Castroviejo D, Escames G, Reiter RJ. Melatonin therapy in fibromyalgia. *J Pineal Res*. 2006;40:98-99.

83. Cordain L, Eaton SB, Sebastian A, et al. Origins and evolution of the Western diet: health implications for the 21st century. *Am J Clin Nutr*. 2005;81:341-354.

84. Rylander R, Remer T, Berkemeyer S, Vormann J. Acid-base status affects renal magnesium losses in healthy, elderly persons. *J Nutr*. 2006;136:2374-2377.

85. Russell IJ, Michalek JE, Flechas JD, Abraham GE. Treatment of fibromyalgia syndrome with Super Malic: a randomized, double blind, placebo controlled, crossover pilot study. *J Rheumatol*. 1995;22:953-958.

86. Rossini M, Di Munno O, Valentini G, et al. Double-blind, multicenter trial comparing acetyl l-carnitine with placebo in the treatment of fibromyalgia patients. *Clin Exp Rheumatol*. 2007;25:182-188.

87. Teitelbaum JE, Johnson C, St Cyr J. The use of D-ribose in chronic fatigue syndrome and fibromyalgia: a pilot study. *J Altern Complement Med*. 2006;12:857-862.

88. Amital D, Vishne T, Rubinow A, Levine J. Observed effects of creatine monohydrate in a patient with depression and fibromyalgia. *Am J Psychiatry*. 2006;163:1840-1841.

89. Watanabe A, Kato N, Kato T. Effects of creatine on mental fatigue and cerebral hemoglobin oxygenation. *Neurosci Res*. 2002;42:279-285.

90. Gaby AR. The role of coenzyme Q10 in clinical medicine, part 1. *Altern Med Rev*. 1996;1:11-17.

91. Gaby AR. The role of coenzyme Q10 in clinical medicine, part 2. *Altern Med Rev*. 1996;1:168-175.

92. Lister RE. An open, pilot study to evaluate the potential benefits of coenzyme Q10 combined with Ginkgo biloba extract in fibromyalgia syndrome. *J Int Med Res*. 2002;30:195-199.

93. Citak-Karakaya I, Akbayrak T, Demirturk F, Ekici G, Bakar Y. Short and long-term results of connective tissue manipulation and combined ultrasound therapy in patients with fibromyalgia. *J Manipulative Physiol Ther*. 2006;29:524-528.

94. Blunt KL, Rajwani MH, Guerriero RC. The effectiveness of chiropractic management of fibromyalgia patients: a pilot study. *J Manipulative Physiol Ther*. 1997;20:389-399.

95. Martin DP, Sletten CD, Williams BA, Berger IH. Improvement in fibromyalgia symptoms with acupuncture: results of a randomized controlled trial. *Mayo Clin Proc*. 2006;81:749-757.

96. Singh BB, Wu WS, Hwang SH, et al. Effectiveness of acupuncture in the treatment of fibromyalgia. *Altern Ther Health Med*. 2006;12:34-41.

97. Deluze C, Bosia L, Zirbs A, Chantraine A, Vischer TL. Electroacupuncture in fibromyalgia: results of a controlled trial. *BMJ*. 1992;305(6864):1249-1252.

98. Sandberg M, Larsson B, Lindberg LG, Gerdle B. Different patterns of blood flow response in the trapezius muscle following needle stimulation (acupuncture) between healthy subjects and patients with fibromyalgia and work-related trapezius myalgia. *Eur J Pain*. 2005;9:497-510.

99. Sandberg M, Lindberg LG, Gerdle B. Peripheral effects of needle stimulation (acupuncture) on skin and muscle blood flow in fibromyalgia. *Eur J Pain*. 2004;8:163-171.

100. Harris RE, Tian X, Williams DA, et al. Treatment of fibromyalgia with formula acupuncture: investigation of needle placement, needle stimulation, and treatment frequency. *J Altern Complement Med*. 2005;11:663-671.

101. Assefi NP, Sherman KJ, Jacobsen C, Goldberg J, Smith WR, Buchwald D. A randomized clinical trial of acupuncture compared with sham acupuncture in fibromyalgia. *Ann Intern Med*. 2005;143:10-19.

102. Mein EA, Greenman PE, McMillin DL, Richards DG, Nelson CD. Manual medicine diversity: research pitfalls and the emerging medical paradigm. *J Am Osteopath Assoc*. 2001;101:441-444.

103. Gamber RG, Shores JH, Russo DP, Jimenez C, Rubin BR. Osteopathic manipulative treatment in conjunction with medication relieves pain associated with fibromyalgia syndrome: results of a randomized clinical pilot project. *J Am Osteopath Assoc*. 2002;102:321-325.

104. Chen KW, Hassett AL, Hou F, Staller J, Lichtbroun AS. A pilot study of external qigong therapy for patients with fibromyalgia. *J Altern Complement Med*. 2006;12:851-856.

105. Ardiç F, Ozgen M, Aybek H, Rota S, Cubukçu D, Gökgöz A. Effects of balneotherapy on serum IL-1, PGE2 and LTB4 levels in fibromyalgia patients. *Rheumatol Int*. 2007;27:441-446.

106. Evcik D, Kizilay B, Gökçen E. The effects of balneotherapy on fibromyalgia patients. *Rheumatol Int*. 2002;22:56-59.

107. Fioravanti A, Perpignano G, Tirri G, et al. Effects of mud-bath treatment on fibromyalgia patients: a randomized clinical trial. *Rheumatol Int*. 2007;27:1157-1161.

108. Dönmez A, Karagülle MZ, Tercan N, et al. SPA therapy in fibromyalgia: a randomised controlled clinic study. *Rheumatol Int*. 2005;26:168-172.

109. Leventhal LJ. Management of fibromyalgia. *Ann Intern Med*. 1999;131:850-858.

110. Merchant RE, Carmack CA, Wise CM. Nutritional supplementation with Chlorella pyrenoidosa for patients with fibromyalgia syndrome: a pilot study. *Phytother Res*. 2000;14:167-173.

111. Pore RS. Detoxification of chlordecone poisoned rats with chlorella and chlorella derived sporopollenin. *Drug Chem Toxicol*. 1984;7:57-71.

112. Morita K, Ogata M, Hasegawa T. Chlorophyll derived from Chlorella inhibits dioxin absorption from the gastrointestinal tract and accelerates dioxin excretion in rats. *Environ Health Perspect*. 2001;109:289-294.

113. Morita K, Matsueda T, Iida T, Hasegawa T. Chlorella accelerates dioxin excretion in rats. *J Nutr*. 1999;129:1731-1736.

114. Nakano S, Noguchi T, Takekoshi H, Suzuki G, Nakano M. Maternal-fetal distribution and transfer of dioxins in pregnant women in Japan, and attempts to reduce maternal transfer with Chlorella (Chlorella pyrenoidosa) supplements. *Chemosphere*. 2005;61:1244-1255.

115. Nakano S, Takekoshi H, Nakano M. Chlorella (Chlorella pyrenoidosa) supplementation decreases dioxin and increases immunoglobulin a concentrations in breast milk. *J Med Food*. 2007;10:134-142.

116. Quigley EM, Flourie B. Probiotics and irritable bowel syndrome: a rationale for their use and an assessment of the evidence to date. *Neurogastroenterol Motil*. 2007;19:166-172.

117. O'Mahony L, McCarthy J, Kelly P, et al. Lactobacillus and bifidobacterium in irritable bowel syndrome: symptom responses and relationship to cytokine profiles. *Gastroenterology*. 2005;128:541-551.

118. Shornikova AV, Casas IA, Mykkänen H, Salo E, Vesikari T. Bacteriotherapy with Lactobacillus reuteri in rotavirus gastroenteritis. *Pediatr Infect Dis J*. 1997;16:1103-1107.

119. Rosenfeldt V, Benfeldt E, Valerius NH, Paerregaard A, Michaelsen KF. Effect of probiotics on gastrointestinal symptoms and small intestinal permeability in children with atopic dermatitis. *J Pediatr*. 2004;145:612-616.

120. Simenhoff ML, Dunn SR, Zollner GP, et al. Biomodulation of the toxic and nutritional effects of small bowel bacterial overgrowth in end-stage kidney disease using freeze-dried Lactobacillus acidophilus. *Miner Electrolyte Metab*. 1996;22(1-3):92-96.

Chapter 6

Clinical Focus: Rheumatoid Arthritis

Introduction

Rheumatoid arthritis is the prototypic inflammatory arthritis, presenting with joint pain and swelling that eventually progresses to variable levels of joint destruction, deformity, and disability in the majority of affected patients. In addition to the musculoskeletal impact of the disease process, rheumatoid arthritis commonly involves internal organs and systemic vasculature to effect pathological changes and serious dysfunction in virtually any tissue or organ. Rheumatoid arthritis is one of the most common autoimmune diseases, with a 1% prevalence across most populations and a 3:1 female-to-male ratio, with typical onset between ages 20 and 40. While acknowledging genetic linkage to HLA-DR4, most medical textbooks still describe the condition as idiopathic,[1] despite the wealth of basic science and clinical research that has clearly defined the contributory roles played by different components of the disease.[2]

Pathophysiology

The historical pathological view of rheumatoid arthritis is that of joint destruction hallmarked by synovial pannus formation, resulting in erosion of bone and cartilage which leads to joint destruction and deformity. Intra-articular inflammation is characterized by the elaboration from neutrophils, monocytes, and synovial cells of prostaglandins (particularly PG-E2), leukotrienes, superoxide anion, peroxynitrite, peroxi and hydroperoxi acids, matrix metalloproteinases, gelatinases, collagenases, tumor necrosis factor-alpha (TNF-α), lymphotoxin, interleukin-1, and interleukin-6. Synovial plasma cells produce the anti-IgG IgM autoantibody known as rheumatoid factor, which has traditionally been used as a serological test to support the diagnosis of rheumatoid arthritis. Intraarticular deposition of rheumatoid factor immune complexes leads to activation of the complement system for further exacerbation and perpetuation of inflammation.

Clinical Presentation

According to the American College of Rheumatology, clinical presentation is generally that of subacute, symmetrical, peripheral polyarthropathy, typically first affecting the wrists, knuckles, and finger joints (metacarpophylangeal, proximal, and distal interphalangeal joints). Systemic manifestations of an inflammatory response (low-grade fever, myalgia, weight loss, malaise) are generally also present. More specific and advanced musculoskeletal findings include gel phenomenon, morning stiffness longer than 1 hour, synovial hypertrophy, radial deviation of the wrists and ulnar deviation of the fingers, swan neck and boutonniere deformities of the fingers, synovitis, and tenosynovitis. Subcutaneous rheumatoid nodules (inflammatory granulomas) are seen in up 30% of patients. Lung (dyspnea, pulmonary nodules, fibrosis), renal, ocular, and pericardial involvement may also occur. Virtually any organ or tissue can be affected by ischemic damage from rheumatoid vasculitis or erosion from inflammatory infiltration. Rheumatoid arthritis patients show increased risk for cardiovascular disease, serious infections, osteoporosis, depression, and adverse effects from drug treatments. Approximately 50% of patients are partially or completely disabled within 5 years of diagnosis.

Diagnosis

Until recently, the diagnosis of rheumatoid arthritis was generally made on clinical grounds, using the criteria of 4 of 7 of the following[3]:

- Morning stiffness longer than 1 hour
- Idiopathic, non-traumatic arthritis of at least 3 joints for more than 6 weeks
- Peripheral arthritis
- Symmetric arthritis (not applicable in patients with peripheral neuropathy, stroke, or hemiplegia)
- Rheumatoid nodules
- Positive rheumatoid factor
- Radiographic manifestations including periarticular erosions or osteoporosis

Reliance upon these clinical criteria was necessary because no accurate and practical laboratory test was available. Within the past few years, however, serological testing for antibodies to cyclic citrullinated proteins (anti-CCP antibodies) have emerged as a new test for the diagnosis of rheumatoid arthritis with high sensitivity and specificity.[4,5,6,7] A recent review concluded that anti-CCP had 67% sensitivity and 95% specificity for rheumatoid arthritis.[8] Typical differentials include genetic hemochromatosis and other forms of iron overload,[9] osteoarthritis, systemic lupus erythematosus (SLE), septic arthritis, Lyme disease, reactive arthritis, gout and other crystal-induced arthropathy, arthritis related to viral infection, psoriatic arthritis, and Adult Still 's disease; occasionally celiac disease (gluten enteropathy) can present as a chronic arthritis that resembles rheumatoid arthritis or SLE.[10,11]

Standard Medical Treatment

When the process leading to rheumatoid arthritis is viewed as idiopathic, the goal of treatment is suppression of the inflammatory pathophysiology with the use of sequential and additive anti-inflammatory drugs. This treatment typically begins with nonsteroidal anti-inflammatory drugs (NSAIDs) and prednisone, then progresses through the disease-modifying antirheumatic drugs (DMARDS) methotrexate, sulfasalazine, and hydroxychloroquine, to finally arrive at the "biologics," which are for the most part cytokine antagonists, including parenterally administered TNF-α antibodies and receptors and interleukin-1 receptor antagonists. Cyclooxygenase-2 (COX-2) -inhibiting drugs have been shown to increase cardiovascular morbidity and mortality and are not appropriate for routine chronic use in the treatment of patients with rheumatoid arthritis, who as a group already have increased risk for cardiovascular disease. Surgical joint replacement and physical and occupational therapy are also used.

Functional Medicine Considerations and Interventions

The functional medicine perspective acknowledges the merits and limitations of the above pathological-pharmaceutical paradigm while further appreciating a broader range of nutritional, hormonal, environmental, and microbial influences that synergize to contribute to the immune dysfunction antedating pathophysiological manifestations. Rather than viewing rheumatoid arthritis as *idiopathic* and thus merely *suppressible*, functional medicine clinicians and their patients are better served by appreciating the disease as *complex, interconnected, and multifactorial*, whereby each component of the disease can be addressed to achieve additive and synergistic clinical benefits. Several of the more pertinent considerations will be described here, separated into the following categories: dietary and nutritional, hormonal, antimicrobial/anti-dysbiotic, and symptomatic.

Dietary and Nutritional Considerations and Interventions

Anti-inflammatory diet — The clinical benefits of a Paleolithic-Mediterranean diet for rheumatoid arthritis patients have been demonstrated in numerous clinical trials.[12,13] The standard American diet is inherently proinflammatory and thus serves to shift the body's internal climate toward one that fosters the development of inflammatory disease. *Direct* mechanisms include the activation of toll-like receptors and nuclear factor-kappa B (NF-κB), while *indirect* mechanisms include depleting the body of anti-inflammatory nutrients and dietary displacement of more nutrient-dense anti-inflammatory foods. Moving away from allergens, sugars, arachidonate, *trans* fats, and chemicals while moving toward fruits, vegetables, berries, nuts, seeds, omega-3 and monounsaturated fatty acids, and lean sources of low-arachidonate protein (possibly including fish, soy, and whey protein) is an absolutely essential foundational component of functional medicine intervention. A health-promoting diet also helps patients avoid overconsumption of chemical preservatives, artificial sweeteners, and carbohydrate-dominant foods such as candies, pastries, breads, potatoes, grains, and other foods with a high glycemic load and high glycemic index. Addition of basic nutritional supplementation (multivitamin, multimineral, combination fatty acids, probiotics, and physiological doses of vitamin D3) complete the supplemented Paleolithic-Mediterranean diet.[14,15] *Failure to implement diet modification undermines all other interventions, whether natural or pharmacological.*[16,17,18]

- **Avoidance of carbohydrate-induced immunosuppression** — Occult infections are widely believed to contribute to the genesis and perpetuation of rheumatoid arthritis and other autoimmune diseases. When inoculated into rats, nasopharyngeal bacteria from rheumatoid arthritis patients induce a rheumatoid arthritis -like disease. Intake of high carbohydrate loads suppresses immune function[19,20] and likely promotes the perpetuation of subclinical infections and dysbiosis. Therefore, avoiding dietary immunosuppression by avoiding high-glycemic foods is proposed to support optimal immune function and the clearing of occult infections.
- **Avoidance of carbohydrate-promoted small intestinal bacterial overgrowth (SIBO)** — At least 40% of rheumatoid arthritis patients have evidence of SIBO.[21] Delivery of a high carbohydrate load to the gastrointestinal lumen promotes SIBO,[22,23] which is inherently proinflammatory.[24,25] Intestinal bacteria are capable of inducing systemic inflammation and chronic, erosive, recurrent polyarthritis in rats that resembles human rheumatoid arthritis,[26,27] and low-carbohydrate diets are well known to alleviate SIBO.[22,28]
- **Avoidance of allergenic foods** — Food allergy avoidance in rheumatoid arthritis patients results in subjective, clinical, and histological improvements.[29,30] Consumption of allergenic foods contributes to the body 's total inflammatory load via immune activation; additionally, allergen consumption can increase intestinal permeability and contribute to dysbiosis, exacerbating systemic inflammation. For these reasons, hypoallergenic/oligoantigenic and rotation diets are foundational components of antirheumatic and anti-inflammatory interventions. Consumption of allergenic foods can result in the formation of immune complexes that deposit in synovium to produce localized joint inflammation; the formation of cross-reacting antibodies to food and articular structures can additionally result in clinical inflammatory arthritis.[31,32] Most patients with inflammatory disorders have numerous food allergies and intolerances which can be identified and treated with the *elimination and challenge* technique. Serological and cytological testing is available, validated, and useful for complex or recalcitrant cases.

Vegan and vegetarian diets — These diets have consistently shown benefit in the treatment of inflammatory disorders such as rheumatoid arthritis.[33,34,35] Implementation of vegan or vegetarian diets (particularly when free of gluten and dense carbohydrate) accomplishes several nutritional and immunologic benefits: (1) avoidance of previously consumed foods to which the patient may have become sensitized (i.e., allergen avoidance), (2) increased consumption of fruits and vegetables that provide balanced natural antioxidants, anti-inflammatory agents, and analgesics and that effect alkalinization for beneficial reductions in cortisol levels, bone resorption, and urinary mineral losses, and (3) qualitative and quantitative changes in gut flora.

Short-term fasting — Fasting is the most hypoallergenic and low-carbohydrate diet available and is suitable for short-term implementation to alleviate numerous chronic health problems, the most responsive of which is chronic hypertension.[36,37] Generally speaking, consumption of food (particularly those high in carbohydrate and saturated fat) induces a systemic inflammatory response[38]; thus, abstinence from food provides a reprieve from dietary inflammatory stimuli for a relative anti-inflammatory effect. Fasting deprives intestinal microbes of substrate, stimulates intestinal B-cell immunity, improves the bactericidal action of neutrophils, raises levels of anti-inflammatory immunomodulatory dehydroepiandrosterone (DHEA), reduces lysozyme release and leukotriene formation, and ameliorates gut permeability. In case reports and clinical trials, short-term fasting (or protein-sparing fasting) has been documented as a safe and effective primary or adjunctive treatment for SLE, rheumatoid arthritis, and non-rheumatic diseases such as chronic hypertension, obesity, type 2 diabetes, and epilepsy.[34,39,40,41,42,43,44,45] Short-term fasting is often used as a precursor to other beneficial dietary changes; it enhances and is sometimes necessary to achieve the benefits of dietary modification.[46]

Combination fatty acid replacement/supplementation — Modernized Western/American diets are notoriously deficient in omega-3 and omega-9 fatty acids and overladen with omega-6 fatty acids (excluding gamma-linolenic acid [GLA]) and *trans*- and saturated fatty acids. These imbalances result in adverse alterations in membrane receptor functions, prostaglandin and leukotrienes synthesis, and genetic expression that favor the genesis and perpetuation of chronic health problems, especially inflammatory phenomenon such as autoimmunity. Diet improvement and supplementation with health-promoting anti-inflammatory fatty acids is therefore a commonly used, well-validated, safe, and highly effective intervention in conditions such as rheumatoid arthritis.

Given at doses of 3000 to 9000 mg/d, alpha-linolenic acid (ALA) from flaxseed oil has impressive anti-inflammatory benefits demonstrated by its ability to halve prostaglandin production in humans.[47] Numerous studies have demonstrated the benefit of GLA from borage, evening primrose, hemp, and blackcurrant seed oils in the treatment of rheumatoid arthritis when used at doses between 500 and 4000 mg/d.[48,49] Fish oil provides omega-3 eicosapentaenoic acid (EPA) and docosahexaenoic acid (DHA), which have proven anti-inflammatory benefits in rheumatoid arthritis.[50,51,52] Combined daily doses of EPA and DHA should generally be in the range of 3000 to 9000 mg/d, consumed in divided doses with food. Omega-9 oleic acid is best sourced from olive oil, which can be used generously in cooking and on raw vegetables; the anti-inflammatory benefits of olive oil are attributable to other fatty acids such as squalene, as well as phenolic antioxidants.

High-dose supplementation with polyunsaturated fatty acids warrants increased intake of antioxidants from the diet, from fruit and vegetable juices, and from properly formulated broad-spectrum antioxidant supplements. Since patients with systemic inflammation are generally in a pro-oxidative state, consideration should be given to the timing and starting dose of fatty acid supplementation and the need for antioxidant protection; some patients should start with a low dose of fatty acid supplementation until inflammation and the hyperoxidative state have been reduced. Fatty acids are not clinically or biochemically interchangeable, and they compete for absorption and metabolism; thus, each of the fatty acids must be supplied (i.e., combination fatty acid therapy, rather than monotherapy) in order for maximum benefits to be obtained.[53]

Vitamin D3 (cholecalciferol) — Epidemiological studies link vitamin D insufficiency with increased risk for numerous chronic health problems, including autoimmunity. Vitamin D deficiency is epidemic in the general population and is even more common in patients with chronic illness and chronic musculoskeletal pain.[54] Correction of vitamin D deficiency supports normal immune protection against infection and provides a clinically significant anti-inflammatory[55] and pain-relieving benefit in patients with musculoskeletal pain.[56] Since the physiological requirement for vitamin D3 in adult men is 3000 to 5000 IU/d, routine use of 1000 to 2000 IU for children and 4000 IU for adults has been recommended.[57] Deficiency and response to treatment are monitored with serum 25-hydroxy vitamin D3 (25[OH]D) while safety is monitored with serum calcium; inflammatory granulomatous diseases and certain drugs such as hydrochlorothiazide increase the propensity for hypercalcemia and warrant incremental dosing and frequent monitoring of serum calcium. Vitamin D2 (ergocalciferol) is not a human nutrient and should not be used in clinical practice because of lesser efficacy and greater propensity for untoward effects. In sum, the immunomodulatory, anti-inflammatory, pain-relieving, osteoporosis-preventing, antidepressant, and health promoting benefits of vitamin D3 warrant its routine inclusion in the treatment of patients with rheumatoid arthritis.

Correction of Hormonal Imbalances

Several hormones, in particular prolactin, cortisol, DHEA, testosterone, and the estrogens, have powerful immunomodulatory actions, and the research literature has delineated patterns of abnormality that typify the hormonal profiles seen in patients with autoimmunity. Specifically, the typical pattern that is seen is that of relative or absolute excesses of prolactin and estrogen(s) and insufficiencies of cortisol, DHEA, and testosterone. Comprehensive hormonal assessment should be a routine component of care for all patients with systemic autoimmunity. The suggested battery of laboratory tests includes serum prolactin, cortisol , serum DHEA-sulfate, free and total testosterone, serum estradiol, and thyroid panel (e.g., TSH, free T4, total T3, reverse T3, and antithyroid antibodies). Abnormalities are treated with effective interventions, whether nutritional, botanical, hormonal (supplementation for insufficiency), or pharmacological (blockade for imbalances or excess production).

Latent and overt hyperprolactinemia — Prolactin is a peptide hormone secreted by the anterior pituitary gland (adenohypophysis); its secretion is inhibited by tonic dopaminergic suppression. Although the hormone is classically associated with lactation, levels of prolactin increase in men and women during times of psychological or physiological stress (including infection) or due to prolactin-secreting pituitary adenoma (prolactinoma). Elevated prolactin affects the immune system in such a way as to promote immune activation, which can promote systemic inflammation and autoimmunity. Patients with rheumatoid arthritis and SLE have higher basal and stress-induced levels of prolactin compared with normal controls.[58,59] Men with rheumatoid arthritis have higher serum levels of prolactin, and these levels correlate with the severity and duration of the disorder.[60,61]

Suppression of prolactin secretion with drug therapy (e.g., bromocriptine or cabergoline) provides clinical benefit in patients with autoimmunity, and a few botanical medicines also lower prolactin levels and might be of benefit via this mechanism. Bromocriptine (2.5 mg/d) was shown to be effective against lupus,[62] and use of bromocriptine appears warranted in patients with rheumatoid arthritis, SLE, reactive arthritis, psoriatic arthritis, and probably multiple sclerosis and uveitis.[63] Cabergoline (0.25 mg twice per week[64]) appears safer and more efficacious than bromocriptine.[65] Cabergoline also provides an antirheumatic benefit in rheumatoid arthritis patients by reducing prolactin secretion.[66] Hypothyroidism commonly causes hyperprolactinemia, and therefore, correction of hypothyroidism can lower prolactin levels for an antirheumatic benefit. *Vitex astus-cagnus* is a botanical medicine that functions like bromocriptine and cabergoline to lower serum prolactin in humans[67,68] via a dopaminergic effect[69]; however, no studies demonstrating an antirheumatic effect of *Vitex* in humans have been published. The botanical *Mucuna pruriens* contains L-dopa and shows clinical dopaminergic activity as evidenced by its effectiveness in Parkinson's disease[70]; however, antirheumatic studies have not yet been performed. High-protein meals stimulate prolactin release,[71] and thus, some of the benefit of vegan and vegetarian diets, as well as fasting, may be derived from reductions in prolactin secretion.

Cortisol insufficiency — Cortisol has immunoregulatory and immunosuppressive actions at physiological concentrations, and low cortisol production is common in patients with chronic immune dysfunction and autoimmunity, according to Jefferies.[72,73] Cortisol production is assessed by 24-hour urine collection or by pre- and post-ACTH challenge, with insufficiency defined as failure of the cortisol level to double after 30 to 60 minutes or failure to rise to at least 18 mcg/dL.[74] Supplementation with 20 mg/d of cortisol is physiological; 10 mg immediately upon waking followed by 5 mg in late morning and 5 mg in midafternoon attempts to replicate the diurnal variation and normal morning peak of cortisol levels. Additional details, rationale, and benefits of cortisol replacement have been reviewed by Jefferies.[75]

Dehydroepiandrosterone insufficiency and supraphysiological supplementation — DHEA is an anti-inflammatory and immunoregulatory hormone that is commonly deficient in patients with autoimmunity and inflammatory arthritis.[76] DHEA levels are suppressed by prednisone,[77] and DHEA supplementation has been shown to reverse the osteoporosis and loss of bone mass induced by corticosteroid treatment.[78] DHEA shows no acute or subacute toxicity when used in supraphysiological doses, even when used in sick patients. For example, in a study of 32 patients with HIV, DHEA doses of 750 to 2250 mg/d were well tolerated and produced no dose-limiting adverse effects.[79] This lack of toxicity compares favorably with DMARDs, nearly all of which show impressive comparable toxicity. Optimal clinical response appears to correlate with serum levels that are supraphysiological,[80] and therefore, treatment dosage is not necessarily dependent on serum DHEA levels, provided that the patient is free of contraindications, particularly sex-hormone-dependent malignancy. Other than mild effects predictable with any androgen (e.g., transient acne, increased facial hair), DHEA supplementation does not appear to cause serious adverse effects and is appropriate for routine clinical use, particularly when used at reasonable doses for appropriate durations in properly selected patients.[81]

When used at doses of 200 mg/d, DHEA has safely provided significant clinical benefit for patients with various autoimmune diseases, including inflammatory bowel disease[82] and SLE,[83] and generally allowed reduction in NSAID and DMARD reliance. In one study. DHEA supplementation allowed for reduced dosing of prednisone (thus avoiding its adverse effects) while providing symptomatic improvement in patients with SLE.[84] In contrast to these favorable results and the practical experience of many clinicians, a small open-label study using DHEA in 11 patients with rheumatoid arthritis failed to show benefit,[85] perhaps due to patient selection, small sample size, concomitant drug use, or failure to correct for DHEA-induced estradiol increase. Fasting and ketogenic diets raise DHEA levels in rheumatoid arthritis patients, and thus, part of the benefit of such dietary interventions is truly endocrinological rather than nutritional or metabolic, as is commonly assumed.[86]

Estrogen excess — Women have higher levels of estrogen than men, and these higher levels correlate with a higher incidence of nearly all autoimmune diseases in women. Generally speaking, estrogens as a group demonstrate proinflammatory effects, and higher estrogen levels (whether from endogenous production or exogenous sources such as oral contraceptives and hormone replacement therapy) correlate with increased risk for autoimmunity. Men with rheumatoid arthritis show an excess of estradiol that is proportional to the degree of inflammation.[87] The estrogen-blocking drugs anastrozole and tamoxifen have demonstrated anti-inflammatory and antirheumatic benefits in case reports of women with autoimmune dermatomyositis.[88] Found in cruciferous vegetables and available as a nutritional supplement, indole-3-carbinol (I3C) promotes preferential production of anti-inflammatory 2-hydroxyestrone while reducing production of proinflammatory and immunodysregulatory 16-alpha-hydroxyestrone. A short-term trial using I3C (375 mg/d) in patients with SLE resulted in modest clinical improvement, as well as favorable modification of estrogen metabolism away from 16-alpha-hydroxyestrone and toward 2-hydroxyestrone.[89] I3C also has anti-inflammatory actions via inhibition of NF-κB, and administration of I3C in an animal model of lupus was shown to significantly prevent disease progression and to prolong life span.[90] Other techniques for reducing estrogen levels include reducing adiposity, avoiding ethanol, surgical correction of varicocele in affected men, and increased consumption of dietary fiber, cruciferous vegetables, and green tea.

Estrogens can be measured in serum and urine samples; in our office, we commonly measure serum estradiol in men and administer the aromatase inhibitor anastrozole at 1 mg (2–7 doses per week) to men whose estradiol level is greater than 30 pg/mL. Although originally designed to lower estrogen levels in women with hormone-responsive breast cancer, anastrozole can be used in men to lower estradiol and raise testosterone[91]; generally, this is exactly the desired result in patients with systemic autoimmunity. Because estrogens are derived from androgens following conversion by aromatase, administration of androgenic hormones may have an estrogenic effect that necessitates modulation via aromatase inhibition.

Testosterone insufficiency — Like DHEA and cortisol, testosterone is immunoregulatory and tends to have an antirheumatic effect. Androgen deficiencies predispose to, are exacerbated by, and contribute to autoimmunity. A large proportion of men with SLE or rheumatoid arthritis have low testosterone[92,93] and suffer the effects of hypogonadism: fatigue, weakness, depression, slow healing, low libido, and difficulties with sexual performance. Testosterone levels may rise following DHEA supplementation (especially in women) and can be elevated by the use of anastrozole or transdermal or intramuscular testosterone. When treated with testosterone, men and women with rheumatoid arthritis show clinical benefit including reduced pain and inflammation, decreased use of NSAIDs, and improved quality of life.[94,95]

Thyroid insufficiency or autoimmunity — Hypothyroidism can cause an inflammatory myopathy that resembles polymyositis, and autoimmune hypothyroidism is a frequent complication of nearly all autoimmune diseases. Hypothyroidism causes reduced intestinal motility, which results in SIBO and thereby contributes to intestinal dysbiosis and the resultant proinflammatory effects. Treatment of hypothyroidism can be accomplished with T4 and/or T3. Supportive measures which may be clinically sufficient and obviate the need for hormone replacement include supplementation with selenium[96,97,98] (reduces thyroid autoimmunity and improves peripheral conversion of T4 to T3), iodine,[99] and tyrosine. Given that thyroid dysfunction and autoimmunity may indicate unrecognized toxic exposure, which can trigger systemic autoimmunity, clinicians are wise to view thyroid dysfunction as a possible sign of previous toxic exposure worthy of direct intervention to ameliorate the underlying cause of immunodysfunction.[100]

Assessment and Treatment for Dysbiosis

Subclinical infections, occult microbial colonization, and other forms of dysbiosis are generally underappreciated causes of autoimmunity induction, perpetuation, and exacerbation. All patients with rheumatoid arthritis have one or more subsets of dysbiosis until proven otherwise by clinical investigation and antimicrobial intervention. Additional details are provided in the excellent overview by Noah[101] (also see *Microbial analysis of mucosal surfaces and environment* in Chapter 2).

Seven types of dysbiosis can be discussed based on location, namely orodental, sinorespiratory, gastrointestinal, parenchymal, genitourinary, cutaneous, and environmental. Of these, sinorespiratory, gastrointestinal, and genitourinary dysbiosis appear most relevant to rheumatoid arthritis in general, but clinicians should remain particularly vigilant for orodental and environmental dysbiosis in difficult cases.

Gastrointestinal dysbiosis — Gastrointestinal dysbiosis is a daily finding in the clinical practice of functional medicine. Specifically relevant to this discussion of rheumatoid arthritis is the association of gastrointestinal microbes such as *Endolimax nana*,[102] *Proteus mirabilis*,[103,104] *Entamoeba histolytica,* and *Giardia lamblia*[105] among patients with rheumatoid arthritis and rheumatoid arthritis-like syndromes. Of lesser notoriety but probably more clinical significance to rheumatoid arthritis patients is induction of systemic inflammation and peripheral arthritis by the ubiquitous bacterium *Eubacterium aerofaciens*, which is increased in the gastrointestinal tracts of rheumatoid arthritis patients and which produces chronic arthritis in animals following administration of its cell wall fragments.[106]

The most significant paradigmatic leap for clinicians to take is the realization that the taxonomy of the microbe is of far less importance than the nature of the interaction between the microbe and the individual patient, as well as that patient's response to the microbe; any individual patient's immune system may have an exaggerated proinflammatory response that manifests clinically as systemic inflammation and autoimmune arthritis, even if the triggering microbe is not classically associated with the disease or if patient population studies have determined that the relationship is statistically insignificant. For this reason, clinicians are justified in searching for and eradicating potentially problematic microbes that may be serving as the immunogenic stimulus for systemic inflammation. For example, while none of the following organisms is classically associated with rheumatoid arthritis, clinicians should realize that *Helicobacter pylori, Klebsiella pneumoniae, Citrobacter freundii, Hafnia alvei, Proteus mirabilis*, and *Candida albicans* have each been shown to induce reactive arthritis or inflammatory autoimmune syndromes that remit following eradication of the microbe.

For practical clinical application, all rheumatoid arthritis patients should have 3-sample comprehensive stool analyses and parasitology assessments performed by a specialty laboratory; dysbiotic microbes are eradicated via pharmacological and botanical antimicrobials supported by dietary interventions (especially a low-carbohydrate diet, discussed above). These tests are critical because they allow for identification (i.e., yeast, bacteria, protozoa, helminths, and their individual identities) and quantification (i.e., amount and combination) of dysbiotic microbes and—very crucially—allow for the performance of the culture and sensitivity tests that are important for guiding treatment; the sensitivity results precisely define which pharmacological and botanical agents can be used (generally in combination) for eradication of the bacteria and yeast. However, performing the tests does not ensure that all microbes will be detected. Because there is a presumptive diagnosis of dysbiosis in rheumatoid arthritis,[107] all patients are treated with an antimicrobial program even in the absence of empiric evidence from the stool tests. The test of dysbiosis is thus in part empiric. Published, peer-reviewed examples of empiric treatment of dysbiosis without microbe identification include the use of rifaximin in the treatment of irritable bowel syndrome and SIBO,[108,109] long-term use of penicillin for the treatment of chronic plaque psoriasis,[110] and use of various antimicrobials, especially sulfamethoxazole-trimethoprim (trimeth-sulfa), against Wegener's granulomatosis.[111] Therefore, patients with unrevealing stool and parasitology assessments may be presumed to have false-negative results and may be treated accordingly for occult bacterial overgrowth.

Clinical Pearl:

It is the author's experience that the culture from stool tests is largely insensitive for anaerobic bacteria. In particular, the anaerobes *Bacteroides fragilis* and *Eubacterium aerofaciens* are not detected on basic or specialized stool tests; only research-based methodology can detect them, and this type of investigation is not performed in routine clinical practice. Overgrowth of both of these species has been associated with dysbiosis.

Sinorespiratory dysbiosis — Sinorespiratory dysbiosis refers to adverse health consequences resultant from microbial colonization of the respiratory tract. The paranasal sinuses and nasopharynx are commonly colonized with bacteria of significant pathogenic potential, and several of these inhabitants are known to be triggers for reactive arthritis and other inflammatory phenomena. Bacteria such as *Staphylococcus aureus, Streptococcus* sp, *Peptococcus/Peptostreptococcus, Klebsiella pneumoniae, Proteus mirabilis, Bacteroides, Haemophilus parainfluenzae,* and *Haemophilus influenzae* are common inhabitants of the upper airways, especially in patients with chronic sinusitis. Essentially, all patients with chronic sinus congestion (chronic rhinosinusitis) have occult fungal colonization to which they are immunologically sensitized (eosinophilic fungal rhinosinusitis).[112] Respiratory tract infections with *Chlamydia pneumoniae* can cause reactive arthritis and undifferentiated oligoarthritis.[113] Other autoimmune/inflammatory disorders such as Wegener's granulomatosis, SLE, dermatomyositis/polymyositis, and psoriasis are also associated with abnormal microbial colonization of the upper respiratory tract. Inoculation of rats with bacteria from the nasopharynx of rheumatoid arthritis patients induces systemic inflammation and chronic arthritis. For practical clinical application, microbiological identification and sensitivity testing can be performed from samples/swabs taken from the nares, nasal cavity, and pharynx; treatment with systemically administered or topically applied antimicrobials can be used specifically or empirically.

Clinical Pearl:

In patients with recalcitrant gastrointestinal dysbiosis, continuous gastrointestinal "seeding" of dysbiotic microbes from the sinorespiratory tract should be suspected and addressed.

Genitourinary dysbiosis — Most patients with chronic, undifferentiated oligoarthritis have evidence of immune response against arthritogenic bacteria.[114] All clinicians were trained to appreciate that genitourinary infection with *Chlamydia trachomatis* can produce inflammatory arthropathy called reactive arthritis, previously known as Reiter's syndrome.[115] In a study of 234 patients with inflammatory arthritis, 44% of patients had genitourinary colonization, mostly due to *Chlamydia, Mycoplasma,* or *Ureaplasma*; the authors concluded, "urogenital swab culture is the only useful diagnostic method for the detection of the arthritogenic infection in extra-articularly asymptomatic patients with undifferentiated oligoarthritis."[116] *Proteus mirabilis* is a pathogenic inhabitant of the genitourinary tract and is a strong candidate for a microbial trigger for rheumatoid arthritis; carriage of *Proteus mirabilis* is increased in the genitourinary tracts of rheumatoid arthritis patients compared to nonarthritic controls, and rheumatoid arthritis patients show clear evidence of immunologic hyperresponsiveness toward *Proteus mirabilis*.[117] Urinary tract infections cause elevations in plasma levels of endotoxins,[118] and men with chronic prostatitis have elevated endotoxin levels in their expressed prostatic secretions[119]; recall that endotoxin is a potent stimulus for immune activation and systemic inflammation.

Practical clinical application begins with history specific for urinary tract infections or symptoms; specific laboratory assessment consists of urinalysis (for leukocytes, mucus, leukocyte esterase, bacteria, culture and sensitivity). Serum tests for sexually transmitted and urogenital pathogens and urethral/vaginal swab for culture, and DNA polymerase chain reaction are generally sufficient for the detection of the majority of urogenital infections. Similar to the protocol evaluation of men with elevated PSA, a clinical trial of antibiotics/antimicrobials may reduce systemic inflammation and thereby implicate a dysbiotic stimulus as a cause of the inflammation. In women, particular attention must be given to correcting gastrointestinal dysbiosis due to the close anatomical proximity and therefore microbiological transfer between the anus and vagina.[120] Assessment of sexual partners is advised in cases of recalcitrant or recurrent genitourinary dysbiosis; barrier methods (e.g., condoms) can be used to prevent transmission/cross-contamination. Nutritional supplements containing *Arctostaphylos uva-ursi*, buchu, and cranberry can be used as urinary antiseptics.

Additional Therapeutic Considerations and Symptomatic Treatments

While the underlying contributors to the proinflammatory state are being investigated and addressed as described above, patients can take advantage of the following therapeutics to slow progression of the disease and alleviate pain and inflammation. In clinical practice, botanicals and other nutritional supplements are commonly used in combination to enhance synergism and reduce the adverse effects and inefficacy that are more commonly seen with high-dose monotherapy.

Uncaria tomentosa, Uncaria guianensis (cat's claw) — Cat's claw has been safely and successfully used in the treatment of osteoarthritis[121] and rheumatoid arthritis. Forty rheumatoid arthritis patients treated with sulfasalazine or hydroxychloroquine received clinical benefit from *Uncaria* extract versus placebo in terms of reduction of the number of painful and swollen joints and the Ritchie Index.[122] High-quality extractions from reputable manufacturers used according to directions are recommended.

Topical *Capsicum annuum, Capsicum frutescens* — Controlled clinical trials have conclusively demonstrated capsaicin's ability to deplete sensory fibers of the neuropeptide substance P and to thus reduce pain. Topical capsaicin has shown effectiveness in relieving the pain associated with diabetic neuropathy, chronic low back pain, chronic neck pain, osteoarthritis, and rheumatoid arthritis.[123] Given the important role of neurogenic inflammation in chronic arthritis, the use of topical *Capsicum* may help break the vicious cycle of neurogenic-immunogenic inflammation.

Oral enzyme therapy with proteolytic/pancreatic enzymes — Oral administration of pancreatic and proteolytic enzymes has a long history of therapeutic use in medicine, particularly in the treatment of inflammatory and malignant diseases. Oral polyenzyme therapy consisting of the between-meal administration of pancreatin, bromelain, papain, amylase, lipase, trypsin, and alpha-chymotrypsin has a wide therapeutic margin and range of clinical applicability. Inter-meal polyenzyme supplementation is rational as an adjunctive treatment in rheumatoid arthritis.[124]

Harpagophytum procumbens (devil's claw) — *Harpagophytum* is a moderately effective. non-anti-inflammatory, centrally acting botanical analgesic with a good track record of safety and efficacy in clinical trials of patients with low back pain and osteoarthritis.[125,126,12/] Products are generally standardized for the content of harpagosides, with a target dose of 60 mg/d when used in isolation. About 8% of patients may experience diarrhea or other mild gastrointestinal effects, and a few patients may experience dizziness.

Willow bark, *Salix* species — Extracts from willow bark have proven safe and effective in the alleviation of moderate/severe low back pain.[128,129] The mechanism of action includes inhibition of prostaglandin formation via inhibition of COX-2 gene transcription by salicylates, phytonutrients which are widely present in fruits, vegetables, herbs, and spices and which are partly responsible for the anticancer, anti-inflammatory, and health-promoting benefits of plant consumption. Vasquez and Muanza[130] pointed out that the only adverse effect that has been documented in association with willow bark was a single case of anaphylaxis in a patient previously sensitized to acetylsalicylic acid (aspirin). The daily dose should not exceed 240 mg of salicin, and products should include other components of the whole plant.

Boswellia serrata — *Boswellia* shows anti-inflammatory and analgesic benefits via inhibition of 5-lipoxygenase and NF-κB[131,132]; positive clinical results have been demonstrated in patients with osteoarthritis of the knees, asthma, and ulcerative colitis.[133,134,135]

Phytonutritional modulation of NF-κB — NF-κB plays a central role in the pathogenesis of the synovitis and joint destruction seen in rheumatoid arthritis.[136] Nutrients and botanicals that either directly or indirectly inhibit NF-κB for an anti-inflammatory benefit include vitamin D, curcumin (requires piperine for absorption[137]), lipoic acid, green tea, rosemary, grape seed extract, propolis, zinc, high-dose selenium, I3C, N-acetyl-L-cysteine, resveratrol, isohumulones, GLA via peroxisome proliferator-activated receptor-gamma, and EPA via peroxisome proliferator-activated receptor-alpha. Several phytonutritional products targeting NF-κB are commercially and clinically available, and many of these phytonutrients, vitamins, and minerals can be consumed in therapeutic doses from foods or nutritional supplements.

Glucosamine sulfate and chondroitin sulfate — Glucosamine and chondroitin sulfates are well tolerated and well documented in the treatment of osteoarthritis. Since these serve as substrate for the rebuilding and preservation of joint cartilage, they serve to help shift the balance toward anabolism and away from catabolism in articular tissues.[138,139,140] Long-term use is necessary for efficacy; glucosamine sulfate is more efficacious than glucosamine hydrochloride.[141]

Creative self-expression, therapeutic writing, and stress management/avoidance. Limited evidence indicates that self-expressive writing can significantly reduce symptomatology in patients with rheumatoid arthritis.[142] Numerous articles have linked stressful life events to the development of systemic inflammatory diseases such as rheumatoid arthritis; mechanistic links include reduction in serum androgens and cortisol, increased serum prolactin, and weakening of mucosal defenses (i.e., reduced secretion of sIgA) for reduction in internal anti-inflammatory hormones, elevation of proinflammatory prolactin, and increases in sinorespiratory, gastrointestinal, and genitourinary dysbiosis, which synergize to promote self-perpetuating systemic inflammation. Stress reduction, stress management, and stress avoidance combined with increased social support and emotional safety and intimacy should be pursued.

Conclusion and Clinical Approach

Peer-reviewed research published in top-tier general medicine and specialty journals substantiates nonpharmacological and nonsurgical treatments for rheumatoid arthritis consisting of dietary, nutritional, botanical, hormonal, and antimicrobial interventions. The first patient visit consists of history, laboratory tests (e.g., serum assays and microbial cultures), dietary intervention, and basic nutritional supplementation. The second and additional follow-up visits refine the treatment plan based on laboratory results and response to treatment. Systemic autoimmune diseases are co-managed with an internist or rheumatologist in case of unpredictable inflammatory exacerbation.

References

1. Merkel PA, Simms RW. Rheumatoid arthritis. In: Andreoli TE, Carpenter CCJ, Griggs RC, Benjamin IJ, eds. *Cecil Essentials of Medicine*. 7th ed. Philadelphia, Pa: Saunders Elsevier; 2007: 804-808.
2. Vasquez A. *Integrative Rheumatology*. 2nd ed. Fort Worth, Tex: Integrative and Biological Medicine Research and Consulting LLC; 2007.
3. Beers MH, Berkow R, eds. *The Merck Manual of Diagnosis and Therapy*. 17th ed. Whitehouse Station; Merck Research Laboratories; 1999: 418.

4. Hill J, Cairns E, Bell DA. The joy of citrulline: new insights into the diagnosis, pathogenesis, and treatment of rheumatoid arthritis. *J Rheumatol*. 2004;31:1471-1473.

5. van Boekel MA, Vossenaar ER, van den Hoogen FH, van Venrooij WJ. Autoantibody systems in rheumatoid arthritis: specificity, sensitivity and diagnostic value. *Arthritis Res*. 2002;4:87-93.

6. Migliorini P, Pratesi F, Tommasi C, Anzilotti C. The immune response to citrullinated antigens in autoimmune diseases. *Autoimmun Rev*. 2005;4:561-564.

7. Mikuls TR, Holers VM, Parrish L, et al. Anti-cyclic citrullinated peptide antibody and rheumatoid factor isotypes in African Americans with early rheumatoid arthritis. *Arthritis Rheum*. 2006;54:3057-3059.

8. van der Woude D, Huizinga TW. The battle between anti-cyclic citrullinated peptide and rheumatoid factor tests: a winner at last? Nat Clin Pract Rheumatol. 2007;3:696-697.

9. Bensen WG, Laskin CA, Little HA, Fam AG. Hemochromatotic arthropathy mimicking rheumatoid arthritis. A case with subcutaneous nodules, tenosynovitis, and bursitis. *Arthritis Rheum*. 1978;21:844-848.

10. Parke AL, Fagan EA, Chadwick VS, Hughes GR. Coeliac disease and rheumatoid arthritis. *Ann Rheum Dis*. 1984;43:378-380.

11. Bourne JT, Kumar P, Huskisson EC, Mageed R, Unsworth DJ, Wojtulewski JA. Arthritis and coeliac disease. *Ann Rheum Dis*. 1985;44:592-598.

12. Skoldstam L, Hagfors L, Johansson G. An experimental study of a Mediterranean diet intervention for patients with rheumatoid arthritis. *Ann Rheum Dis*. 2003;62:208-214.

13. McKellar G, Morrison E, McEntegart A, et al. A pilot study of a Mediterranean-type diet intervention in female patients with rheumatoid arthritis living in areas of social deprivation in Glasgow. *Ann Rheum Dis*. 2007;66:1239-1243.

14. Vasquez A. A five-part nutritional protocol that produces consistently positive results. *Nutritional Wellness*. September 2005. Available online at: http://optimalhealthresearch.com/protocol.

15. Vasquez A. Implementing the five-part nutritional wellness protocol for the treatment of various health problems. *Nutritional Wellness*. November 2005. Available online: http://optimalhealthresearch.com/protocol.

16. Vasquez A. Common oversights and shortcomings in the study and implementation of nutritional supplementation. *Naturopathy Digest*. June 2007. Available online at: http://www.naturopathydigest.com/archives/2007/jun/vasquez.php.

17. Seaman DS. The dietary pursuit of disease overwhelms the power of nutritional supplements. *Nutritional Wellness*. August 2007. Available online at: http://www.nutritionalwellness.com/archives/2007/aug/08_seaman.php.

18. Seaman DR. The diet-induced proinflammatory state: a cause of chronic pain and other degenerative diseases? *J Manipulative Physiol Ther*. 2002;25:168-179.

19. Sanchez A, Reeser JL, Lau HS, et al. Role of sugars in human neutrophilic phagocytosis. *Am J Clin Nutr*. 1973;26:1180-1184.

20. Rasmussen A, Segel E, Hessov I, Borregaard N. Reduced function of neutrophils during routine postoperative glucose infusion. *Acta Chir Scand*. 1988;154(7-8):429-433.

21. Henriksson AE, Blomquist L, Nord CE, Midtvedt T, Uribe A. Small intestinal bacterial overgrowth in patients with rheumatoid arthritis. *Ann Rheum Dis*. 1993;52:503-510.

22. Ramakrishnan T, Stokes P. Beneficial effects of fasting and low carbohydrate diet in D-lactic acidosis associated with short-bowel syndrome. *JPEN J Parenter Enteral Nutr*. 1985;9:361-363.

23. Gottschall E. *Breaking the Vicious Cycle: Intestinal Health Through Diet*. Revised edition. Kirkton Press; 1994.

24. Lin HC. Small intestinal bacterial overgrowth: a framework for understanding irritable bowel syndrome. *JAMA*. 2004;292:852-858.

25. Lichtman SN, Wang J, Sartor RB, et al. Reactivation of arthritis induced by small bowel bacterial overgrowth in rats: role of cytokines, bacteria, and bacterial polymers. *Infect Immun*. 1995;63:2295-2301.

26. Severijnen AJ, van Kleef R, Hazenberg MP, van de Merwe JP. Chronic arthritis induced in rats by cell wall fragments of Eubacterium species from the human intestinal flora. *Infect Immun*. 1990;58:523-528.

27. Stimpson SA, Brown RR, Anderle SK, et al. Arthropathic properties of cell wall polymers from normal flora bacteria. *Infect Immun*. 1986;51:240-249.

28. Mayne AJ, Handy DJ, Preece MA, George RH, Booth IW. Dietary management of D-lactic acidosis in short bowel syndrome. *Arch Dis Child*. 1990;65:229-231.

29. van de Laar MA, Aalbers M, Bruins FG, van Dinther-Janssen AC, van der Korst JK, Meijer CJ. Food intolerance in rheumatoid arthritis. II. Clinical and histological aspects. *Ann Rheum Dis*. 1992;51:303-306.

30. Hafstrom I, Ringertz B, Spangberg A, et al. A vegan diet free of gluten improves the signs and symptoms of rheumatoid arthritis: the effects on arthritis correlate with a reduction in antibodies to food antigens. *Rheumatology (Oxford)*. 2001;40:1175-1179.

31. Hvatum M, Kanerud L, Hallgren R, Brandtzaeg P. The gut-joint axis: cross reactive food antibodies in rheumatoid arthritis. *Gut*. 2006;55:1240-1247.

32. Inman RD. Antigens, the gastrointestinal tract, and arthritis. *Rheum Dis Clin North Am*. 1991;17:309-321.

33. Kjeldsen-Kragh J. Rheumatoid arthritis treated with vegetarian diets. *Am J Clin Nutr*. 1999;70(Suppl 3):594S-600S

34. Kjeldsen-Kragh J, Haugen M, Borchgrevink CF, et al. Controlled trial of fasting and one-year vegetarian diet in rheumatoid arthritis. *Lancet*. 1991;338(8772):899-902.

35. Tanaka T, Kouda K, Kotani M, et al. Vegetarian diet ameliorates symptoms of atopic dermatitis through reduction of the number of peripheral eosinophils and of PGE2 synthesis by monocytes. *J Physiol Anthropol Appl Human Sci*. 2001;20:353-361.

36. Goldhamer A, Lisle D, Parpia B, Anderson SV, Campbell TC. Medically supervised water-only fasting in the treatment of hypertension. *J Manipulative Physiol Ther*. 2001;24:335-339.

37. Goldhamer AC, Lisle DJ, Sultana P, et al. Medically supervised water-only fasting in the treatment of borderline hypertension. *J Altern Complement Med*. 2002;8:643 650.

38. Aljada A, Mohanty P, Ghanim H, et al. Increase in intranuclear nuclear factor kappaB and decrease in inhibitor kappaB in mononuclear cells after a mixed meal: evidence for a proinflammatory effect. *Am J Clin Nutr*. 2004;79:682-690.

39. Goldhamer AC. Initial cost of care results in medically supervised water-only fasting for treating high blood pressure and diabetes. *J Altern Complement Med*. 2002;8:696-697.

40. Fuhrman J, Sarter B, Calabro DJ. Brief case reports of medically supervised, water-only fasting associated with remission of autoimmune disease. *Altern Ther Health Med*. 2002;8(4):112, 110-1.

41. Müller H, de Toledo FW, Resch KL. Fasting followed by vegetarian diet in patients with rheumatoid arthritis: a systematic review. *Scand J Rheumatol.* 2001;30:1-10.

42. Kjeldsen-Kragh J, Rashid T, Dybwad A, et al. Decrease in anti-Proteus mirabilis but not anti-Escherichia coli antibody levels in rheumatoid arthritis patients treated with fasting and a one year vegetarian diet. *Ann Rheum Dis.* 1995;54:221-224.

43. Bergqvist AG, Schall JI, Gallagher PR, Cnaan A, Stallings VA. Fasting versus gradual initiation of the ketogenic diet: a prospective, randomized clinical trial of efficacy. *Epilepsia.* 2005;46:1810-1819.

44. Yudkoff M, Daikhin Y, Nissim I, et al. Short-term fasting, seizure control and brain amino acid metabolism. *Neurochem Int.* 2006;48(6-7):650-656.

45. Kim DW, Kang HC, Park JC, Kim HD. Benefits of the nonfasting ketogenic diet compared with the initial fasting ketogenic diet. *Pediatrics.* 2004;114:1627-1630.

46. McCarty MF. A preliminary fast may potentiate response to a subsequent low-salt, low-fat vegan diet in the management of hypertension - fasting as a strategy for breaking metabolic vicious cycles. *Med Hypotheses.* 2003;60:624-633.

47. Adam O, Wolfram G, Zollner N. Effect of alpha-linolenic acid in the human diet on linoleic acid metabolism and prostaglandin biosynthesis. *J Lipid Res.* 1986;27:421-426.

48. Brzeski M, Madhok R, Capell HA. Evening primrose oil in patients with rheumatoid arthritis and side-effects of non-steroidal anti-inflammatory drugs. *Br J Rheumatol.* 1991;30:370-372.

49. Rothman D, DeLuca P, Zurier RB. Botanical lipids: effects on inflammation, immune responses, and rheumatoid arthritis. *Semin Arthritis Rheum.* 1995;25:87-96.

50. Adam O, Beringer C, Kless T, et al. Anti-inflammatory effects of a low arachidonic acid diet and fish oil in patients with rheumatoid arthritis. *Rheumatol Int.* 2003;23:27-36.

51. Lau CS, Morley KD, Belch JJ. Effects of fish oil supplementation on non-steroidal anti-inflammatory drug requirement in patients with mild rheumatoid arthritis: a double-blind placebo controlled study. *Br J Rheumatol.* 1993;32:982-989.

52. Kremer JM, Jubiz W, Michalek A, et al. Fish-oil fatty acid supplementation in active rheumatoid arthritis. A double-blinded, controlled, crossover study. *Ann Intern Med.* 1987;106:497-503.

53. Vasquez A. Reducing pain and inflammation naturally, part 2: New insights into fatty acid supplementation and its effect on eicosanoid production and genetic expression. *Nutritional Perspectives.* January 2005: 5-16.

54. Plotnikoff GA, Quigley JM. Prevalence of severe hypovitaminosis D in patients with persistent, nonspecific musculoskeletal pain. *Mayo Clin Proc.* 2003;78:1463-1470.

55. Timms PM, Mannan N, Hitman GA, et al. Circulating MMP9, vitamin D and variation in the TIMP-1 response with VDR genotype: mechanisms for inflammatory damage in chronic disorders? *QJM.* 2002;95:787-796.

56. Al Faraj S, Al Mutairi K. Vitamin D deficiency and chronic low back pain in Saudi Arabia. *Spine.* 2003;28:177-179.

57. Vasquez A, Manso G, Cannell J. The clinical importance of vitamin D (cholecalciferol): a paradigm shift with implications for all healthcare providers. *Altern Ther Health Med.* 2004;10:28-36.

58. Dostal C, Moszkorzova L, Musilova L, Lacinova Z, Marek J, Zvarova J. Serum prolactin stress values in patients with systemic lupus erythematosus. *Ann Rheum Dis.* 2003;62:487-488.

59. Moszkorzova L, Lacinova Z, Marek J, Musilova L, Dohnalova A, Dostal C. Hyperprolactinaemia in patients with systemic lupus erythematosus. *Clin Exp Rheumatol.* 2002;20:807-812.

60. Mateo L, Nolla JM, Bonnin MR, Navarro MA, Roig-Escofet D. High serum prolactin levels in men with rheumatoid arthritis. *J Rheumatol.* 1998;25:2077-2082.

61. Seriolo B, Ferretti V, Sulli A, Fasciolo D, Cutolo M. Serum prolactin concentrations in male patients with rheumatoid arthritis. *Ann N Y Acad Sci.* 2002;966:258-262.

62. Alvarez-Nemegyei J, Cobarrubias-Cobos A, Escalante-Triay F, Sosa-Munoz J, Miranda JM, Jara LJ. Bromocriptine in systemic lupus erythematosus: a double-blind, randomized, placebo-controlled study. *Lupus.* 1998;7:414-419.

63. McMurray RW. Bromocriptine in rheumatic and autoimmune diseases. *Semin Arthritis Rheum.* 2001;31:21-32.

64. Serri O, Chik CL, Ur E, Ezzat S. Diagnosis and management of hyperprolactinemia. *CMAJ.* 2003;169:575-581

65. Sabuncu T, Arikan E, Tasan E, Hatemi H. Comparison of the effects of cabergoline and bromocriptine on prolactin levels in hyperprolactinemic patients. *Intern Med.* 2001;40:857-861.

66. Erb N, Pace AV, Delamere JP, Kitas GD. Control of unremitting rheumatoid arthritis by the prolactin antagonist cabergoline. *Rheumatology* (Oxford). 2001;40:237-239

67. Wuttke W, Jarry H, Christoffel V, Spengler B, Seidlova-Wuttke D. Chaste tree (Vitex agnus-castus)--pharmacology and clinical indications. *Phytomedicine.* 2003;10:348-357.

68. Milewicz A, Gejdel E, Sworen H, et al. Vitex agnus castus extract in the treatment of luteal phase defects due to latent hyperprolactinemia. Results of a randomized placebo-controlled double-blind study. *Arzneimittelforschung.* 1993;43:752-756.

69. Meier B, Berger D, Hoberg E, Sticher O, Schaffner W. Pharmacological activities of Vitex agnus-castus extracts in vitro. *Phytomedicine.* 2000;7:373-381.

70. Katzenschlager R, Evans A, Manson A, et al. Mucuna pruriens in Parkinson 's disease: a double blind clinical and pharmacological study. *J Neurol Neurosurg Psychiatry.* 2004;75:1672-1677.

71. Ishizuka B, Quigley ME, Yen SS. Pituitary hormone release in response to food ingestion: evidence for neuroendocrine signals from gut to brain. *J Clin Endocrinol Metab.* 1983;57:1111-1116.

72. Jefferies WM. Mild adrenocortical deficiency, chronic allergies, autoimmune disorders and the chronic fatigue syndrome: a continuation of the cortisone story. *Med Hypotheses.* 1994;42:183-189.

73. Jefferies WM. The etiology of rheumatoid arthritis. *Med Hypotheses.* 1998;51:111-114.

74. Wilson TA. Adrenal hypoplasia. Updated June 16, 2006. Available online at: http://www.emedicine.com/PED/topic45.htm.

75. Jefferies W McK. *Safe Uses of Cortisol.* 3rd ed. Springfield, Ill: Charles C. Thomas; 1996.

76. Dessein PH, Joffe BI, Stanwix AE, Moomal Z. Hyposecretion of the adrenal androgen dehydroepiandrosterone sulfate and its relation to clinical variables in inflammatory arthritis. *Arthritis Res.* 2001;3:183-188.

77. Rittmaster RS, Givner ML. Effect of daily and alternate day low dose prednisone on serum cortisol and adrenal androgens in hirsute women. *J Clin Endocrinol Metab.* 1988;67:400-403.

78. Mease PJ, Ginzler EM, Gluck OS, et al. Effects of prasterone on bone mineral density in women with systemic lupus erythematosus receiving chronic glucocorticoid therapy. *J Rheumatol.* 2005;32:616-621.
79. Dyner TS, Lang W, Geaga J, et al. An open-label dose-escalation trial of oral dehydroepiandrosterone tolerance and pharmacokinetics in patients with HIV disease. *J Acquir Immune Defic Syndr.* 1993;6:459-465.
80. Barry NN, McGuire JL, van Vollenhoven RF. Dehydroepiandrosterone in systemic lupus erythematosus: relationship between dosage, serum levels, and clinical response. *J Rheumatol.* 1998;25:2352-2356.
81. Gaby AR. Dehydroepiandrosterone: biological effects and clinical significance. *Altern Med Rev.* 1996;1:60-69.
82. Andus T, Klebl F, Rogler G, Bregenzer N, Scholmerich J, Straub RH. Patients with refractory Crohn's disease or ulcerative colitis respond to dehydroepiandrosterone: a pilot study. *Aliment Pharmacol Ther.* 2003;17:409-414.
83. Chang DM, Lan JL, Lin HY, Luo SF. Dehydroepiandrosterone treatment of women with mild-to-moderate systemic lupus erythematosus: a multicenter randomized, double-blind, placebo-controlled trial. *Arthritis Rheum.* 2002;46:2924-2927.
84. Petri MA, Lahita RG, Van Vollenhoven RF, et al. Effects of prasterone on corticosteroid requirements of women with systemic lupus erythematosus: a double-blind, randomized, placebo-controlled trial. *Arthritis Rheum.* 2002;46:1820-1829.
85. Giltay EJ, van Schaardenburg D, Gooren LJ, et al. Effects of dehydroepiandrosterone administration on disease activity in patients with rheumatoid arthritis. *Br J Rheumatol.* 1998;37:705-706.
86. Fraser DA, Thoen J, Djoseland O, Forre O, Kjeldsen-Kragh J. Serum levels of interleukin-6 and dehydroepiandrosterone sulphate in response to either fasting or a ketogenic diet in rheumatoid arthritis patients. *Clin Exp Rheumatol.* 2000;18:357-362.
87. Tengstrand B, Carlstrom K, Fellander-Tsai L, Hafstrom I. Abnormal levels of serum dehydroepiandrosterone, estrone, and estradiol in men with rheumatoid arthritis: high correlation between serum estradiol and current degree of inflammation. *J Rheumatol.* 2003;30:2338-2343.
88. Sereda D, Werth VP. Improvement in dermatomyositis rash associated with the use of antiestrogen medication. *Arch Dermatol.* 2006;142:70-72.
89. McAlindon TE, Gulin J, Chen T, Klug T, Lahita R, Nuite M. Indole-3-carbinol in women with SLE: effect on estrogen metabolism and disease activity. *Lupus.* 2001;10:779-783.
90. Auborn KJ, Qi M, Yan XJ, et al. Lifespan is prolonged in autoimmune-prone (NZB/NZW) F1 mice fed a diet supplemented with indole-3-carbinol. *J Nutr.* 2003;133:3610-3613.
91. Leder BZ, Rohrer JL, Rubin SD, Gallo J, Longcope C. Effects of aromatase inhibition in elderly men with low or borderline-low serum testosterone levels. *J Clin Endocrinol Metab.* 2004;89:1174-1180.
92. Karagiannis A, Harsoulis F. Gonadal dysfunction in systemic diseases. *Eur J Endocrinol.* 2005;152:501-513.
93. Gordon D, Beastall GH, Thomson JA, Sturrock RD. Androgenic status and sexual function in males with rheumatoid arthritis and ankylosing spondylitis. *Q J Med.* 1986;60(231):671-679.
94. Booji A, Biewenga-Booji CM, Huber-Bruning O, Cornelis C, Jacobs JW, Bijlsma JW. Androgens as adjuvant treatment in postmenopausal female patients with rheumatoid arthritis. *Ann Rheum Dis.* 1996;55:811-815.
95. Cutolo M, Balleari E, Giusti M, Intra E, Accardo S. Androgen replacement therapy in male patients with rheumatoid arthritis. *Arthritis Rheum.* 1991;34:1-5.
96. Duntas LH, Mantzou E, Koutras DA. Effects of a six month treatment with selenomethionine in patients with autoimmune thyroiditis. *Eur J Endocrinol.* 2003;148:389-393.
97. Gartner R, Gasnier BC, Dietrich JW, Krebs B, Angstwurm MW. Selenium supplementation in patients with autoimmune thyroiditis decreases thyroid peroxidase antibodies concentrations. *J Clin Endocrinol Metab.* 2002;87:1687-1691.
98. Gartner R, Gasnier BC. Selenium in the treatment of autoimmune thyroiditis. *Biofactors.* 2003;19(3-4):165-170.
99. Wright JV. Why you need 83 times more of this essential, cancer-fighting nutrient than the "experts" say you do. *Nutrition and Healing.* 2005;12.
100. Schmidt MA, Bland JS. Thyroid gland as sentinel: interface between internal and external environment. *Altern Ther Health Med.* 1997;3:78-81.
101. Noah PW. The role of microorganisms in psoriasis. *Semin Dermatol.* 1990;9:269-276.
102. Burnstein SL, Liakos S. Parasitic rheumatism presenting as rheumatoid arthritis. *J Rheumatol.* 1983;10:514-515.
103. Ebringer A, Rashid T, Wilson C. Rheumatoid arthritis: proposal for the use of anti-microbial therapy in early cases. *Scand J Rheumatol.* 2003;32:2-11.
104. Rashid T, Darlington G, Kjeldsen-Kragh J, Forre O, Collado A, Ebringer A. Proteus IgG antibodies and C-reactive protein in English, Norwegian and Spanish patients with rheumatoid arthritis. *Clin Rheumatol.* 1999;18:190-195.
105. Galland L. Intestinal protozoan infection is a common unsuspected cause of chronic illness. *J Advancement Med.* 1989;2:539-552.
106. Severijnen AJ, Kool J, Swaak AJ, Hazenberg MP. Intestinal flora of patients with rheumatoid arthritis: induction of chronic arthritis in rats by cell wall fragments from isolated Eubacterium aerofaciens strains. *Br J Rheumatol.* 1990;29:433-439.
107. Galland L, Barrie S. Intestinal dysbiosis and the causes of disease. *Journal of Advancement in Medicine.* 1993;6:67-82. Available online at: http://www.ei-resource.org/articles/candida-and-gut-dysbiosis-articles/intestinal-dysbiosis-and-the-causes-of-disease.
108. Pimentel M, Park S, Mirocha J, Kane SV, Kong Y. The effect of a nonabsorbed oral antibiotic (rifaximin) on the symptoms of the irritable bowel syndrome: a randomized trial. *Ann Intern Med.* 2006;145:557-563.
109. Sharara AI, Aoun E, Abdul-Baki H, Mounzer R, Sidani S, Elhajj I. A randomized double-blind placebo-controlled trial of rifaximin in patients with abdominal bloating and flatulence. *Am J Gastroenterol.* 2006;101:326-333.
110. Saxena VN, Dogra J. Long-term use of penicillin for the treatment of chronic plaque psoriasis. *Eur J Dermatol.* 2005;15:359-362.
111. Popa ER, Stegeman CA, Kallenberg CG, Tervaert JW. Staphylococcus aureus and Wegener's granulomatosis. *Arthritis Res.* 2002;4:77-79.
112. Ponikau JU, Sherris DA, Kern EB, et al. The diagnosis and incidence of allergic fungal sinusitis. *Mayo Clin Proc.* 1999;74:877-884.
113. Braun J, Laitko S, Treharne J, et al. Chlamydia pneumoniae: a new causative agent of reactive arthritis and undifferentiated oligoarthritis. *Ann Rheum Dis.* 1994;53:100-105.
114. Weyand CM, Goronzy JJ. Clinically silent infections in patients with oligoarthritis: results of a prospective study. *Ann Rheum Dis.* 1992;51:253-258.
115. Kobayashi S, Kida I. Reactive arthritis: recent advances and clinical manifestations. *Intern Med.* 2005;44:408-412.
116. Erlacher L, Wintersberger W, Menschik M, et al. Reactive arthritis: urogenital swab culture is the only useful diagnostic method for the detection of the arthritogenic infection in extra-articularly asymptomatic patients with undifferentiated oligoarthritis. *Br J Rheumatol.* 1995;34:838-842.
117. Rashid T, Ebringer A. Rheumatoid arthritis is linked to Proteus: the evidence. *Clin Rheumatol.* 2007;26:1036-1043.
118. Goto T, Makinose S, Ohi Y. Plasma endotoxin concentrations in patients with urinary tract infections. *Int J Urol.* 1995;2:238-242.

123

119. Dai YP, Sun XZ, Zheng KL. Endotoxins in the prostatic secretions of chronic prostatitis patients. *Asian J Androl*. 2005;7:45-47.

120. Miles MR, Olsen L, Rogers A. Recurrent vaginal candidiasis. Importance of an intestinal reservoir. *JAMA*. 1977;238:1836-1837.

121. Piscoya J, Rodriguez Z, Bustamante SA, Okuhama NN, Miller MJ, Sandoval M. Efficacy and safety of freeze-dried cat 's claw in osteoarthritis of the knee: mechanisms of action of the species Uncaria guianensis. *Inflamm Res*. 2001;50:442-448.

122. Mur E, Hartig F, Eibl G, Schirmer M. Randomized double blind trial of an extract from the pentacyclic alkaloid-chemotype of uncaria tomentosa for the treatment of rheumatoid arthritis. *J Rheumatol*. 2002;29:678-681.

123. Deal CL, Schnitzer TJ, Lipstein E, et al. Treatment of arthritis with topical capsaicin: a double-blind trial. *Clin Ther*. 1991;13:383-395.

124. Galebskaya LV, Ryumina EV, Niemerovsky VS, Matyukov AA. Human complement system state after wobenzyme intake. *Vestnik Moskovskogo Universiteta. Khimiya*. 2000;41(Supplement):148-149.

125. Leblan D, Chantre P, Fournie B. Harpagophytum procumbens in the treatment of knee and hip osteoarthritis. Four-month results of a prospective, multicenter, double-blind trial versus diacerhein. *Joint Bone Spine*. 2000;67:462-467.

126. Chrubasik S, Junck H, Breitschwerdt H, Conradt C, Zappe H. Effectiveness of Harpagophytum extract WS 1531 in the treatment of exacerbation of low back pain: a randomized, placebo-controlled, double-blind study. *Eur J Anaesthesiol* 1999;16:118-129.

127. Chrubasik S, Model A, Black A, Pollak S. A randomized double-blind pilot study comparing Doloteffin and Vioxx in the treatment of low back pain. *Rheumatology* (Oxford). 2003;42:141-148.

128. Chrubasik S, Eisenberg E, Balan E, Weinberger T, Luzzati R, Conradt C. Treatment of low-back pain exacerbations with willow bark extract: a randomized double-blind study. *Am J Med*. 2000;109:9-14.

129. Chrubasik S, Kunzel O, Model A, Conradt C, Black A. Treatment of low-back pain with a herbal or synthetic anti-rheumatic: a randomized controlled study. Willow bark extract for low-back pain. *Rheumatology* (Oxford). 2001;40:1388-1393.

130. Vasquez A, Muanza DN. Comment: Evaluation of presence of aspirin-related warnings with willow bark. *Ann Pharmacotherapy*. 2005;39:1763.

131. Takada Y, Ichikawa H, Badmaev V, Aggarwal BB. Acetyl-11-keto-beta-boswellic acid potentiates apoptosis, inhibits invasion, and abolishes osteoclastogenesis by suppressing NF-kappa B and NF-kappa B-regulated gene expression. *J Immunol*. 2006;176:3127-3140.

132. Singh S, Khajuria A, Taneja SC, Johri RK, Singh J, Qazi GN. Boswellic acids: A leukotriene inhibitor also effective through topical application in inflammatory disorders. *Phytomedicine*. 2008 Jan 26 [Epub ahead of print].

133. Kimmatkar N, Thawani V, Hingorani L, Khiyani R. Efficacy and tolerability of Boswellia serrata extract in treatment of osteoarthritis of knee: a randomized double blind placebo controlled trial. *Phytomedicine*. 2003;10:3-7.

134. Gupta I, Parihar A, Malhotra P, et al. Effects of Boswellia serrata gum resin in patients with ulcerative colitis. *Eur J Med Res*. 1997;2:37-43.

135. Gupta I, Gupta V, Parihar A, et al. Effects of Boswellia serrata gum resin in patients with bronchial asthma: results of a double-blind, placebo-controlled, 6-week clinical study. *Eur J Med Res*. 1998;3:511-514.

136. Foell D, Kane D, Bresnihan B, et al. Expression of the pro-inflammatory protein S100A12 (EN-RAGE) in rheumatoid and psoriatic arthritis. *Rheumatology* (Oxford). 2003;42:1383-1389.

137. Shoba G, Joy D, Joseph T, Majeed M, Rajendran R, Srinivas PS. Influence of piperine on the pharmacokinetics of curcumin in animals and human volunteers. *Planta Med*. 1998;64:353-356.

138. Reginster JY, Deroisy R, Rovati LC, et al. Long-term effects of glucosamine sulphate on osteoarthritis progression: a randomised, placebo-controlled clinical trial. *Lancet*. 2001;357(9252):251-256.

139. Bruyere O, Pavelka K, Rovati LC, et al. Glucosamine sulfate reduces osteoarthritis progression in postmenopausal women with knee osteoarthritis: evidence from two 3-year studies. *Menopause*. 2004;11:138-143.

140. Mazières B, Hucher M, Zaïm M, Garnero P. Effect of chondroitin sulphate in symptomatic knee osteoarthritis: a multicentre, randomised, double-blind, placebo-controlled study. *Ann Rheum Dis*. 2007;66:639-645.

141. Vlad SC, LaValley MP, McAlindon TE, Felson DT. Glucosamine for pain in osteoarthritis: why do trial results differ? *Arthritis Rheum*. 2007;56:2267-2277.

142. Smyth JM, Stone AA, Hurewitz A, Kaell A. Effects of writing about stressful experiences on symptom reduction in patients with asthma or rheumatoid arthritis: a randomized trial. *JAMA*. 1999;281:1304-1309.

Chapter 7

Case Reports

The following 3 case reports provide representative examples of the clinical assessments and interventions that might be used in the treatment of neuromusculoskeletal disorders when approached from a functional medicine perspective. These are neither the best nor worst examples, but rather practical results and experiences that might be seen in clinical practice. These cases represent 3 divergent clinical conundrums: idiopathic relapsing-remitting peripheral neuropathy, recalcitrant rheumatoid arthritis, and the presentation of widespread musculoskeletal pain consistent with a diagnosis of fibromyalgia. For the sake of ease and brevity, lab results provided are those that are significant to the case and available at the time of this writing; values are given when relevant and are otherwise described as normal or abnormal.

Idiopathic Relapsing-Remitting Peripheral Neuropathy

March 2003: Initial Presentation

This patient was a 40-year-old Caucasian male with a 5-year history of recurrent numbness in his feet and to a lesser extent in his hands. He reported that the numbness was slightly worse on the right than the left and that it felt as though his hands and feet were "asleep." He had 9 episodes of this numbness in the past 2.5 years, each lasting for about 7 days. He experienced mostly peripheral sensory disturbance; however, one episode was associated with weakness of the right ankle. The experiences of extremity paresthesia were noted to occur with consumption of shellfish and seafood; they also were associated with fever of 102°F that lasted for 24 to 48 hours and occurred before the onset of numbness. The patient also desired weight loss, cardiovascular disease prevention, and treatment for fatigue, which he rated at a severity of 7/10.

The review of systems was significant for fatigue, allergies, chemical sensitivity, dyscognition, work stress, and mild gastrointestinal discomfort. Previous evaluations in January and February 2002 included magnetic resonance imaging (MRI) of the brain, neck, and spinal cord, as well as lumbar puncture for cerebrospinal fluid (CSF) analysis; results of these studies were normal. The patient had been assessed by several neurologists with no results. Family history was significant for insulin-dependent diabetes mellitus. Screening physical examination was normal except for +1/4 patellar reflexes and +0/4 Achilles reflexes (normal = +2/4); patient was 5'9" and 170 pounds.

Previous lab results in 2002 included the following:

- Serum protein electrophoresis: normal
- Comprehensive metabolic panel: normal
- Complete blood count (CBC): normal except for slightly low hemoglobin and hematocrit
- Erythrocyte sedimentation rate: slightly high at 16 mm/hr (normal < 15)

- Antinuclear antibody screen (ANA): low positive at 1:40 (normal = negative)
- Serum complement levels: normal

Due to the coincidence of the fever and neuropathy with the consumption of shellfish, I advised the patient of the probability of gastrointestinal dysbiosis and recommended stool analysis and comprehensive parasitology assessment, which the patient refused. Two weeks later, the patient completed follow-up labs and (per patient request) comprehensive cardiovascular risk assessment, which were significant for the following results:

- Thyroid stimulating hormone (TSH): normal at 2 µIU/L
- Ferritin: normal at 88 ng/mL
- ANA: negative (normal)
- Total cholesterol: normal at 143 mg/dL
- Triglycerides: normal at 77 mg/dL
- Low-density lipoprotein: normal at 93 mg/dL
- Homocysteine: normal at 6.9 µmol/L
- C-reactive protein (CRP): markedly elevated at 11.1 mg/L (normal < 1.69)
- Fibrinogen: high at 441 mg/dL (normal < 350)

I advised the patient that the combination of elevated CRP and fibrinogen reflected evidence of mild-moderate systemic inflammation and that, given his clinical presentation and lab results, stool analysis and comprehensive parasitology assessment were advised. He again refused stool analysis and comprehensive parasitology assessment; however, he was now willing to perform a lactulose-mannitol test to assess gastrointestinal mucosal permeability.

April 2003: Intestinal Permeability Results

Lactulose recovery (high at 1.51%; normal < 0.80%) and mannitol recovery (low-normal at 8%; normal = 5–30%) resulted in an extremely elevated lactulose-to-mannitol ratio at 0.19 (normal < 0.03). Consistent with my impression on the first visit, these results indicated markedly increased gastrointestinal mucosal permeability. The patient was advised of this and was now willing to undergo stool analysis and comprehensive parasitology assessment. To facilitate mucosal repair, the patient was advised to consume glutamine, 6 g three times daily, zinc, 40 mg three times daily, and a medical food product containing low doses of vitamins and minerals, in addition to inulin and fructooligosaccharides for probiotic support.

May 2003: Stool Analysis and Comprehensive Parasitology Results

Results were significant for the following:

- *Bifidobacterium*: low at 1+ (optimal = = 3–4+)
- *Lactobacillus*: low at 0+ (optimal = 3–4+)
- *Proteus mirabilis*: high at 4+ (optimal = negative or 0+)
- Ova and parasites: negative (normal)
- *Giardia*: negative (normal)
- *Cryptosporidium*: negative (normal)
- *Campylobacter*: negative (normal)
- Enterohemorrhagic *Escherichia coli*: negative (normal)
- Lysozyme: normal
- Lactoferrin: normal
- Fecal secretory IgA: moderately high at 358 ng/mL (normal = 40–204)

These results were consistent with 2-component gastrointestinal dysbiosis (probiotic insufficiency and hypersensitivity dysbiosis). *Proteus mirabilis* is a gram-negative bacterium implicated as a microbial trigger for autoimmune conditions such as rheumatoid arthritis,[1] and in this case, it appeared that hypersensitivity toward *Proteus mirabilis* (as evidenced by the elevated sIgA) was resulting in increased intestinal permeability secondary to local mucosal inflammation and was promoting immune sensitization to dietary and peripheral nerve (neuronal and/or myelin) antigens. The lack of beneficial flora would be expected to facilitate immune hypersensitivity, as well as the persistent dysbiotic colonization.[2] Culture and sensitivity results showed that the patient's *Proteus mirabilis* was resistant to all natural agents, so the patient was started on a 7-day course of ciprofloxacin, to which his *Proteus mirabilis* was sensitive.

July 2003: Symptomatic and Laboratory Results of Treatment

The patient noted improved energy and reduced fatigue, with no events of numbness. He was now able to consume shellfish without fever or neuropathy. His CRP normalized to 1.26 mg/L (normal < 1.69) within 6 weeks of treatment for dysbiosis. The patient remained completely asymptomatic until a recurrence in 2007; he was very pleased with the results and lamented the expenditure of more than $10,000 with neurologists who could provide neither explanations nor solutions for his health concerns.

March 2007: Recurrence of Fatigue and Neuropathy Following Work and Family Stress

The patient reported a very significant recurrence of peripheral neuropathy and fatigue following several months of increased work-related stress and family stress, which included the death of a parent-in-law and relocation to a new city. Due to the sustained success of the previous treatment plan, I recommended reassessment for stool dysbiosis, along with a few additional tests. Significant results included:

- CBC: normal except for elevated leukocytes due to resolving upper respiratory infection
- Lipid panel: normal
- Comprehensive metabolic panel: normal
- TSH: normal
- Free T4: normal
- Ferritin: normal
- High-sensitivity C-reactive protein (hsCRP): high but otherwise uninterpretable relevant to patient's overall health status due to resolving upper respiratory infection
- Dehydroepiandrosterone sulfate (DHEA-S): high-normal
- 25-hydroxy vitamin D3 (25[OH]D): normal at 42 ng/mL (normal = 30–100)
- Prolactin: normal
- ANA: negative
- Estradiol: low "normal" at < 15 pg/mL (normal = 0–53)
- Protein electrophoresis: normal
- Urinalysis: normal
- *Bifidobacterium*: 4+ (optimal = 3–4+)
- *Lactobacillus*: 2+ (optimal = 3–4+)
- *Pseudomonas*: high at 4+ (optimal = negative or 0+)
- *Candida glabrata*: 1+ (optimal = negative or 0+)
- *Rhodotorula*: 1+ (optimal = negative or 0+)
- Lysozyme: normal
- Lactoferrin: normal
- Fecal secretory IgA: high-normal at 203 ng/mL (normal = 40–204)

The most important findings were the low estradiol and the high *Pseudomonas*. Although the estradiol was reported as normal, this was a major clue for endocrine imbalance and thus a probable contributor to inflammatory imbalance. Testosterone was not measured with the first order of tests; however, I ordered it immediately upon receipt of the undetectable estradiol. *Pseudomonas aeruginosa* is a gram-negative bacterium implicated as a possible microbial trigger for neuroautoimmune conditions such as multiple sclerosis (MS).[3,4] Based on the relationship between *Pseudomonas* dysbiosis and neuroautoimmunity, therapeutic eradication of the *Pseudomonas* was warranted.

Results of testosterone measurements were:

- Testosterone, total: low at 175 ng/dL (normal = 241–827)
- Testosterone, free: low-normal 7.6 pg/mL (normal = 6.8–21.5)

Testosterone has positive immunomodulatory effects that counteract inflammation and autoimmunity, as demonstrated in animal models of immune-mediated peripheral neuropathy[5] and in humans with autoimmune disease.[6,7] In addition to basic dietary improvement and foundational supplementation (see *Dietary Interventions* in Chapter 2), the patient was treated with a combination of botanical and pharmaceutical antimicrobials (antibacterial and antifungal), along with transdermal testosterone. Follow-up testing showed estradiol, testosterone, and CRP to be within their normal ranges, and the patient responded with improved energy and quality of life and complete alleviation of peripheral neuropathy for the following year (as of this writing in March 2008).

Case Summary and Conclusion

This case demonstrates the successful treatment of an idiopathic peripheral neuropathy that defied standard assessment by several neurologists. In this case, the neuropathy appeared to be immune mediated, triggered by a combination of dietary antigen exposure (shellfish and seafood), increased intestinal permeability (documented by the lactulose-mannitol assay), and gastrointestinal colonization (dysbiosis) due to bacteria known to be associated with human autoimmunity. Anti-dysbiosis interventions effected normalization of inflammatory status (normalization of CRP levels), long-term improvement in quality of life, and sustained alleviation of neuropathy. When stressful life events and patient noncompliance with the previously successful treatment plan allowed recolonization and a return of symptoms, anti-dysbiosis interventions and hormonal correction again provided consistent and persistent benefit.

Recalcitrant Rheumatoid Arthritis

July 2005: Initial Presentation

This patient was a 51-year-old man with a 4-year history of rheumatoid arthritis (diagnosis confirmed by 2 medical specialists) which had not responded to pharmaceutical drugs ranging from prednisone and methotrexate to the "biologics" such as infliximab. Complicating his clinical picture was high cardiovascular risk due to his concomitant obesity, hypertension (140/100 mm Hg), hypercholesterolemia, and severe systemic inflammation evidenced by high hsCRP. The patient habitually consumed a proinflammatory diet marked by sugared drinks, hamburgers, and fried potatoes. When I asked what he thought caused his disease, the patient replied, "The specialist told me this was a genetic disease," to which I responded, "You have the same genes now that you've had all your life. Your genes did not change 4 years ago, so something else must have happened. Let's see if we can discover what that was."

Blood samples were drawn for basic laboratory evaluation, and the patient submitted samples for a partial stool analysis and parasitology examination within the first few weeks of assessment. Results included:

- Comprehensive metabolic panel: normal except for slightly elevated alanine aminotransferase (ALT) consistent with the patient's obesity

Peripheral Neuropathy Patient Narrative, March 2008

In September 2000, I experienced extremely numb feet for the first time. I thought that I was getting a cold or the flu since I had a fever, but nothing ever materialized. However, the numbness continued, so… the doctor took my temperature and blood pressure and told me to get some exercise. No blood test was performed.

My feet eventually returned to normal after about a week. However, the numbness returned around Christmas 2000. Once again, the numbness subsided after about 1 week.

I continued to have these episodes of fever, followed by numbness, every 3 to 6 months. Episodes 3 and 4 were in May and November 2001. However, in January 2002, things got worse.… Again, I had a high fever and flu-like symptoms. The numbness was bad, but I went to the doctor for primarily treatment of the flu. The doctor suggested that I see a neurologist.

The neurologist's first thought was that I had signs of MS. He recommended an MRI of my brain. The good news was that the results were negative. I was very relieved to hear that I did not have MS. However, the doctor and neurologist could not provide an answer to my extreme numbness. I returned to normal after about 10 days.

One month later in February 2002, I had my 6th case, which was even worse than case 5. This time, the numbness was so severe that I lost all strength in my right foot. I literally could not use it. After I fell down in my home office, I decided that I better get some help. I was so paralyzed that my wife had to help me walk. Otherwise, I had to hop on my left foot, which was also numb. The neurologist tested my reflexes, and I basically had none in my right foot. I did have some response in my left. Due to the severity, the neurologist then reverted back to his MS theory. I had 2 MRIs on my neck and spine and a spinal tap in order to positively prove or disprove the MS theory. Much to my relief, all tests yielded negative results. The neurologist, however, was at a loss on what to do next. By the time the MRI results were back, I was getting stronger. The neurologist said to call him if it ever happened again, and he would refer me to another neurologist in the medical center.

Case 7 was in June 2002, but it was very mild compared to 5 and 6. Again, the symptoms lasted for about a week. I was fine until October 2002, when I endured case number 8. I ate a lot of seafood on a business trip in California. I flew home and the numbness began again. The pattern of fever followed by numbness seemed to be related to the consumption of shellfish. So I eliminated shellfish from my diet and was pretty cautious about what I ate.

Case number 9 was in January 2003. We went to a party on a Friday night, and I ate a lobster empanada. I didn't realize that it was lobster until after I ate it. By the time we got home that night, I had a fever, and by morning, my feet were numb again. This time, my wife took me to see Dr. Alex Vasquez. My wife had been searching for a naturopathic doctor for quite some time, and she found Dr. Vasquez. She was very happy with the results she was getting for a variety of issues. Thanks to my wife, she insisted that I see Dr. Vasquez.

Dr. Vasquez first did a cardiovascular profile and found extremely elevated levels of CRP.… While this news was not good, I was thrilled that Dr. Vasquez had found this problem and we could do something about my situation before it was too late.

Why did I have such high levels of CRP? Dr. Vasquez suspected that I had a malabsorption issue, so he suggested that I take an intestinal permeability ("leaky gut") test. Sure enough, I was extremely leaky. No wonder I was so tired all of the time. My body was not absorbing any of the nutrients from my food and vitamins but it was absorbing all of the toxins. Very interesting.

Our next step was to determine why I had such a leaky gut. It was a safe bet that malnutrition, alcoholism, and drug addiction were not the causes, so we had to focus on food allergies and parasites/bacteria. He did find 2 kinds of bacteria.… Dr. Vasquez treated me with antibiotics to kill the bacteria and supplemented my system with probiotics. He also put me on a strong supplementation program to rebuild my weakened body. Within a month, I felt much better. The supplementation program has certainly given me more energy and strength. The most exciting news has been that my CRP has come down to 1.26 mg/L, which is below the high-risk threshold.

I had been feeling fine until late February 2007. I came down with a cold with a low-grade fever and could tell that the numbness was gradually returning to my feet. Within 48 hours of the initial fever, I had full-blown numbness in both of my feet and some numbness in my fingers. I had almost no strength in my right foot. I had slightly more strength in my left foot; however, I had to hold on to something or someone in order to walk. This was perhaps my most severe case ever. I was pretty well immobilized for about a week, and the numbness gradually went away over the course of the following week.

When I got back to Dallas, I had pretty well recovered on my own, but I did seek out Dr. Vasquez again for guidance. We did more blood work on April 12, 2007, and found extremely high levels of CRP of 29.70 mg/L which was quite alarming. While I had recovered from the numbness, I had developed bronchitis in early April, and this was probably affecting my CRP levels to some degree.

Dr. Vasquez then suggested a testosterone test, which was done on April 18, 2007. My testosterone level was 175 ng/dL, which was below the normal range of 241 to 827. We immediately started to use testosterone gel on a daily basis. We tested again on June 7, 2007, and my testosterone was now up to 376 ng/dL which is a normal level. [Repeated stool test also found dysbiosis, which was treated with a combination of nutritional, botanical, and pharmaceutical antibiotics.]

Since then, I have used probiotics on a daily basis, as well as fish oil, vitamin D, and vitamin C. I continued to take testosterone gel through January 2008 and have felt fine. I have been healthy with no signs of numbness.

- Lipid panel: hypercholesterolemia of 250 mg/dL
- hsCRP: extremely high at 124 mg/L (normal = 0–3)
- Ferritin: 294 ng/mL (normal = 22–322; optimal = 40–70)
- Testosterone, total: low-normal at 283 ng/dL (normal = 241–827)
- Testosterone, free: low-normal at 10.4 pg/mL (normal = 7.2–24.0)
- Estradiol: high-normal at 41 pg/mL (normal = 0–53; optimal = 15–30)
- DHEA-S: low at 65 mcg/dL (normal = 70–310)
- Ova and parasites: negative
- *Bifidobacterium*: 0+ (optimal = 3–4+)
- *Lactobacillus*: 0+ (optimal = 3–4+)
- *Citrobacter freundii*: 1+ (optimal = 0+)

Given the patient's extremely high cardiovascular risk, I referred him to an internal medicine specialist for at least short-term pharmacological immunosuppression of inflammation, hypertension, and hypercholesterolemia. (The patient refused the referral and added, "Those drugs have not worked for me, and I am not going back to drugs.") I also advised the patient to reduce his intake of beef and wheat. A simple plan of nutritional supplementation consisted of the following:

- A high-potency multivitamin-multimineral supplement
- Combination fatty acid supplementation with modest doses of alpha-linolenic acid (ALA), gamma-linolenic acid (GLA), eicosapentaenoic acid (EPA), and docosahexaenoic acid (DHA) (anti-inflammation and cardio-protection)
- Vitamin D, 4000 IU/d (anti-inflammation, cardioprotection, antihypertension)
- Micronized DHEA, 50 mg/d (correction of deficiency and hormonal immunomodulation)
- Anastrozole, 1 mg twice weekly (slightly lower estrogens and raise androgens[8] for hormonal immunomodulation)
- Emulsified oil of oregano,[9] 150 mg three times daily, and undecylenic acid derived from castor bean oil,[10] 200 mg twice daily, to address the *Citrobacter* dysbiosis.

August 2005: Progress Evaluation

Approximately 1 month after the receipt of initial laboratory results and the implementation of the initial treatment plan, the patient reported marked relief of joint pain and swelling, both of which recurred following consumption of his formerly habitual fast-food lunch. Reassessment of hsCRP showed a reduction to 7.5 mg/L; this was considered powerful objective documentation of the success of the intervention. The patient remarked that these results were far better than what had been achieved previously with prednisone and infliximab. We repeated HsCRP testing again the following month and found it stable at 7 mg/L despite imperfect compliance with the successful dietary, nutritional, and botanical interventions.

Case Summary and Conclusion

This case demonstrates the initial success of simple nutritional and hormonal interventions in treating an idiopathic inflammatory disease, which was completely unresponsive to some of the most powerful anti-inflammatory drugs on the medical market. The sustained reduction in hsCRP provides clear evidence of therapeutic anti-inflammatory efficacy despite the complete avoidance of anti-inflammatory drugs and the sole reliance upon safe and simple nutritional interventions. In sum, the patient's proinflammatory lifestyle, along with the gastrointestinal dysbiosis and hormonal imbalances, were synergizing to create such marked systemic inflammation that his overall status had become pathological and consistent with the diagnosis of a rheumatoid arthritis; simple, safe, and gentle correction of these synergistic imbalances provided powerful anti-inflammatory and symptomatic benefit, while also facilitating weight loss, cardioprotection, and avoidance of the financial costs and clinical risks associated with pharmaceutical and biologic anti-inflammatory drugs. Even with only moderate compliance, the plan demonstrated tremendous success for the observed period of several months.

Widespread Musculoskeletal Pain Consistent with a Diagnosis of Fibromyalgia

July 2005: Initial Presentation

This patient was a 55-year-old woman with a long-term history of hypertension, multiple chemical sensitivity, and other complaints, which were managed with little success by numerous specialists. Although her diet and life-style were strict and health promoting (e.g., organic foods, numerous supplements, regular exercise, supportive long-term relationship, positive outlook), she had developed widespread, nonspecific musculoskeletal pain, which reached a level of severity that adversely impacted her quality of life and efforts to remain physically active. Her mother's medical history was significant for Hashimoto's autoimmune thyroiditis and polymyalgia rheumatica.

Physical examination revealed normal strength, reflexes, and sensation, numerous positive tender points consistent with fibromyalgia, and hypertension of 145/100 mm Hg. Over the next several weeks, laboratory assessments were performed, with the following results:

- Comprehensive metabolic panel: normal
- Lipid panel: normal
- hsCRP: normal
- Ferritin: normal
- DHEA-S: normal
- TSH, free T4, and free T3: normal
- Serum 25(OH)D: normal
- Aldolase: normal
- Erythrocyte sedimentation rate (ESR): normal
- Phosphorus: normal
- Rheumatoid factor: normal
- Lyme disease serology: normal (negative)
- Ova and parasites: negative
- *Bifidobacterium*: 3+ (optimal = 3–4+)
- *Lactobacillus*: 3+ (optimal = 3–4+)
- Fecal secretory IgA: normal

Before the receipt of the stool analysis and parasitology results, I treated the patient empirically for gastrointestinal dysbiosis and small bowel bacterial overgrowth; this intervention provided no benefit. Fine-tuning of the patient's nutritional program also provided no benefit. All lab results were within normal limits, and physical examination was unrevealing and nonspecific. The patient met the tender point criteria for fibromyalgia, and no clinical or laboratory evidence of pathological or functional disorder was discovered. I referred the patient to a medical internist for evaluation and second opinion; no disease was found, and the diagnosis of fibromyalgia was confirmed.

October 2005: Re-evaluation

The patient appeared sincere about her complaints despite the lack of objective clinical and laboratory findings. Although she met the positive and negative criteria for fibromyalgia, this diagnosis was considered unsatisfactory in the context of this patient's healthy lifestyle, age (>50), lack of response to vitamin D 4000 IU/d, and lack of clinical or laboratory evidence of gastrointestinal dysbiosis, particularly occult bacterial overgrowth of the small bowel.

Pathological, myopathic, or inflammatory processes had been largely excluded by clinical examination and laboratory testing. Testing for toxic heavy metals was therefore performed following oral administration of the chelating agent dimercaptosuccinic acid (DMSA), 10 mg/kg, and urine collection. Results were significant for the following:

- Lead: 30 mcg/g creatinine (normal < 5)
- Mercury: 21 mcg/g creatinine (normal < 3)

The lead and mercury levels were extremely elevated; in fact, the bar graph of the mercury level extended off the page of the laboratory report. The combined toxicity of lead and mercury is synergistic and "exponential" rather than merely additive; therefore, the finding of combined elevations of lead and mercury was considered significant, though not necessarily causative, for the patient's musculoskeletal pain. I advised the patient of these findings and offered treatment for toxic metal accumulation, with the hope that this might provide at least some symptomatic relief.

The patient was begun on a regimen that included the following treatments, which were directed simultaneously toward promotion of overall health and the facilitated urinary and fecal excretion of toxic heavy metals.

- Healthy diet and regular exercise: Maintenance of her previous diet, nutritional supplement program, and regular exercise (to the extent tolerated due to pain).
- DMSA, 10 mg/kg: DMSA is approved by the FDA for the treatment of lead accumulation (i.e., lead poisoning). It is also effective for mercury poisoning. DMSA has a good record of safety and efficacy in adults and children when used in doses ranging from 10–30 mg per kilogram of body weight. For this patient, the lower dose was used due to her long-standing history of multiple chemical sensitivity and our desire to avoid immunologic sensitization or other idiosyncratic reaction. Treatment was continued for several months, with the patient consuming DMSA only on alternating weeks; this approach is used to avoid toxicity in general and any myelosuppresion in particular.
- Phytochelatins: Phytochelatins are peptides produced by some plants to bind to and thus protect the plant from toxic heavy metals.[11] Oral suppelementation of phytochelatin concentrates is used to bind heavy metals in the gut during physiological enterohepatic recirculation; a pharmacologically analogous practice is the use of cholestyramine to bind cholesterol and prevent its (re)uptake in the gut. Phytochelatin supplementation appears safe and effective based on clinical utilization, although no controlled trials have been published supporting its use. However, given its safety, phytochelatin supplementation was used in this patient to facilitate fecal excretion of toxic metals.
- Selenium, 800 µg/d: Selenium is a multifunctional mineral that provides antioxidant benefits and helps increase elimination of toxic metals. A safe but relatively high dose was used in this patient to facilitate lead and mercury excretion.
- Potassium citrate: Potassium citrate increases mercury excretion. This was provided via generous consumption of fruit and vegetable juices.

August 2006: Progress and Reassessment

Symptomatic improvement was noted following the implementation of the aforementioned protocol for enhancing the clearance of lead and mercury. Follow-up DMSA-provoked urine collection testing for heavy metals provided the following significant results:

- Lead: 15 mcg/g creatinine (normal < 5)
- Mercury: 8.3 mcg/g creatinine (normal < 3)

Coincident with this significant reduction in toxic metals was the subjective and sustained reduction in pain experienced by the patient.

July 2007: Completion of Treatment

Via e-mail in July 2007, 2 years following the initiation of investigation and treatment, the patient stated, "I don't have the noticeable symptoms of soreness and aches." The patient was offered a third heavy metal test but did not follow through, owing at least in part to her lack of concern over this matter now that her symptoms had been alleviated.

Case Summary and Conclusion

Lead and mercury are ubiquitous in the environment and accumulate at different rates among patients based on diet, lifestyle, and genetic influences. Lead contributes to the population burden of hypertension,[12] and levels of mercury high enough to warrant concern are seen in at least 8% of American women, even when accurate yet insensitive analyses are used.[13] It is possible that lead and mercury could synergize to impair muscle metabolism and result in diffuse musculoskeletal pain; the pain may also be mediated centrally as a unique manifestation of heavy metal neurotoxicity. Following the exclusion of inflammatory and myopathic disease, the clinical diagnosis of fibromyalgia was confirmed in this patient, yet therapeutic success was achieved by searching for and effectively treating occult heavy metal toxicity due to lead and mercury.

References

1. Rashid T, Ebringer A. Rheumatoid arthritis is linked to Proteus: the evidence. *Clin Rheumatol.* 2007;26:1036-1043.
2. Drisko JA, Giles CK, Bischoff BJ. Probiotics in health maintenance and disease prevention. *Altern Med Rev.* 2003;8:143-155.
3. Hughes LE, Bonell S, Natt RS, et al. Antibody responses to Acinetobacter spp. and Pseudomonas aeruginosa in multiple sclerosis: prospects for diagnosis using the myelin-acinetobacter-neurofilament antibody index. *Clin Diagn Lab Immunol.* 2001;8:1181-1188.
4. Hughes LE, Smith PA, Bonell S, et al. Cross-reactivity between related sequences found in Acinetobacter sp., Pseudomonas aeruginosa, myelin basic protein and myelin oligodendrocyte glycoprotein in multiple sclerosis. *J Neuroimmunol.* 2003;144(1-2):105-115.
5. Yeo SW, Chang KH, Park SN, Suh BD. Effects of testosterone in the treatment of immune-mediated sensorineural hearing loss. *Eur Arch Otorhinolaryngol.* 2003;260:316-319.
6. Cutolo M. Sex hormone adjuvant therapy in rheumatoid arthritis. *Rheum Dis Clin North Am.* 2000;26:881-895.
7. Cutolo M, Sulli A, Capellino S, et al. Sex hormones influence on the immune system: basic and clinical aspects in autoimmunity. *Lupus.* 2004;13:635-638.
8. Leder BZ, Finkelstein JS. Effect of aromatase inhibition on bone metabolism in elderly hypogonadal men. *Osteoporos Int.* 2005;16:1487-1494.
9. Force M, Sparks WS, Ronzio RA. Inhibition of enteric parasites by emulsified oil of oregano in vivo. *Phytother Res.* 2000;14:213-214.
10. Undecylenic acid. Monograph. *Altern Med Rev.* 2002;7:68-70.
11. Cobbett CS. Phytochelatins and their roles in heavy metal detoxification. *Plant Physiol.* 2000;123:825-832.
12. Nash D, Magder L, Lustberg M, et al. Blood lead, blood pressure, and hypertension in perimenopausal and postmenopausal women. *JAMA.* 2003;289:1523-1532.
13. Schober SE, Sinks TH, Jones RL, et al. Blood mercury levels in US children and women of childbearing age, 1999-2000. *JAMA.* 2003;289:1667-1674.

About the Author

Alex Vasquez, DC, ND, OMSII, began his professional training at Texas Chiropractic College and later graduated from Western States Chiropractic College in Portland, Oregon. He then attended and graduated from the Naturopathic Medicine Program at Bastyr University near Seattle, Washington. Over the next few years, Dr. Vasquez maintained a private practice (first in Seattle, then in Houston, Texas), taught orthopedics and rheumatology at Bastyr University, and pursued his constant review of MEDLINE for the continuous compilation of his biomedicine, nutrition, and physiology database. Dr. Vasquez has published more than 70 articles and letters in magazines, newspapers, and peer-reviewed journals including *Alternative Therapies in Health and Medicine, JAMA, The Lancet, BMJ, The Annals of Pharmacotherapy, Journal of the American Osteopathic Association, Integrative Medicine: A Clinician's Journal, Evidence-based Complementary and Alternative Medicine,* and *Arthritis & Rheumatism* (official journal of the American College of Rheumatology). Dr. Vasquez has written two textbooks, *Integrative Orthopedics* and *Integrative Rheumatology,* both of which were revised in 2007 for their second editions. Dr. Vasquez's current affiliations include National University of Health Sciences (Adjunct Professor), The Institute for Functional Medicine (Forum Consultant), and Biotics Research Corporation (Researcher and Lecturer). He is currently a student at University of North Texas Health Science Center–Texas College of Osteopathic Medicine, where he will graduate in 2010 as a Doctor of Osteopathic Medicine.